DIABETES SELF-MANAGEMENT'S HIDDEN SECRETS OF NATURAL HEALING

Using foods, supplements, and more to slow or even reverse the complications of diabetes

D1379039

DIABETES SELF-MANAGEMENT'S HIDDEN SECRETS OF NATURAL HEALING

by Diana W. Guthrie Ph.D., A.R.N.P., F.A.A.N., C.D.E., B.C.-A.D.M., A.H.N.-B.C., C.H.T.P.

Using foods, supplements, and more to slow or even reverse the complications of diabetes

with an overview of diabetes care by Richard A. Guthrie M.D., F.A.C.E., C.D.E.

DIABETES SELF-MANAGEMENT BOOKS
NEW YORK

Library of Congress Cataloging-in-Publication Data
Guthrie, Diana W.
    Diabetes self-management's hidden secrets of natural healing using foods, supplements, and more to slow and even reverse the complications of diabetes / by Diana W. Guthrie; with an overview of diabetes care by Richard A. Guthrie.
    p. cm.
    Includes bibliographical references and index.
    ISBN 0-9631701-8-X
    1. Diabetes—Alternative treatment. I. Title. II. Title: Hidden secrets of natural healing using foods, supplements, and more to slow and even reverse the complications of diabetes.
    RC661.A47G89 2006
    616.4'62—dc22   2006016046

PROJECT EDITOR
Ingrid Strauch
DESIGN AND ILLUSTRATION
Richard Boland

Our thanks to Cynthia Payne, M.S., R.D., C.D.E., and Charlotte Eliopolous, Ph.D., for their careful reviewing, and to Miri Rotkovitz, M.A., R.D., for preparing the "Super Foods" appendix.

Diabetes Self-Management Books is an imprint of R.A. Rapaport Publishing, Inc., 150 West 22nd Street, New York, NY 10011.
Printed in the United States of America.
10 9 8 7 6 5 4 3 2 1

CONTENTS

APPENDICES

PREFACE

Controlling blood glucose and blood pressure levels has definitively been shown to prevent or delay the progression of numerous complications associated with diabetes, including kidney disease (nephropathy), eye disease (retinopathy), nerve damage (neuropathy), and heart disease. The question for all people with diabetes is how best to achieve the goals of blood glucose and blood pressure control with the fewest negative side effects.

Research has shown that performing regular physical activity and losing excess body weight can go a long way toward getting to both of these goals. Certain dietary patterns have been shown to help with blood glucose control, blood pressure control, and weight loss. Stress reduction helps, too. But no single diet, exercise, or stress reduction program works for all people with diabetes. So again, the question for people with diabetes is how best to incorporate more physical activity into their lives, reduce their stress, and eat better without feeling controlled by diabetes or deprived in their food choices.

This book cannot give you all the answers to these questions, but it will give you some new ideas about individualizing your diabetes control program and perhaps trying some new techniques for achieving the best health possible. In the following pages you'll read about both alternative medical systems and complementary therapies that might be of use to you.

Alternative medicine refers to medical and health care systems, practices, and products used in place of conventional Western medicine. Complementary therapies are practices and products that are used along with conventional therapies. Some therapies once considered to be alternative or complementary are now considered conventional because they have been shown to be safe and effective. Others, however, may be ineffective or even harmful under certain circumstances. For this reason, people with diabetes are encouraged to discuss their use of any complementary or alternative therapy with their conventional health-care provider.

As a holistic nurse who is certified in diabetes education and management and a healing touch practitioner, I realize the responsibility I am taking in sharing the information found on these pages. I do not wish to lead anyone into doing something that might be harmful rather than helpful. Nor do I wish for anyone to replace their conventional diabetes treatment with an alternative without the assistance of a qualified practitioner.

This book's major purpose is to act as a starting place—to expose you to some of the many choices out there, guide you to additional resources, and help you ask the right questions and share the correct information with your health-care professional.

The more you inform and educate yourself about any alternative or complementary therapy you'd like to try, the better chance you have of avoiding the ineffective ones and making the best use of therapies that can help you attain and maintain a high degree of diabetes control.

By opening this book, you have taken the first step on a path of discovery. This path may not necessarily be a straight one, but it should be a rewarding one. As you read, keep in mind that what might work for one person might not work as well for another. Take time in making any decisions, and enjoy the possibilities.

Diana W. Guthrie

Diana W. Guthrie, PhD, ARNP, FAAN, CDE, BC-ADM, AHN-BC, CHTP

1. DIABETES: AN OVERVIEW

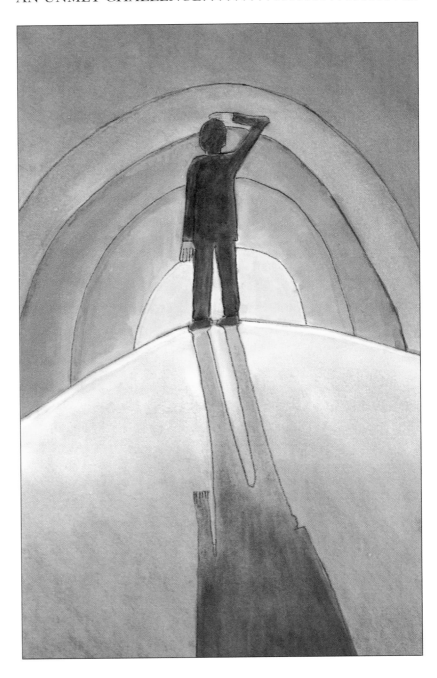

1.
DIABETES:
AN OVERVIEW
by Richard A. Guthrie, M.D., C.D.E.

Diabetes is a common metabolic disease affecting both adults and children that is becoming more common each year. According to the U.S. Centers for Disease Control and Prevention, there are now 20.8 million people in the United States with diabetes, and that number is increasing by 7% per year. The World Health Organization estimates that there are nearly 200 million people in the world with diabetes and projects over 300 million in another few years.

More than 400,000 Americans die from diabetes every year, and the estimated annual cost to the U.S. economy is over $156 billon and rising. Most of this money is spent in treating the complications of diabetes rather than the day-to-day management of it. This is tragic since almost all of the complications are preventable.

What is diabetes?

Diabetes is actually a group of diseases, all characterized by high blood glucose levels. Most cases of diabetes are divided into three main groups: Type 1 diabetes, Type 2 diabetes, and gestational diabetes.

Type 1 diabetes, previously known as juvenile diabetes or insulin-dependent diabetes, is most common in children and is thought to be due to an inherited defect in the immune system causing the destruction of the insulin-producing beta cells of the pancreas. Once diagnosed, people with Type 1 diabetes must take insulin throughout their lifetime. Type 1 diabetes represents about 10% of the total cases of diabetes.

Type 2 diabetes, which constitutes 90% of the people with diabetes, was once called non-insulin-dependent diabetes or adult-onset diabetes. Now, however, it occurs in children as well as adults. In addition, people with Type 2 diabetes often eventually use insulin to control their blood glucose levels.

Initially, people with Type 2 diabetes tend to have higher-than-normal blood insulin levels, and they also tend to be insulin-resistant, meaning their cells are resistant to the action of insulin, so that more is needed to get glucose into the cells to be used for energy. When the insulin-producing cells of the pancreas are forced to overwork because of this insulin resistance, it causes the cells to die and eventually results in insulin deficiency. This type of diabetes is increasing rapidly in adults as well as children.

Gestational diabetes is diabetes diagnosed during pregnancy. It may disappear after childbirth, but it is likely to develop again during subsequent pregnancies. Women with gestational diabetes are also at a higher risk of developing Type 2 diabetes later in life.

When the body doesn't have enough insulin, as in Type 1 diabetes, or the body cannot use its insulin properly, as in Type 2 diabetes, glucose accumulates in the bloodstream and cannot get into the cells to be used for fuel. The system works a lot like the fuel pump on a car. The fuel pump takes the fuel from the tank and pumps it into the cylinder to be burned but the engine won't work if the pump is broken. Insulin takes the glucose from the blood and pumps it into cells (muscle, fat, liver, etc.) to be burned for fuel. When there is no insulin or the insulin doesn't work right,

Diagnosing Diabetes and Prediabetes

A blood test is necessary to diagnose diabetes and prediabetes. Prediabetes is a condition in which blood glucose levels are higher than normal but not high enough for a diagnosis of diabetes. Having prediabetes raises the risk of developing Type 2 diabetes. This table shows the tests used and the blood glucose levels at which diabetes and prediabetes are diagnosed. For a firm diagnosis of diabetes, a second blood test should be done on a separate day to confirm the first.

TEST	DIAGNOSIS OF DIABETES	DIAGNOSIS OF PREDIABETES
Fasting plasma glucose test	126 mg/dl	100–125 mg/dl
Oral glucose tolerance test	200 mg/dl or higher two hours after consuming the equivalent of 75 grams of glucose	140–199 mg/dl two hours after consuming the equivalent of 75 grams of glucose
Random plasma glucose test	200 mg/dl or higher and symptoms of diabetes such as increased thirst, increased urination, and unexplained weight loss	

the glucose cannot get out of the bloodstream and into the cells and then the cells can't work.

When glucose accumulates in the blood, the kidneys attempt to excrete it into the urine. This causes the loss of water and salt, leading to the classic symptoms of Type 1 diabetes: excessive urination, dehydration, and excessive thirst. The lack of fuel to the cells then causes the cells to want more food, causing hunger, another typical symptom of Type 1 diabetes. People with undiagnosed Type 2 diabetes also sometimes experience these symptoms, but they may also experience no symptoms or just vague symptoms, such as a feeling of tiredness most of the time.

What causes diabetes?

The different types of diabetes have different causes. Most cases of Type 1 diabetes are believed to be caused by an autoimmune reaction, in which the immune system mistakenly destroys the insulin-producing beta cells of the pancreas. The cause of this beta cell destruction is unknown, although there are many theories, some of which are currently being studied. It seems likely that genetics are involved and also likely that certain environmental factors, such as viruses, are necessary to trigger the autoimmune process in susceptible individuals. One area of current study is whether being fed cow's milk very early in life may trigger Type 1 diabetes in the offspring of parents with Type 1 diabetes. Other factors also have been proposed as causes or triggers of Type 1 diabetes, but none have been proven at this time.

The cause of Type 2 diabetes is also unclear, but genetics also appear to be a factor, with obesity being a common, triggering environmental risk factor. Obesity, age, and a sedentary lifestyle all appear to promote insulin resistance, one of the key underlying causes of high blood glucose levels in Type 2 diabetes. This is why the initial treatment of Type 2 diabetes is often diet and exercise, with the goal of lowering weight, increasing muscle mass, and lowering insulin resistance.

During pregnancy, a woman's insulin

needs naturally rise, and she also naturally becomes more insulin-resistant because of hormones produced by the placenta for the baby's growth. If her pancreas cannot keep up with her body's increased needs, her blood glucose level will rise, and she will be diagnosed with gestational diabetes. In some cases, the stress, weight gain, and hormonal changes of pregnancy will reveal a previously undiagnosed case of Type 1 or Type 2 diabetes.

Acute complications

There are three major acute complications of diabetes and its treatment: hypoglycemia, diabetic ketoacidosis, and hyperosmolar hyperglycemic state. In hypoglycemia, blood glucose levels are too low. In diabetic ketoacidosis and hyperosmolar hyperglycemic state, blood glucose levels are too high.

Hypoglycemia

Hypoglycemia occurs when there is too much insulin in the blood relative to the amount of glucose. This can happen for a number of reasons, including skipping a meal, eating less food than usual, or taking more insulin than necessary for the amount of food eaten. It can also happen if a person does more physical activity or exercises more vigorously than normal without eating more food or taking less insulin or other blood-glucose-lowering drugs. And it can happen if a person has an illness that causes vomiting or diarrhea (although most illnesses raise rather than lower blood glucose levels). Hypoglycemia is a common side effect of injected insulin and the sulfonylurea class of oral medicines, which includes glipizide (brand names Glucotrol, Glucotrol XL), glyburide (DiaBeta, Glynase, Micronase), and glimepiride (Amaryl).

Common signs and symptoms of hypoglycemia include shakiness, sweating, a fast heartbeat, looking pale, weakness and fatigue, a headache sometimes accompa-

Treating Hypoglycemia

To treat hypoglycemia, follow the "rule of 15":

1. Check your blood glucose level with your meter, and treat a blood glucose level under 70 mg/dl by consuming 15 grams of carbohydrate. The following items have about 15 grams of carbohydrate:

- 3–4 glucose tablets
- 1 dose of glucose gel (in most cases, 1 small tube is 1 dose)
- ½ cup of orange juice or regular soda (not sugar-free)
- 1 tablespoon of honey or syrup
- 1 tablespoon of sugar or 5 small sugar cubes
- 6–8 LifeSavers
- 8 ounces of skim (nonfat) milk

2. Wait about 15 minutes, then re-check your blood glucose level with your meter. If your blood glucose level is still low (below 80 mg/dl), consume another 15 grams of carbohydrate and check again in about 15 minutes.

3. If your next planned meal is more than an hour away, you may need to eat a small snack in addition to your hypoglycemia treatment.

4. Since blood glucose levels may begin to drop again about 40–60 minutes after treatment, it's a good idea to recheck your blood glucose level about an hour after treating a low.

nied by nausea, impaired vision, difficulty communicating, difficulty absorbing new information, dizziness, numbness or tingling, and unusual behavior. However, a person may have symptoms that do not appear on this list. Each person should be aware of his unique set of symptoms of hypoglycemia. Because mild hypoglycemia can progress quickly to moderate hypoglycemia, in which a person would need

Goals for Blood Glucose Control

Both the American Diabetes Association and the American College of Endocrinology have established goals for blood glucose control for healthy, nonpregnant adults with diabetes. Both sets of recommendations are based on studies showing the benefits of intensive blood glucose control. Talk to your diabetes care team about the target blood glucose range and the HbA_{1c} level that is right for you.

	AMERICAN DIABETES ASSOCIATION RECOMMENDATIONS	AMERICAN COLLEGE OF ENDOCRINOLOGY RECOMMENDATIONS
HbA_{1c}*	Less than 7% or as close to normal as possible	6.5% or lower
Fasting or before-meal plasma glucose levels	90–130 mg/dl	Less than 110 mg/dl
Plasma glucose levels after meals	Less than 180 mg/dl	Less than 140 mg/dl

* The HbA_{1c} test measures the percentage of hemoglobin in the blood that is *glycosylated*, or permanently bound to glucose. The higher the percentage, the higher the average blood glucose level over the previous two to three months.

help treating himself, or severe hypoglycemia, in which a person loses consciousness or has a seizure, it's important to treat hypoglycemia as quickly as possible.

Some people experience symptoms of hypoglycemia when their blood glucose level is above 70 mg/dl, the level at which adults are usually advised to take action. In fact, this is quite common among people who have had elevated blood glucose levels for a long time and whose brains have become accustomed to high blood glucose levels. In this case, treatment for hypoglycemia is not necessary, although finding a distracting activity may be. Treating for hypoglycemia when the blood glucose level is not low can contribute to chronic high blood glucose levels as well as cause weight gain.

Some people experience no symptoms of hypoglycemia when their blood glucose is low or do not notice any symptoms that occur. This is called *hypoglycemia unawareness,* and it is fairly common among people with Type 1 diabetes who normally keep their blood glucose levels very close to normal. In many cases, people with hypo-glycemia unawareness can regain their symptoms of hypoglycemia by maintaining higher-than-normal blood glucose levels for a week or longer and being very careful to avoid even mild hypoglycemia during this time. A training program called blood glucose awareness training, or BGAT, has also been shown to improve blood glucose control and awareness of hypoglycemia in people with Type 1 diabetes. People with hypoglycemia unawareness may also benefit from wearing a wristwatch-like device such as the Sleep Sentry, which sounds an alarm in response to perspiration or a drop in skin temperature, or the GlucoWatch G2 Biographer, which measures the glucose level in the interstitial fluid (the fluid between cells) and can be set to sound an alarm at a particular glucose level.

Diabetic ketoacidosis

Very high blood glucose can lead to diabetic ketoacidosis, a very serious, life-threatening condition. When the blood glucose level is extremely high, the kidneys attempt to rid the body of the excess glucose by increasing urination, which can lead to dehydration. At the same time, with no glucose entering the cells for energy, the body begins to break down fat for energy. The by-products of fat metabolism are called ketones. If ketones are formed faster than the body can get rid of them in urine, they build up in the bloodstream and poison it. Treatment in a hospital is necessary for anyone with diabetic ketoacidosis.

Signs and symptoms of diabetic ketoacidosis include a lack of appetite, stomach pain, nausea and vomiting, blurry vision, a fever or warm, dry, flushed skin, difficulty breathing, feelings of weakness, sleepiness, and a fruity odor to the breath.

Diabetic ketoacidosis can affect anyone with diabetes, although it more commonly affects those with Type 1 diabetes. The most common trigger for diabetic ketoacidosis is an infection. Other potential triggers include stroke, heart attack, trauma, alcohol abuse, certain drugs such as corticosteroids, and skipping or lowering one's insulin doses. Very high blood glucose could also be caused by an insulin pump malfunction that interferes with insulin delivery.

Diabetic ketoacidosis takes some time to develop, so with regular blood glucose monitoring and ketone testing when blood glucose levels are high, it should be preventable. Every person with diabetes should know what to do about higher-than-normal blood glucose levels and have a set of sick-day guidelines, which often include instructions to use more—not less—insulin or diabetes medicines.

Hyperosmolar hyperglycemic state

Very high blood glucose can also lead to a hyperosmolar hyperglycemic state. In this condition, the person becomes dehydrated, but there is usually no buildup of ketones in the blood. However, like diabetic ketoacidosis, hyperosmolar hyperglycemic state is life-threatening and requires treatment in a hospital. Also like diabetic ketoacidosis, it is commonly triggered by illness, trauma, or skipping insulin doses. It most commonly occurs in elderly people with Type 2 diabetes.

Signs and symptoms of a hyperosmolar hyperglycemic state are a dry, parched mouth, extreme thirst, sleepiness or confusion, and warm, dry skin with no sweating. This condition takes days or even weeks to develop, so like diabetic ketoacidosis, it should be preventable with regular blood glucose monitoring.

Long-term complications

Chronic high blood glucose can damage the blood vessels and nerves of the body, leading to long-term complications including retinopathy (eye disease), nephropathy (kidney disease), neuropathy (nerve damage), and cardiovascular disease.

Retinopathy

Damage to the tiny blood vessels of the retina can cause them to swell and leak or can cause new, weak blood vessels to grow on the retina's surface. Untreated, retinopathy can lead to decreased vision or blindness. Diabetes also raises the risk of several other vision-threatening eye conditions.

Nephropathy

Damage to the kidneys can eventually lead to kidney failure and the need for dialysis or a kidney transplant.

Neuropathy

Any nerve in the body can be affected by high blood glucose levels. The most common type of nerve damage associated with diabetes is called peripheral diabetic neuropathy, because it affects the nerves in the feet, legs, hands, and sometimes arms. Peripheral neuropathy can cause pain, tingling, or numbness in the affected body parts. Numbness or loss of sensation in the feet raises the risk of developing a foot ulcer, since small cuts or abrasions may go unnoticed and untreated.

Drugs Used to Treat Diabetes

This chart shows the drugs currently prescribed to treat diabetes. All are approved for use in people with Type 2 diabetes. The only drugs approved for use by people with Type 1 diabetes are insulin and amylin, which are also approved for use by people with Type 2 diabetes.

DRUG CLASS AND EXAMPLES	HOW IT LOWERS BLOOD GLUCOSE
Alpha-glucosidase inhibitors acarbose (Precose) miglitol (Glyset)	Inhibits absorption of some types of carbohydrate in the small intestine
Amylin pramlintide (Symlin)	Reduces postmeal release of glucose by the liver, slows the rate of stomach emptying
Biguanides metformin (Glucophage, Glucophage XR)	Decreases glucose production by the liver, reduces insulin resistance in muscle and liver cells
D-Phenylalanine derivatives nateglinide (Starlix)	Stimulates the pancreas to release more insulin when blood glucose levels are high
Incretin mimetics exenatide (Byetta)	Enhances insulin secretion in response to elevated blood glucose levels, suppresses secretion of glucagon (a hormone that raises blood glucose levels), and slows stomach emptying
Insulin	Directly lowers blood glucose
Meglitinides repaglinide (Prandin)	Stimulates the pancreas to release more insulin when blood glucose levels are high
Sulfonylureas glimepiride (Amaryl) glipizide (Glucotrol, Glucotrol XL) glyburide (DiaBeta, Glynase, Micronase)	Stimulates the pancreas to release more insulin
Thiazolidinediones pioglitazone (Actos) rosiglitazone (Avandia)	Reduces insulin resistance in muscle and fat cells

Autonomic neuropathy is damage to the nerves that control automatic functions, such as heartbeat and digestion. Autonomic neuropathy can cause bladder problems, loss of sexual function, orthostatic hypotension (blood pressure that drops when a person stands up), delayed stomach emptying, constipation or frequent diarrhea, and abnormal sweating.

Cardiovascular disease

Cardiovascular disease is the leading cause of death among people with diabetes. In most cases, cardiovascular disease is associated with atherosclerosis, the buildup of fatty deposits in the inner linings of artery walls. Atherosclerosis raises the risk of heart attack, stroke, and peripheral artery disease, which can cause leg pain and raise the risk of developing a foot ulcer if blood circulation to the foot is diminished.

Large studies have definitively shown that controlling blood glucose levels can decrease the risk of developing any of these complications and can slow the progression of existing complications. Controlling blood pressure levels has been shown to reduce the risk of cardiovascular diseases.

Controlling diabetes

In conventional Western medicine, the three cornerstones of diabetes treatment are diet, exercise, and insulin or other medicines, if needed. The goal of treatment is to keep blood glucose, blood pressure, and blood lipid (cholesterol and triglyceride) levels as close to normal as possible.

Diet is a cornerstone of treatment not least because a body that is well nourished functions and feels better than one that is not. In addition, to maintain blood glucose in the normal range, people with diabetes must learn to match their carbohydrate intake to their level of available insulin. Carbohydrate raises blood glucose, while insulin lowers it. For people who inject insulin, this means matching insulin doses to grams of carbohydrate in a meal or snack. For people who don't take insulin, checking blood glucose level before and one to two hours after a meal gives an idea of how much carbohydrate the pancreas can handle at one sitting, given the current medication.

For people who are overweight or obese, diet is also an important weight-loss tool. Losing excess body fat can help to lower insulin resistance and blood pressure and can improve blood cholesterol and triglyceride levels.

Exercise can improve general fitness, lower insulin resistance by lowering body fat and increasing muscle mass, lower blood pressure, and improve blood cholesterol and triglyceride levels. It also has positive effects on mood. Because exercise usually lowers blood glucose levels immediately, it has the potential to cause hypoglycemia. People who use insulin, especially, must learn to adjust their insulin doses or carbohydrate intake to avoid hypoglycemia with exercise.

Insulin and the other drugs approved for the treatment of diabetes all lower blood glucose levels, although they may do it by different means. Which drug is appropriate for which individual depends on the type of diabetes he has and any other medical conditions he may have.

An unmet challenge

The need to control diabetes is obvious, but actually doing it can be a challenge, as demonstrated by the large number of Americans with diabetes whose blood glucose levels are not in the recommended range. Sticking to a meal plan, getting regular physical activity, and carrying out a complicated medication regimen are difficult for many people. For some, the emotional hurdle of accepting the diagnosis of a chronic condition gets in the way of adequate diabetes self-care. For others, depression is a barrier.

For all of its advances in the treatment of diabetes—from the discovery of insulin in 1921 to the development of home blood glucose meters in more recent decades—Western medicine clearly doesn't have all the answers. And that's what makes an exploration of alternative and complementary medicine so intriguing. Perhaps what we can learn from other cultures and other approaches will help lead to the ultimate goal: a long and healthy life with diabetes.

2. WHAT IS COMPLEMENTARY AND ALTERNATIVE MEDICINE?

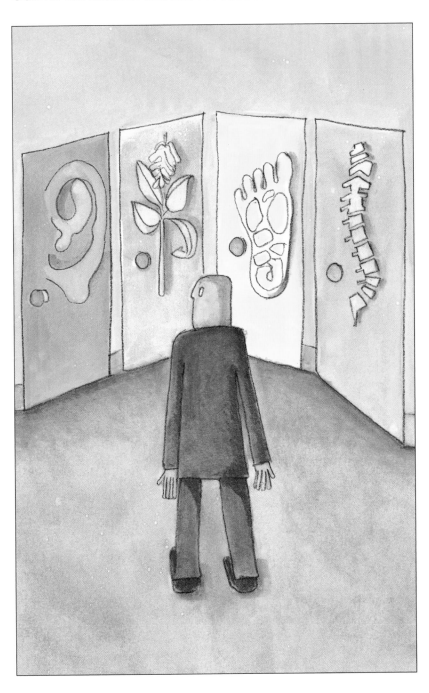

2.
WHAT IS COMPLEMENTARY AND ALTERNATIVE MEDICINE?

Complementary medicine and alternative medicine are terms used to describe approaches to health care that are outside the realm of conventional Western medicine. As defined by the National Center for Complementary and Alternative Medicine (part of the National Institutes of Health), they are diverse medical and health-care systems, practices, and products that are not presently considered to be part of conventional medicine.

Although the terms are often used interchangeably, complementary medicine and alternative medicine are not exactly the same thing. Complementary medicine refers to practices that are used along with conventional medicine, while alternative medicine is used in place of conventional medicine. An example of complementary medicine would be using acupuncture along with diet, exercise, and medicine to treat diabetes. An example of alternative medicine would be using acupuncture in place of diet, exercise, and medicine to treat diabetes.

For the most part, conventional medicine is considered "evidence-based" medicine, because its practices are based on both a doctor's clinical experience as well as scientific evidence gathered from clinical trials. Such trials analytically evaluate the outcomes of medical treatments in terms of life span, symptoms, disease complications, and overall quality of life. For example, the advice to maintain blood glucose levels in the near-normal range was evaluated in a clinical trial known as the Diabetes Control and Complications Trial. The results of this trial clearly showed that following this advice lowers the incidence of long-term complications affecting the eyes, kidneys, and nerves.

One of the main roles of the National Center for Complementary and Alternative Medicine is to support scientific research on complementary and alternative healing practices and products. Another is to integrate scientifically proven complementary and alternative practices into conventional medicine.

As more studies are done and more evidence accumulates on the benefits of some therapies, more and more practices once considered unconventional are entering mainstream medicine. For example, many hospitals now have stress-reduction programs that include the teaching of relaxation methods and meditation. The practice of tai chi, a Chinese exercise system that originated as a martial art, has become almost commonplace and is now often recommended by conventional health-care professionals to older people and those with balance problems.

But not all forms of complementary and alternative medicine that are subjected to scientific scrutiny stand up to the test. The National Center for Complementary and Alternative Medicine also publishes alerts and advisories to let the public know about practices and products that have not been proven effective or that have been shown to be unsafe. And many therapies have not yet been studied in clinical trials.

Types of CAM therapies

The National Center for Complementary and Alternative Medicine has grouped complementary and alternative medicine therapies into five categories, as follows:

Alternative medical systems. These are systems of medicine built on a complete system of theory and practice. This category includes both systems that originated thousands of years ago, such as traditional Chinese medicine and Ayurveda, the traditional medical system of India, and the more recently developed medical systems, such as homeopathy and naturopathy.

Mind–body interventions. These interventions are based on the theory that mental and emotional factors can influence physical health, and they use techniques intended to enhance the mind's capacity to affect bodily functions and symptoms. Some, such as cognitive-behavioral therapy, patient support groups, and prayer, are now considered mainstream because of the abundance of evidence backing their benefits. Others, including guided imagery and therapies that use art, music, or dance, are still considered complementary and alternative medicine.

Biologically based therapies. These therapies use products found in nature such as foods, herbs, other botanical products, and nonbotanical dietary supplements such as vitamins, glucosamine, melatonin, and even animal parts to influence health. Some of these therapies may overlap with the conventional medical use of vitamins and minerals.

Manipulative and body-based methods. These methods treat various conditions through movement, touch, and body manipulation. They include chiropractic, massage, Rolfing, reflexology, the Alexander Technique, the Feldenkrais Method, and others.

Energy therapies. Energy therapies involve the use of energy fields. There are two types. *Biofield therapies* are based on the belief that energy fields exist in and around the body. Practitioners typically place their hands on or near the body and use their own energy to affect the energy field of the person. Examples include Reiki and Therapeutic Touch. *Bioelectromagnetic-based therapies* involve unconventional uses of electromagnetic fields to influence health and healing.

CAM therapies for diabetes

Research on complementary therapies that might be of use to people with diabetes have focused both on day-to-day blood glucose control and on preventing or alleviating the symptoms of various complications. Numerous botanical products, for example, have been noted to have a blood-glucose-lowering effect, and some have now been tested in clinical trials. The antioxidant alpha-lipoic acid has been tested as a treatment for the pain of peripheral neuropathy (nerve damage in the feet and legs). The effects of yoga on blood glucose control, nerve function, cardiac function, and lung function have been examined in numerous studies. Biofeedback-assisted relaxation has been studied for pain relief and increased circulation to the feet.

Many of these studies have had encouraging results, so why hasn't your doctor added any herbal supplements or complementary therapies to your diabetes regimen? Frustrating as it may seem, good scientific research takes a long time. Studies with promising results may be followed by studies with ambiguous or weaker results. Different researchers may use different doses of a substance or slightly different forms of a substance or practice, making it difficult to draw generalized conclusions. They may also choose to study a treatment in, say, only men, making it difficult to apply the study results to women. In addition, different experts may analyze study results differently and draw different conclusions. And even when a product or practice does well under study conditions, it can be difficult to replicate those conditions in the real world.

In the case of dietary supplements with a blood-glucose-lowering effect, many have not been tested in enough people or for long enough for many conventional health-care providers to feel comfortable recommending them. When new drugs are tested for safety and effectiveness, thousands of people take them under experimental conditions before they are approved for marketing by the U.S. Food and Drug Administration (FDA). In addition, some herbs can interact with other herbs, foods, and drugs, and many of these effects are still being discovered. If dietary supplements are going to be used like drugs for diabetes control, it makes sense to hold them to the same standards as drugs.

Even if the use of dietary supplements is a long way from entering mainstream diabetes treatment, it has been well established that anything that lowers stress levels can lower blood glucose levels, and many of the complementary therapies discussed in this book can have a stress-reducing effect.

Exploring CAM therapies

Surveys show that Americans are most likely to use complementary and alternative medicine for conditions such as pain, colds, anxiety or depression, gastrointestinal disorders, and sleeping problems. When considering using CAM therapy for these conditions or for improved diabetes control, consider the pros, cons, cost, and, most important, safety.

Safety first

Safety is a concern when using conventional medicine, and it's no less a concern when using complementary and alternative practices. After all, if a product or practice is strong enough to have a positive effect on your body, it can also have side effects. Here are some steps for keeping yourself safe:

■ Do your research. Find out as much as you can about the practice or product you'd like to try. Consider the arguments of both skeptics and believers. Look for information about use of the treatment specifically in people with diabetes. Pay attention to the source of any information you find, and be wary of any "experts" who sell the products or services they recommend. If you come across scientific studies, note whether the subjects were animals or people. While animal studies are useful in developing certain treatments, they do not prove the effectiveness of a treatment in humans.

■ Talk to your health-care provider. Ask if he has any knowledge about the practice or product you'd like to try. Share what you've learned in your research, and ask if he knows of any contraindications (medical reasons not to use a particular treatment) or circumstances in which a normally safe treatment might become unsafe. If your health-care provider has concerns, ask if he knows of any other options to achieve your treatment goal.

■ If you intend to change your diet significantly, talk to a registered dietitian, who can tell you if your proposed eating plan provides adequate nutrients and whether and how it may affect your blood glucose control. Many dietitians who work with people with diabetes are also becoming knowledgeable about herbal supplements and their effects on blood glucose levels.

■ Talk to your pharmacist. Many pharmacists are knowledgeable about herbal products and other dietary supplements and the possible ways in which they may interact with prescription or nonprescription drugs.

■ Make sure the practitioner you've chosen has the appropriate license or certification to practice (but be aware that some certification programs are voluntary and require very little education to acquire). Anyone offering health-related services should be willing to tell you where he was educated, what kind of degree or certification he has, and how his practice is regulated by the state in which he practices.

■ Monitor your blood glucose levels. Any practice that involves physical activity (such as yoga or tai chi) or causes you to relax (such as massage or meditation) can lower your blood glucose levels. While this is generally a good thing, it can lead to hypoglycemia in some people, and it may signal a need to have a snack or lower the amount of insulin or diabetes medicines you take before you engage in this practice again.

In the case of dietary supplements taken with the goal of lower blood glucose levels, regular monitoring will let you know if the product is working or whether you might be better off spending your money elsewhere.

■ If you are susceptible to hypoglycemia, carry a source of carbohydrate with you at all times.

Questions for your CAM practitioner

As you explore the world of complementary therapies, it may help to remember that other cultures often perceive health and illness differently from how Western medicine perceives it. Many traditional healing systems believe, for example, that there are vital energies that run through the body on established channels, or pathways, called meridians. Illness occurs when there is a blockage in the flow of vital energy, so treatment—whether in the form of acupuncture, massage, diet, or use of herbs—is aimed at clearing such blockages.

If you're not familiar with the theory behind the practice, it can be difficult to assess how a given therapy might help you. Asking a CAM practitioner some of the following questions may help you to get a better sense of what to expect when trying something new:

■ What are the benefits of this treatment, practice, or type of therapy?
■ Will this treatment lower (or raise) my blood glucose levels?
■ Will this treatment reduce the amount of pain I'm feeling?
■ What percentage of people who try this therapy reap the benefits?
■ Do I have to believe in the treatment or the philosophy behind it to benefit from it?
■ How soon should I begin to feel the effects?
■ How long must I continue this treatment?

■ What are the side effects and how common are they?
■ Are any of the side effects permanent?
■ How much will this cost me?

Checking your blood glucose level before and after any treatments and keeping a symptom log can help you to assess whether a given therapy is having any benefit. Be wary of practitioners who encourage you to continue treatments that don't appear to be having any benefit. While there are many honest practitioners of complementary therapies out there, there are also unscrupulous ones who are mainly out to take your money.

Price and quality

In most cases, you'll be paying for complementary therapies out of your own pocket, although certain "wellness" programs offered through hospitals may be covered by insurance. If the service you're seeking is more mainstream, you should be able to compare prices to establish the going rate in your geographic area. However, it's important to consider quality as well as price. A therapist or teacher with more experience and expertise may charge more than one just starting out, but you may also get more for your money with the more experienced person, making it worth paying more. Similarly, if both group sessions and individual sessions are offered, the group sessions are likely to be less expensive, and they may be the better option if you decide you enjoy the group interaction and opportunity to meet others. However, if you prefer more individual attention or privacy, you may want to pay more for one-on-one classes or sessions. How you feel about a practitioner and how well you can communicate with this person may also influence your selection.

When shopping for dietary supplements, price may not reflect quality. The government does not regulate these products the way it regulates prescription and over-the-counter drugs. It does not require supplement manufacturers to perform any tests of product composition, quality, strength, or effectiveness. However, there are some independent companies that test herbal products and other supplements for quality. (Note that none of these companies tests the effectiveness of supplements on any disease or body function.)

■ The "USP-verified" label mark indicates that the U.S. Pharmacopeia, an independent, not-for-profit organization, has tested the supplement to assure that what's on the label is in the bottle, the supplement does not contain harmful levels of contaminants, the supplement will break down and release its ingredients in the body, and the supplement was made under good manufacturing practices.

■ The National Nutritional Foods Association, a trade organization for retailers and suppliers of natural products, administers the TruLabel program, which recognizes products that have passed tests to assess the purity and safety of their ingredients. Products are also evaluated to see whether they contain the ingredient amount listed on the label.

■ ConsumerLab.com is a private company that tests consumer products relating to health, wellness, and nutrition, including herbal products, vitamins, minerals, and other supplements for quality, strength, purity, and availability, or whether the supplement will break down and release its ingredients in the body. ConsumerLab.com allows manufacturers and distributors to use specific "CL Seals" to identify products that have met ConsumerLab.com standards.

Using common sense

Some complementary and alternative medicine practices have much potential to improve health and quality of life, but caution is in order to choose and use therapies that work for you rather than against you. Be sure you are making educated choices, and use common sense:

■ Do not substitute complementary medical practices for conventional treatment. This is an unsafe use of CAM.

■ Keep your conventional health-care provider informed about your use of complementary therapies. Even if he can't tell you whether it will help, he can probably tell you whether and how it could hurt or negatively interact with other treatments you may be using.

■ Watch out for unrealistic promises and sensational claims. If something sounds too good to be true, it probably is. No one has found a "natural" cure for diabetes (or AIDS or all types of cancer), so if they say they have, look for treatment or products elsewhere.

■ Remember that "natural" doesn't necessarily mean "safe."

■ Watch out for claims based on a single scientific study. A single study almost never proves anything.

■ Avoid practitioners who are secretive about their methods or who suggest that a government or medical community conspiracy prevents their therapy from being widely used.

■ Don't take megadoses of any dietary supplement, including vitamins and minerals, unless you do so under the supervision of a physician. At best you'll be wasting your money, but at worst you could do serious harm: Some substances that are helpful in small doses become toxic in large doses.

■ Monitor your blood glucose levels when trying something new, and keep records to determine the effect the treatment is having. If a CAM therapy is having a positive effect, you may need to lower your doses of diabetes medicines to avoid low blood glucose.

■ Pay attention to how you feel. Don't ignore the signals your body is sending you. If something feels wrong, it probably is. Don't let your desire for a particular therapy to work for you cloud your good judgment.

3. FIRST THINGS FIRST: SELF-ASSESSMENT

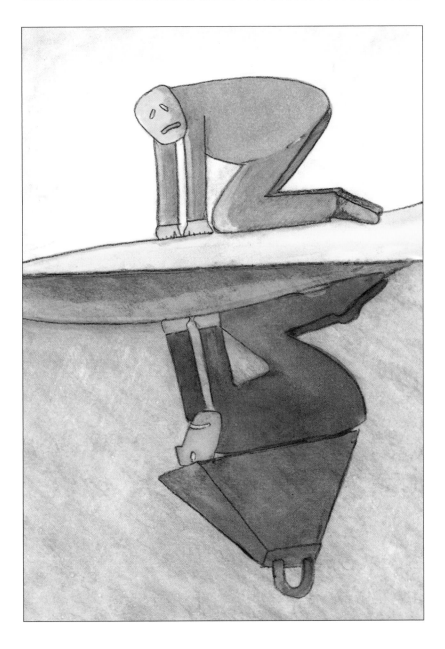

3.
FIRST THINGS FIRST: SELF-ASSESSMENT

Diabetes affects more than just your body. It can affect how you feel about your body, yourself, your life, and your place in the world. Upon being diagnosed with diabetes, many people go through the same emotional stages identified by psychiatrist Elisabeth Kübler-Ross in the 1960's as typical for people just diagnosed with a terminal illness: denial, anger, bargaining, depression, and acceptance. It has also been noted that people with diabetes have a much higher rate of depression than the rest of the population—even long after being diagnosed with diabetes.

This chapter gives you an opportunity to assess whether you might be depressed, how you deal with stress, whether more diabetes education might help to lower your stress levels, and whether your spiritual needs are being met. While people experiencing major depression should seek conventional help immediately, many complementary practices are useful for dealing with everyday stress and for getting in closer touch with your spiritual side.

Responding to the diagnosis

The order in which these stages occur, how long each stage lasts, and the number of times a person repeats each stage is unique to the individual. Often, it's not just the person who has been diagnosed with diabetes who experiences these feelings but also his close friends and family members.

Denial. To a certain degree, denial is protective: If you deny that you have diabetes or that it is having or will have any effect on your life, you don't have to feel the fear, anger, or guilt that often come with acknowledging the serious effects diabetes can (and maybe already has had) on your health and lifestyle. However, denial has a high price if it prevents you from caring for your diabetes. The longer your blood glucose goes uncontrolled, the likelier you are to develop long-term diabetes complications.

One way to get past denial is to truthfully assess whether diabetes has already affected your life in some way. Before the diagnosis, did you take frequent naps? Did you curtail your normal activities so you could be sure to be near a bathroom when you needed one? Did small cuts and scrapes take a long time to heal? Did you have frequent infections of any kind?

Low energy, blurry vision, frequent thirst, the need to urinate more than usual, slow-healing wounds, and frequent infections can all be side effects of high blood glucose—and they can all make your life miserable. Bringing your blood glucose levels into the near-normal range can have positive effects on your life now, not just in 10 or 15 years when you might develop diabetes complications.

Anger. Anger at God or fate, friends and relatives who don't have diabetes (particularly those who seem less attentive to their health than you are), seemingly insensitive healthcare professionals, as well as anger at oneself is common after a diagnosis of diabetes. While it isn't pleasant to have these feelings, it also isn't constructive to deny that you're having them. Nor is it constructive to lash out at those around you. It can help, however, to describe your feelings to a sympathetic listener, to find a safe place—such as a support group or a therapist's office—to express them, or to write them down in a journal.

If you're feeling guilty or angry at yourself over past behavior, such as eating too much and not exercising, remind yourself that you can't change the past; you can only affect the future. It simply doesn't help to blame yourself over what you should have done to prevent getting diabetes (if that was even possible). The fact that you're still alive means it's not too late to change your lifestyle.

Bargaining. A person in the bargaining stage might have thoughts such as, "If I do this, can I put off having diabetes for a while?" While there's no way to undo the diagnosis, in a sense, everything that falls under the heading of diabetes self-care is a bargain of sorts. Changing your diet and getting more physical activity will help you prevent both the short-term and long-term consequences of high blood glucose. In addition, people who are able to lower their insulin resistance through dietary changes and exercise are sometimes able to lower the amount of medicine they need to take.

Certain types of complementary practices can also help with blood glucose control, but they should be used as complements to conventional care, not alternatives. Learning to meditate is a great idea, but meditation cannot take the place of following a meal plan designed to control your blood glucose.

Bargaining may help you begin to appreciate what you will have to do to control your diabetes, even if the bargains you try to make initially aren't the ones you ultimately carry out.

Depression. Periods of depression are normal in adjusting to a big life change. Mild depression may respond to self-care, such as getting regular exercise and seeking out support from friends. But depression that becomes pervasive or long-lasting may require more than self-care efforts. If you are unable to accomplish daily tasks for days on end, find no pleasure in any activities, or are having thoughts of suicide, seek professional help from your usual health-care provider or a mental health-care provider.

Reacting to the Diagnosis

In her groundbreaking 1969 book *On Death and Dying*, psychiatrist Elisabeth Kübler-Ross described the psychological stages terminally ill people typically go through when confronted with their own death. It has since been noted that many people go through similar stages when diagnosed with diabetes or some other chronic disease. The stages that Kübler-Ross identified are as follows:

Denial and isolation: "This can't be happening to me."
Anger: "Why me?"
Bargaining: "If I do this, can I put off death (or diabetes) for a while?"
Depression: "I feel hopeless."
Acceptance: "I accept my fate and am ready to die (or live with diabetes and the self-care it requires)."

These stages don't necessarily happen in this order, and most people cycle through them more than once, with varying intensity of emotion.

Acceptance. Accepting diabetes does not mean that you like having it. It means you are willing to take responsibility for following a regimen to stay healthy. People who have accepted their diabetes still sometimes feel discouraged or stressed about having diabetes and still need help from others in controlling it. In fact, accepting diabetes often means accepting that you need to ask for help and support at times.

Are you depressed?

Even if you accepted your diabetes long ago, you can still become depressed. For reasons that are not entirely understood, people with diabetes have double the likelihood of developing depression as people who don't have diabetes. How do you know if you or someone you know is depressed?

Specific criteria for major depression are listed in the DSM-IV (Diagnostic and Statistical Model of Mental Disorders, fourth edition), a tool used by physicians to identify and classify psychiatric illnesses such as depression. A major depressive episode is defined by the DSM-IV as "a period of at least two weeks during which there is either depressed mood or the loss of interest or pleasure in nearly all activities."

In addition to these two cardinal symptoms, people with depression also tend to have several of the following symptoms and signs: sleep problems (sleeping too much, being unable to get to sleep, or being unable to stay asleep), impaired concentration or memory, an increase or decrease in appetite and accompanying weight gain or weight loss, either restlessness and irritability or having everything seem in slow motion, a lack of energy, feelings of guilt or worthlessness, a dramatic decrease in sex drive, and negative thoughts of oneself and the future that may be tied to thoughts of death or suicide. Depression can also manifest itself physically in a number of ways, including backaches, diarrhea, constipation, headaches, excessive sweating, dry mouth, generalized itching, or blurry vision.

If you think you might be depressed, see your health-care provider. While mild or moderate depression can clear up with time and self-care, major depression has been known to lead to suicide, and in that sense, it is life-threatening.

Conventional treatment for depression includes antidepressant drugs and/or psychotherapy, or "talk therapy." One form of psychotherapy that has been studied for the treatment of depression is called cognitive-behavioral therapy, or CBT. CBT is a method for teaching an individual different ways of thinking in response to stressful situations. It is intended to replace habitual, negative thinking patterns with more realistic responses. CBT focuses more on present ways of thinking and behaving rather than exploring the origins of one's thought patterns and behavior. (In contrast, psychodynamic therapy is based on the theory that exploring past traumas is important to psychological healing.) At least one study has shown that people who undergo CBT are less likely to have a recurrence of depression—at least in the short term—than people who only take antidepressants.

Although CBT is effective for treating depression, not all psychotherapists are trained in this specific method. You may have to ask around a bit to find one. Your health-care provider, your state's psychological or psychiatric association, or your local mental health clinic may be able to help. Also, in practice, many psychotherapists use both cognitive-behavioral and psychodynamic techniques.

Whether you and your health-care team select antidepressants, psychotherapy, or a combination to treat your depression, it is important to know that the majority of people who have one episode of major depression are likely to have a recurrence. One small study of people with depression and diabetes suggests that the recurrence rate within five years of the first episode can be as high as about 90%. Because of the high risk of a relapse, it is important not to discontinue therapy as soon as the immediate symptoms resolve and to discuss an appropriate maintenance plan with your therapist or health-care provider. People who experience several episodes of depression may be advised to take long-term antidepressant therapy.

While self-care efforts alone cannot treat depression, they are important to regaining good health. Here are some self-care guidelines:

■ Because high blood glucose levels have been associated with depression, make an effort to keep your blood glucose levels in target range. Seek help from your diabetes care team if necessary.

■ Exercise has been found to improve mood and lower stress levels. Engage in moderately vigorous activity on most if not all days of the week.

■ Eating right will support your recovery and also help keep your blood glucose levels in control.

■ Participate in normal social activities or join a support group to help keep feelings of isolation at bay.

■ Learn and practice a stress-reduction technique such as the relaxation response.

A few dietary supplements, including St. John's wort and SAM-e, have been studied for their effects on depression. At this point, neither could be recommended over prescription antidepressants for major depression.

St. John's wort. Some studies have suggested that this herbal preparation is helpful for mild depression; others have shown that it is not effective at treating major depression. St. John's wort can have side effects similar to those of prescription antidepressants, including dry mouth, dizziness, digestive problems, fatigue, headache, and sexual problems. In addition, it can interact with numerous types of prescription drugs, including antidepressants.

SAM-e. Short for S-adenosyl-methionine, this chemical substance is found in all human cells. Some studies have found SAM-e effective for symptoms of depression but not more effective than prescription antidepressants. Side effects can include nausea and constipation.

Dealing with stress

Some people humorously define stress as the difference between the way you'd like your life to be and the way it is. However you define it, diabetes can cause it. It can be a physical stressor if symptoms of diabetes or its complications cause pain or lack of sleep. It can be a psychological stressor if it causes emotions such as anger, sadness, or fear. At times it can be a source of acute stress if, for example, you suddenly realize you're out of needed supplies and the pharmacy is closed. And it can be a source of

Quick Cool-Down

When something stressful happens, your heart pounds, your breathing quickens, and you feel upset. By taking a few minutes to focus only on your breathing, you can slow your heart rate, lower your blood pressure, and also feel calmer and more ready to deal with the situation. Here's what to do:

1. Sit or lie down, and place one hand on your chest and one on your abdomen.

2. Close your eyes.

3. Breathe in through your nose for a count of three and out through your mouth for a count of five. Continue for several minutes.

If you're performing deep relaxation breathing correctly, you should feel the hand on your abdomen move out and in, while the hand on your chest stays relatively still. This exercise can be done almost anywhere, any time you feel stressed.

chronic stress if symptoms or feelings continue for days at a time.

Many people deal with stress by overeating, drinking alcohol, or smoking. Some cope by pretending the problem doesn't exist, and some respond by taking on more and more responsibilities, even while their heads or backs ache and their relationships suffer. None of these coping methods works well in any situation, and when you have diabetes, it can seriously disrupt your blood glucose control.

Better coping skills can be learned, however. Some simple methods of short-term coping include counting to 10 backward when a stressful situation comes up or focusing only on your breathing for several minutes, until your heart stops racing. Repeating an affirmation, such as "It's only a number" or "I'll get through this," or saying a prayer can help you to feel calmer and better able to handle the situation. It may also help to make a list of people you can call in a crisis and keep it in a place where you can find it easily.

Over the longer term, prioritizing what needs to be done can keep you from getting overwhelmed. Ask your health-care team for help in prioritizing your diabetes care. If you feel overwhelmed by the amount of information or number of tasks you're being asked to perform, ask which you absolutely must do now and which could wait for a few weeks, when you're better able to absorb more information or work on adopting a new habit.

Assess your readiness to change. Your health-care team may have suggested numerous lifestyle changes to help your diabetes control, but you're likely to be most successful when you work on something that you want to change and feel confident that you can change, not just something you feel you should change. As important as it is to work on diabetes self-care tasks, sometimes there are other issues, such as job stress or relationship issues, that must be dealt with first. Review your health-care team's recommendations and the barriers that stand in your way of reaching them, then choose an area you feel ready and able to work on.

Set realistic goals. This is key to feeling confident that you can make the changes you want to make. One way to make large goals more manageable is to break them into smaller tasks. Starting a new walking program, for example, could be broken down into shopping for walking shoes and socks, planning one or more routes for your walks, marking the days and times on your calendar that you will walk, and calling some friends to see if anyone will join you on your walks. As you see that you can accomplish the smaller tasks, you are likely to feel more confident about achieving the larger goal.

Ask for help when you need it. Most people want to help; they just don't know how.

If you're specific about what you want and ask politely, friends, relatives, and even strangers will often be willing to lend a hand. However, it's better to spread your requests among a few people rather than loading up one person, such as a spouse, with all of them. That can lead to burnout and possibly cause you to miss out on other, more effective sources of help.

Learn to say no. You can help others best when you've first taken care of yourself. So find polite but direct ways to say no to requests or demands that seem unreasonable or that you just can't handle right now. Many people are afraid of hurting others when they say no or making another person angry, but in truth, most people are able to deal with the idea that you sometimes are busy or have other priorities.

Another technique for dealing with stressful situations, although usually not in the heat of the moment, is called "reframing." Reframing involves finding a different way to view a situation. So, for example, if you feel that having diabetes is a bummer, you could look for something good that has come out of the diagnosis and perhaps come up with, "This diagnosis has motivated me to take better care of myself." You may still feel that having diabetes is a bummer, but with reframing, the picture is not all dark.

Yet another way to reduce the amount of stress caused by your diabetes is to view diabetes control as an experiment, not a test that you pass or fail. Many diabetes-related problems have no single right or wrong answer. After all, medical researchers are still looking for the best way to control blood glucose levels, so it should come as no surprise that your efforts don't always produce exactly the results you wished for. With experimentation, however, you can learn more about how your body works and what best controls your blood glucose levels. The problem-solving process involves five basic steps:
■ Identify the problem.

■ Decide what you will do to solve it.
■ Put your thoughts into action.
■ Evaluate whether your action helped.
■ If it didn't, decide what to try next time.

Change only one thing at a time so you know what did or didn't help. If none of your efforts resolve blood glucose control or other diabetes problems, don't hesitate to ask for help from your diabetes care team.

The experimental approach can be used for many types of problems. If your friends nag you about what to eat, for example, brainstorm some responses, and try them out. It's also useful when trying new complementary practices and therapies. If you decide to try a dietary supplement, for example, add only one at a time and evaluate its effect before adding another. This may take some time, since some herbs or practices may require a few weeks rather than a few days to see results.

Finally, set aside time to relax. Find an activity that calms you, such as reading a book, doing tai chi, or using aromatherapy, and do it regularly. If you are accustomed to smoking, drinking, or eating for relaxation, explore some other options, such as taking a walk.

Assessing your diabetes knowledge

Lacking the information you need about diabetes and how to control it can make trying to manage your diabetes more stressful than it needs to be. After all, monitoring your blood glucose levels is just frustrating if your readings are always high and you don't know what to do to bring them down. Similarly, carefully planning meals can seem like a waste of time if your blood glucose is always high after eating.

Studies show that people who understand their treatment do better at carrying it out. To assess your knowledge of diabetes control, ask yourself the following questions:

■ Do you know what the purpose of your meal plan is?
■ Do you know which foods contain carbohydrate?
■ Do you know how the medicines you take work?
■ Do you know what to do if you miss a dose?
■ Should you take your medicine even if you skip a meal?
■ Do you know why exercise usually lowers blood glucose? Do you know why it can sometimes raise it?
■ Do you know what to do when your blood glucose reading is above the target range identified by your physician?
■ Do you know how to care for your diabetes when you're ill?

If you don't know the answers to these questions or if you have other questions about your diabetes control plan, ask the members of your diabetes care team. Be sure you have basic knowledge about diabetes, the way it is treated, your responses to treatment, and any problems you have in dealing with your diabetes before you try any type of complementary therapy. Be sure you know how to use your blood glucose meter; you will need it to determine the effects of complementary therapies on your blood glucose levels. Since many complementary therapies are aimed at pain relief and stress reduction, take note of the effect that pain and stress have on your blood glucose levels. (Chances are, they raise them.)

Attending to your spiritual needs

Spirituality is not often addressed by conventional medical practitioners, but it can have an effect on both your physical and mental health. While many people associate spirituality with religion, it can also be defined as experiencing the presence of a greater power or presence and experiencing a closeness to that presence. It may mean taking time to contemplate your place in the ultimate order of things or focusing on the things that give life meaning. It may or may not mean being involved in organized religion.

In recent years, scientists have begun to research the role of spirituality on health and illness. Researchers have studied both *intrinsic religiosity* (a personal sense of the importance of spirituality and religion) and *extrinsic religiosity* (which includes frequent attendance at religious services) and have found physical and mental health benefits from both.

People who report higher levels of intrinsic religiosity have been found to have better survival rates after severe illness, less depression in older age, less disability and mortality when faced with chronic disease, and possibly stronger immune systems.

Frequent attendance at religious services has been found to be associated with a longer life, lower blood pressure, and fewer symptoms of depression. At least one study found that people who engage in volunteer work as well as attending church live even longer.

The diagnosis of diabetes may have caused you to question your spiritual beliefs and may have altered what you consider the meaning and purpose of your life. Your initial response may have included feelings of anger, betrayal, or loss of faith. Eventually, however, many people are able to see diabetes as an opportunity to find new meaning in life. For example, it can be the beginning of a new commitment to your own health or to helping others with diabetes or other chronic problems. Diabetes may also be the motivator you've needed to try something you've always wanted to do but never dared to before.

Several of the complementary practices described in this book—including prayer, walking the labyrinth, and yoga—can help to explore the spiritual side of life.

Taking the driver's seat

Taking responsibility for your health can be frightening, but it can also be empowering.

When you are empowered, you work with the health-care providers and specialists that you choose rather than just being told by them what to do when.

Being empowered starts with being knowledgeable—about diabetes, any complementary therapies you'd like to try, and about yourself. To become empowered in your diabetes management, keep records of your blood glucose readings, with notes about what you ate, physical activity, and stressful occurrences, and bring these records to your appointments. If what you're currently doing to manage your blood glucose isn't working well, take the reins by asking what you could do differently. If your health-care provider doesn't refer you for a yearly eye exam or perform regular foot examinations, go ahead and ask for them.

If you're thinking of trying a CAM therapy and wish to talk to your health-care provider about fitting it in with your regular diabetes care, do your research first. This will enable you to ask more questions and also to be assertive and keep the dialogue going with health-care professionals who are dismissive (or worse) when the subject of alternative medicine is raised.

Knowing yourself requires an honest self-assessment of your strengths, weaknesses, and state of mind. This can be a painful process if it forces you to acknowledge that you're depressed, have a low quality of life, or have difficulty communicating with others, but it also empowers you to seek help in areas where you need it most. Joining a diabetes support group or making an appointment with a psychotherapist is not a sign of weakness but rather a sign of strength and courage to change.

Assessing your diabetes knowledge and your personal strengths and weaknesses can also help you determine what's motivating you to try a particular complementary therapy. Is it because you're burned out on controlling your diabetes and hope that there's an alternative, easier way? Or is it because you're interested in exploring the mind–body connection, something that alternative therapies tend to emphasize more than conventional medicine?

Complementary therapies can make your diabetes control easier in the long run. But finding the practice or treatment that suits you, learning to use it, and using it regularly takes time and effort. With that in mind, pick something that appeals to you or intrigues you in some way. With luck, you will begin to look forward to your practice, whatever it may be, and learn to enjoy the journey as much as the end result.

4. WHAT'S OUT THERE: AN INTRODUCTION TO ALTERNATIVE MEDICAL SYSTEMS

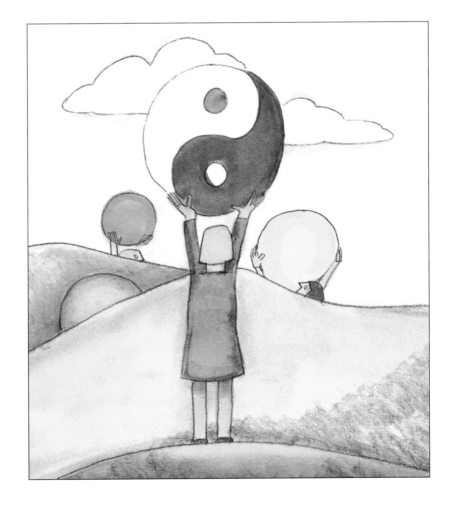

4.
WHAT'S OUT THERE: AN INTRODUCTION TO ALTERNATIVE MEDICAL SYSTEMS

The National Center for Complementary and Alternative Medicine, the part of the National Institutes of Health that supports research into complementary therapies, defines an alternative medical system as a system of medicine built on a complete system of theory and practice. While the medical systems described here fit that definition, most are used in a complementary way, or along with Western medicine, in the United States as well as in their country of origin.

Traditional Chinese medicine

Traditional Chinese medicine, or TCM, is one of the oldest medical practices, with archeological evidence of its existence dating back thousands of years. Obviously, the practice of Chinese medicine evolved over the years, with discoveries, such as the fact that herbs could be preserved through drying or that a person's pulse revealed information about his health, moving it forward.

As it evolved over the centuries, one of the main theories of TCM became that maintaining health depends on maintaining the balance of yin and yang in the body. In this system, all things, including the body, are composed of opposing but complementary forces called yin and yang. Traditionally, yin is dark, passive, feminine, cold, moist, negative, and moving downward or inward, while yang is light, active, male, warm, positive, and moving upward or outward. In the world, earth and water are yin, while sun and fire are yang. In the body, many of the major organs are classified as yin-yang pairs, which must be kept in balance for good health.

Another of the main theories of TCM is that of the five elements, namely water, wood, fire, earth, and metal. These elements can be related to different seasons of the year, colors, sounds, emotions, tastes, and bodily organs. In this way, the body is viewed as a reflection of the world. The elements also have yin and yang characteristics. Like the seasons of the year, the elements are believed to occur in phases, with each one generating the next and all of them affected in some way by the others. When applied to medicine, the phases of the five elements may help explain the progression of an illness and its prognosis.

Yet another fundamental belief in Chinese medicine is that an energy called qi (pronounced "chee") flows along pathways in the body called meridians. If the flow of qi along these meridians is blocked or unbalanced, illness can occur. Causes of qi imbalance may include external forces such as cold or heat, strong emotions, or lifestyle factors such as poor diet, too little sleep, or too much alcohol.

To make a diagnosis and determine a course of treatment, a doctor of Chinese medicine would assess the balance of body, mind, and spirit by taking a history and performing various physical examinations.

The tools of TCM include acupuncture, acupressure, moxibustion, cupping, herbal therapy, massage, diet, and exercise, particularly the practice of tai chi and qigong, which incorporates meditation as well as movements and breathing techniques.

■ Acupuncture is performed by placing thin metal needles along the body's meridians.

■ Acupressure uses the hands or fingers to

apply pressure to points along the body's meridians.

■ Moxibustion is done by burning dried mugwort, an herb, over a specific acupuncture point to expel cold, warm the meridians, and increase the flow of energy.

■ Cupping is done by heating the air in a cup or flask to create suction and placing it on the skin to stimulate the qi in that area.

■ Massage removes blockages of energy and promotes movement of energy.

■ Dietary advice might include choosing foods that are either yin or yang to help restore the yin-yang balance of the body.

■ Mixtures of Chinese herbs, roots, minerals, and animal parts are most often prepared as teas, by boiling them in water and drinking the resulting brew. Sometimes they are supplied in pill form.

■ Tai chi is a form of exercise that is performed with smooth, flowing movements. It not only tones the muscles and improves balance, but it calms the mind and promotes mental and physical relaxation.

■ Active qigong also involves performing sequences of smooth, flowing movements similar to or the same as those done in tai chi. Passive, or sitting, qigong involves doing breathing exercises and meditation. A practice called external qigong involves transferring the practitioner's qi to another person for healing purposes.

A visit to a TCM practitioner would most likely include a history-taking, including questions about your eating, sleeping, and working habits. Your tongue, tone and strength of voice, general appearance, and pulses might also be assessed. The practitioner might also assess your breath or body odor. Your back, chest, and other body parts might be palpated (felt with the fingers) for tenderness or irregularities.

On the basis of this examination and the complaint that brought you to the practitioner's office in the first place, you might receive a course of acupuncture (or a referral to an acupuncturist), a massage or some other form of physical manipulation, a pre-

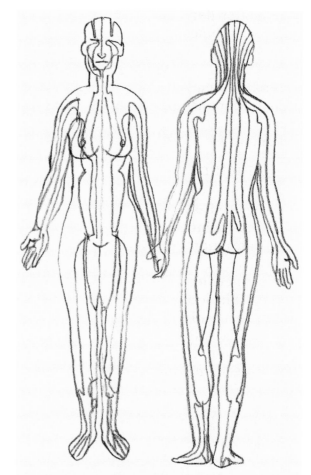

Meridians

A key concept in traditional Chinese medicine is that there is vital energy, called qi, that runs through the body on established pathways called meridians. Illness can occur when there is a blockage in the flow of vital energy, so treatment—whether in the form of acupuncture, massage, diet, or use of herbs—is aimed at clearing such blockages.

scription for some sort of herbal medicine, and recommendations for dietary changes and exercise.

Over 50 schools are accredited by the Accreditation Commission for Acupuncture and Oriental Medicine, the national accrediting agency recognized by the United States Department of Education. Some offer degrees only in acupuncture;

others offer degrees in acupuncture and traditional Chinese or Oriental medicine. A typical master's degree program lasts four years.

Certain Chinese medicine practices, particularly acupuncture and tai chi, have been studied and found to be helpful for certain conditions.

Acupuncture

Acupuncture is generally done by inserting very fine needles (usually 1 to 15 at any one time) into points along the meridians. In most states, nonphysician acupuncturists are required by law to use disposable, one-time-use needles to prevent disease transmission. (Physicians are not required to use disposable needles since they are assumed to be familiar with sterilization procedures.) The insertion of acupuncture needles is usually quick, relatively painless, and, when done correctly, bloodless. Once in place, the acupuncturist may twirl the needles manually or send a weak electrical current through them to aid in increasing or unblocking energy flow. The needles are then left in place for about 15–40 minutes.

For people who can't stand needles, electroacupuncture or laser acupuncture may provide alternatives. Electroacupuncture uses a small electric current and conductive pads to stimulate acupuncture points. Laser acupuncture uses low-level laser for the same purpose. When applied to the skin, low-level lasers produce no sensation and do not burn the skin. However, it is hypothesized that the laser light can penetrate into the tissues where it has a stimulative effect.

Many scientific studies have been done to determine the effectiveness of acupuncture, with mixed results. Among those showing promising results were studies on adult postoperative and chemotherapy nausea and vomiting and in postoperative dental pain. Acupuncture also appears to be a useful adjunct to treatment, or even an alternative treatment, for conditions such as addiction, headache, menstrual cramps, nausea related to pregnancy, tennis elbow, fibromyalgia, myofascial pain, osteoarthritis, low back pain, carpal tunnel syndrome, and asthma, as well as for stroke rehabilitation. It has also been shown to relieve pain and improve functionality in people with osteoarthritis of the knee.

Some people feel energized by an acupuncture session, while others feel relaxed. The most common side effect is fainting upon insertion of the needles. While a person may feel immediate symptom relief after an acupuncture session, it may take several sessions to complete the healing process. On the other hand, if no improvement is noted after five sessions, other avenues of treatment may need to be sought.

There is no real Western explanation for how acupuncture works, but it has been proposed that it somehow regulates the nervous system, possibly increasing the activity of pain-killing chemicals and immune system cells at particular sites in the body. It may also affect the release of neurotransmitters and neurohormones in the brain, consequently affecting the parts of the central nervous system related to sensation and involuntary body functions, such as the processes that affect blood pressure and body temperature.

Acupuncture was little known in the United States until the early 1970's. Since then, more than 8 million American adults are believed to have used acupuncture, and there are an estimated 13,000 licensed and certified acupuncturists in the United States, including many conventional physicians. Most states have established training standards for acupuncture certification, but they have varied requirements for obtaining a license to practice acupuncture.

If you're curious about whether acupuncture might help a symptom or health condition that you have, speak to your conventional health-care provider first. He may know whether there's any evidence for using acupuncture in your situation and, if so, may be able to refer you to an acupuncturist (or know someone who can). If your own health-care team cannot provide a referral, there are organizations that can. To find a physician with training in acupuncture, check the listings on the Web site of the American Academy of Medical Acupuncture, www.medicalacupuncture.org. To find acupuncturists who may or may not be physicians, search on the Web site www.acufinder. com or on the Web site of the National Certification Commission for Acupuncture and Oriental Medicine, www.nccaom.org.

Ayurveda

Ayurveda is the ancient health-care system of India. Some 5,000 years old, it is believed to originate from divine sources. Many consider Ayurveda more of a way of life than a medical system. It is based on the belief that the natural state of the body is one of balance. Illness is a result of imbalance, so any treatments or changes in lifestyle are aimed at restoring balance. However, there is no healing, or balance, without addressing the needs of body, mind, and spirit.

Similar to the Chinese concept of qi, Ayurveda holds that all life is based on an underlying force, or vital energy. In Ayurveda, this vital energy is called prana, and it is centered around energy centers in the body called chakras. Prana is the source of all manifested matter, including the five elements—earth, water, fire, air, and space (or ether)—of which every living thing is made. These elements constitute the three doshas, or primary life forces.

All three doshas are found in each cell of every human being, but in a unique combination. The one or two that dominate determine the dosha type of the person. Each type has characteristic physical and mental tendencies, as well as tendencies to develop certain illnesses. Identifying a person's dosha type helps a doctor to diagnose what's wrong with the person and recommend the correct treatment. Diagnostic

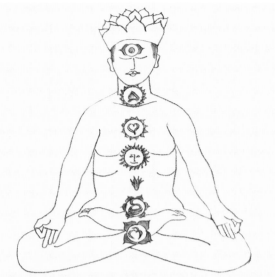

The Seven Major Chakras

According to some Eastern philosophies, the chakras are hubs of physical or spiritual energy in the body. Each chakra is associated with different levels of consciousness, bodily functions, and archetypal elements such as earth, fire, time, space, etc. Each is also associated with a particular color and believed to vibrate at a different frequency. Numerous medical systems focus on "opening," "clearing," and "energizing" the various chakras as a means of achieving physical and psychological health. The seven major chakras are as follows:

7. Crown chakra (purple)—chakra of consciousness

6. Brow or "third eye" chakra (indigo) —chakra of time, awareness, and light

5. Throat chakra (blue)—chakra of communication and growth

4. Heart chakra (green)—chakra of love, equilibrium, and well-being

3. Solar plexus chakra (yellow)— chakra of personal power, self-esteem, and personality

2. Sacral chakra (orange)—chakra of emotion, sexuality, and creativity

1. Root chakra (red)—chakra of security, survival, and basic human potentiality

methods also include a detailed technique of pulse diagnosis, examination of tongue, voice, eyes, skin, urine, stools, and general appearance.

"Detoxification" is an important means of treatment and may include purging the system by way of fasting, steam baths, enemas, laxatives, vomiting, nasal washing, and blood-letting. A person may also be instructed to purge the mind of negative thoughts and feelings.

Ayurveda places a heavy emphasis on personal responsibility. Although certain procedures, such as blood-letting, would be performed by a medical professional, other parts of a treatment recommendation would be up to the patient to carry out. For example, he might be advised to follow a particular diet, do yoga exercises, meditate, take certain herbs, or perform breathing exercises or self-massage. A person might also be advised to listen to certain music or surround himself with a particular color or certain aromas.

Some aspects of Ayurveda are already widely practiced in the United States. Transcendental meditation, for example, was introduced to the Western world by Maharishi Mahesh Yogi in the 1950's. More recently, Deepak Chopra, a Western-trained endocrinologist, helped to popularize the use of yoga, breathing, and massage therapy to regain balance in life.

Certain noninvasive practices are available through spas in the United States. Treatments may include massage with certain oils or herbal powders, steam baths, facials using Indian herbs and spices. Relaxation, clear skin, and enhanced beauty are the main goals, although some believe the application of certain oils and powders can draw out toxins from the body.

Ayurvedic practitioners are not currently licensed to practice medicine in the United States (unless they also have a recognized medical degree), nor is the practice of Ayurveda regulated by state or federal agencies. Standards of competency are set by individual schools that have received state approval. However, with the establishment of the National Ayurvedic Medical Association, one of whose stated missions is "to establish and maintain standards of education, ethics, professional competency, and licensing," this situation may be changing.

Tibetan medicine

Tibetan medicine is another medical system that dates back thousands of years. It is rooted in Buddhism with shamanistic influences. According to the Buddhist perspective, physical illness is inextricably bound with mental, social, and spiritual illness.

In this system, disorders are thought to arise from four sources:
- Actions in past lives
- Actions taken earlier in this life
- Spirits
- Imbalanced eating or behavior, which can give rise to superficial disorders.

The aim of Tibetan medicine is to restore the balance of three physical factors, translated as wind, bile, and phlegm. However, the meanings of these words are different from and much broader than their English meanings. A Tibetan doctor bases his diagnosis, at least in part, on questioning the person seeking care, observing the person, and taking his pulse.

Treatment, or restoration of a balance of wind, bile, and phlegm, may include spiritual practices as well as medication. If the spirits are involved, exorcism may be necessary.

While Tibetan medicine is an interesting field of study, there are very few trained practitioners of Tibetan medicine and even fewer licensed to practice in the United States, so it would be unlikely for a Westerner to have the opportunity to consult a Tibetan doctor. Some Tibetan herbal medicines have been tested in Western laboratories, but it is difficult to evaluate their efficacy since many Western ailments are not recognized in Tibetan medicine and vice versa.

Homeopathy

Homeopathy was developed in the early 1800's by a German physician named Samuel Hahnemann, who believed that a substance that caused symptoms similar to those caused by a disease would cure that disease. For example, if an herbal preparation caused nasal congestion in a person who was not sick, very small amounts of that herb might be used to treat a cold. This is the homeopathic principle that "like cures like."

A second homeopathic principle is that an illness is specific to the individual, so that two people with the same ailment might be treated differently, depending on physical characteristics, emotional state, or some other variable.

A third, and the most controversial of Dr. Hahnemann's principles, is that the more a remedy is diluted, the greater its potency. Homeopathic remedies are made by diluting a small amount of an active substance in distilled water (or sometimes alcohol) until there's only one molecule of active ingredient per thousand, million, or even billion molecules of water. These mixtures are shaken vigorously at various points of the dilution process. The belief is that shaking causes the "energy" of the active ingredient to "imprint" on the water molecules, so that the resulting substance can have an effect, even if there's only one molecule or even no molecules of the active ingredient left.

Homeopathic remedies are made from numerous substances, including plant parts such as bark, roots, leaves, fruits, flowers, and resins; minerals; and animal parts. Remedies may be taken orally in pill, powder, or drop form, rubbed topically, or injected. The standards for the ingredients and the preparation of homeopathic remedies are contained in the Homeopathic Pharmacopeia of the United States. However, this compilation of documents does not provide information on the uses of these remedies.

The Food and Drug Administration (FDA) regulates homeopathic remedies differently from how it regulates conventional prescription and nonprescription (over-the-counter) medicines. For example, homeopathic remedies are exempted by law from meeting the "safe and effective" requirements that drugs must meet. However, the FDA guidelines do state that if a homeopathic drug claims to treat a serious disease such as cancer, it can be sold by prescription only. Only products sold for self-limiting conditions such as colds, headaches, and other minor health problems that eventually go away on their own can be sold without a prescription. The guidelines also state that homeopathic product labels must include an ingredients list, adequate directions for use and the dilution factor.

Homeopathy is practiced by some medical doctors as well as acupuncturists, chiropractors, naturopaths, osteopaths, and others. Because of the principle that an illness is specific to the individual, a visit to a practitioner of homeopathy would likely include a detailed history-taking, including questions about feelings, thoughts, and lifestyle as well as physical symptoms. Hahnemann believed that simply allowing a person to tell his own story of the problem brought the person some relief. Based on a person's story and symptoms, a remedy would be prescribed. In classical homeopathy, the practitioner prescribes only one remedy at a time. In complex homeopathy, more than one remedy is given at once.

The expectation in homeopathy is that symptoms get worse before they get better. This is sometimes called the "healing crisis." The explanation for how healing takes place, called "Hering's Law of Cure" after Constantine Hering, M.D., an early homeopath, has three parts: Symptoms move from vital organs to less vital parts of the body; healing progresses from the upper part of the body to the lower part; and symptoms disappear in the reverse order of appearance.

While homeopathy has become more popular in recent years, most conventional medical professionals remain skeptical of its premise. Supporting this attitude are research studies that suggest the main effects of homeopathic remedies are due to the placebo effect, in which improvement of symptoms cannot be attributed to the treatment but rather to a person's belief that the treatment is helping.

Because the amount of active ingredients in homeopathic remedies is so small, the risks associated with taking them are likely to be low. However, delaying seeking treatment for a serious illness or relying on homeopathic remedies for serious conditions for which there are effective conventional treatments would not be advisable.

Osteopathic medicine

Osteopathic medicine is actually a recognized system of conventional Western medicine, not a form of alternative medicine. However, many Americans are not familiar with this type of medicine. Osteopathic physicians (D.O.'s) are licensed to practice the full scope of medicine in all 50 states, just like medical doctors (M.D.'s). Their training is very similar, but students of osteopathy receive extra training in the musculoskeletal system and in techniques for manipulating the musculoskeletal system.

The reason for this extra training is that osteopathic medicine views the musculoskeletal system as central to a person's well-being. Diagnosis and treatment, therefore, start with attention to the bones, muscles, tendons, tissues, nerves, and spinal column. A visit to an osteopath might include as assessment of how you walk, sit, and stand as well as how you move, extend, and rotate your limbs, hands, and feet.

A key concept in osteopathy is that structure affects function. So, for example, if the structure of the upper spine is somehow abnormal, the function of the lungs might be affected. The resulting breathing problems might lead to less oxygen getting to the heart, leading to heart problems. Treatment of all of these problems might start with correcting the structure of the upper spine.

Another central tenet of osteopathy is that the body has an innate ability to heal itself. The manipulation techniques used by osteopaths to align the body's musculoskeletal components are aimed at encouraging self-healing.

Osteopathic medicine was founded in 1874 by Andrew Taylor Still, M.D. Today there are 20 osteopathic medical schools in the United States. Many osteopaths work as primary-care physicians and use a holistic approach in their practice. It's worth noting, however, that some doctors of osteopathy rarely if ever use osteopathic manipulative techniques in their practice. They function exactly like M.D.'s. If you would like to see a D.O. who uses manipulative techniques, it's a good idea to ask about a physician's approach before you make an appointment.

Chiropractic

The main form of treatment offered by chiropractors is manipulation of the joints and adjacent tissues, particularly the joints of the spinal column. The theory behind this practice is that interference with the muscular, nervous, and skeletal systems of the body impairs normal function and lowers resistance to disease. While some applications of chiropractic remain unproven, this approach has been found effective at treating some cases of chronic low back pain—and for a lower cost than conventional medical treatment.

Although the practice of spinal manipulation has existed since ancient times, the modern profession of chiropractic was founded in 1895 by Daniel Palmer, a magnetic healer who sought to find the cause of all disease. An experience that strongly influenced his thinking was his near-miraculous curing of a man's deafness by manipulating a vertebra that appeared to be out of place. From this and other experiences, Palmer came to believe that decreased nerve flow was the cause of all disease and that misplaced spinal vertebrae caused pressure on the nerves, interfering with their flow and function.

Some chiropractors still believe as Palmer did that misaligned vertebrae resulting in nerve interference causes disease, and that spinal adjustments can effectively treat disease and ill health. For example, some recommend spinal adjustments for problems such as asthma or digestive problems. Others limit their practice to musculoskeletal problems of a mechanical origin and offer modes of treatment besides spinal adjustments, such as massage or physical therapy techniques to relax muscles and increase joint mobility.

Today's chiropractors must graduate from an accredited four-year chiropractic college, usually following two to four years of undergraduate education. Chiropractic education includes course work in anatomy, physiology, biochemistry, microbiology, public health, and pathology. Chiropractors must have a state license to practice.

Each state determines the scope of clinical procedures that chiropractors may legally perform in that state. Providing care for musculoskeletal conditions using manipulation as a primary intervention is within the legal scope of chiropractic practice in all 50 states. All currently exclude prescribing drugs and performing major surgery from chiropractic practice. In some states, chiropractors with relevant training may be allowed to perform pelvic or rectal exams, do acupuncture, prescribe herbal medicine, offer advice on nutrition, dispense nutritional supplements, perform minor surgery, put on casts, and do manipulation under anesthesia.

A visit to a chiropractor typically includes a history-taking followed by a physical exam. Other diagnostic tools used by chiropractors include x-rays, ultrasound, electromyography (a test in which a needle electrode is inserted into a muscle to measure the muscle's response to electrical activity), and applied kinesiology (a method of manual muscle testing).

Spinal adjustments, if deemed necessary, may be performed either as quick thrusts or as slow, sustained pressure. Some chiropractors use a handheld hammer-like device called an activator to manipulate the spine, although others frown on its use, saying it is ineffective. Chiropractors may also be able to offer advice on self-help measures, such as using hot or cold packs and exercising, that may relieve or prevent aches and pains. Occasionally, chiropractic manipulations will aggravate symptoms or cause soreness that lasts for a few days.

While chiropractic manipulations may offer relief from some types of back and neck pain, it is not appropriate treatment for all cases of back or neck pain. For that reason, it's important to have an accurate diagnosis, either from your conventional medical care provider or from the chiropractor. If chiropractic care does reduce symptoms, it generally need not be continued once symptoms have disappeared and you are feeling well.

Naturopathy

While the concept of "natural medicine" has been around for a long time, the practice of naturopathy (and coining of the term) as a distinct system of medicine emerged in the United States in the late 1800's and flourished in the early 1900's. After several decades of less visibility, naturopathy is regaining popular interest today.

Naturopathic medicine is a system of primary care that focuses on prevention of disease and disability and optimal health through the use of the body's self-healing process. A familiar example of self-healing is the ability of a strong immune system to fight off a cold, even if the cold virus has entered your system. Another is the ability of the skin to heal after being cut. When the body is stressed, however, its ability to self-heal may be impaired. Naturopathy works on removing obstacles to self-healing and creating an environment conducive to self-healing.

Doctors of Naturopathic Medicine (N.D.s) base their treatment of patients on the following six principles:

1. Make use of the healing power of nature.

2. Identify and treat the causes of the problem rather than just suppressing the symptoms, such as pain or fever.

3. First, do no harm. Use methods and substances that have the fewest side effects, avoid suppressing symptoms that might help the person heal, and work with the person's self-healing process.

4. The doctor is the teacher. Naturopaths educate their clients and encourage self-responsibility for health care.

5. Treat the whole person. At a person's initial visit, a naturopath asks about his physical, mental, and emotional state, genetic and environmental influences, social life, spiritual health, and nutrition practices. All of these can affect a person's health.

6. Prevent disease. Naturopaths assess their patients' risk factors for certain diseases, including their family history and lifestyle, to better counsel them on prevention.

Many of the principles followed by naturopaths are the same as those followed by medical doctors (M.D.s). The two differ, however, in their approaches to treatment. Some of the approaches that an N.D. might use (and an M.D. most likely would not) include botanical medicine (the use of herbs), manipulative therapy (such as chiropractic), homeopathy, and acupuncture. (To practice therapies such as chiropractic or acupuncture, a naturopath would have to hold the relevant credentials and licensures.) A naturopath is also more likely to perform nutrition assessments and education, toxicity assessments, and allergy assessments.

There are currently three schools of naturopathy in the United States that are accredited through the same body that oversees conventional medical schools: Bastyr University in Seattle, National College of Naturopathic Medicine in Portland, Oregon, and South West College of Naturopathic Medicine, in Tempe, Arizona. Other accredited universities—for example the University of Bridgeport in Connecticut—have N.D. degree programs.

Schooling for a Doctor of Naturopathic Medicine degree takes four years to complete and is considered graduate-level education. Students must have completed an undergraduate degree before enrolling. During the first two years of training, the curriculum in a naturopathic school is nearly the same as that in medical school. The next two years also cover the same diagnostic tests and skills as would be covered in medical school. However, there is a greater emphasis in these two years on the recognition of toxicity, nutrition, and lifestyle assessment. Herbal use, psychological counseling, and physical medicine make up the rest of naturopathic studies.

Not all states in the United States recognize the N.D. degree. In those that do, naturopaths often practice as primary-care physicians. In those that don't, naturopaths cannot prescribe treatments that are considered to be conventional medicine but they may offer other health-care services.

While naturopaths may offer the broadest range of naturopathic medical therapies, various naturopathic remedies are also offered by other health-care providers, including chiropractors, nutritionists, holistic nurses, and massage therapists. To find an N.D., look in the Yellow Pages of the phone book, or call the American Association of Naturopathic Physicians.

Orthomolecular medicine

The term orthomolecular was coined in the late 1960's by Linus Pauling, Ph.D., an American chemist who won the Nobel Prize for Chemistry in 1954 and the Nobel Prize for Peace in 1963 for his work to ban nuclear testing. "Ortho" means normal, and "molecular" relates to small amounts. The term describes a medical approach that uses "naturally occurring substances normally present in the body." The goal in this approach is to balance the chemistry of the body through the use of vitamins, minerals, trace elements, essential fatty acids, and amino acids. Because large doses of vitamins and minerals are sometimes prescribed, orthomolecular medicine is sometimes called megavitamin therapy.

Pauling first applied his idea to psychiatry, suggesting that schizophrenia might be treated with nutrients such as niacin. While that suggestion was largely criticized or ignored, his 1971 book *Vitamin C and the Common Cold* received much public interest, as well as much criticism from the medical community. The practice of orthomolecular medicine remains controversial today but has its supporters.

The following are the basic principles of orthomolecular medicine:
■ Nutrition comes first in diagnosis and treatment.
■ Because each living organism is unique, each requires different amounts of nutrients for optimum health.
■ Drug treatment should be used sparingly and only for specific reasons.
■ Environmental pollution and food poisoning are hindrances to optimum health and must be investigated when determining the cause of an illness.
■ Blood tests do not necessarily reflect the levels of nutrients found in the tissues of the body.
■ Hope is the indispensable ally of the physician and the absolute right of the patient.

In an initial visit to a doctor or clinic that practices orthomolecular medicine, you would most likely be asked to fill out a detailed nutrition history. Various blood tests would be done as part of the initial assessment and redone as needed as treatment progressed. Some of these blood tests would be the same as those typically ordered by conventional physicians, and some would be different (and therefore probably not covered by most health insurance plans).

Depending on the specifics of your nutrition history, you might be counseled on how to improve your diet. Orthomolecular medicine discourages consumption of fast foods, refined sugar, and food additives and encourages consumption of whole foods that are high in fiber and low in fat. Certain vitamins and minerals might be prescribed, possibly in doses much higher than the recommended dietary allowance. In some cases, injections of vitamins might be recommended.

Practitioners of orthomolecular therapy include physicians, psychiatrists, nurses, and nutritionists. Some belong to organizations such as the Society of Orthomolecular Health Medicine or the International Society for Orthomolecular Medicine, while others may have no organizational affiliation.

Holistic medicine

Holistic medicine, which is also known as integrative medicine, is an approach to healing that integrates conventional and complementary practices and that addresses the whole person—body, mind, and spirit. Any medical professional, whether conventional or alternative, can take a holistic approach. In addition to treating disease, holistic practitioners attempt to educate their patients on how to better care for themselves through lifestyle changes, nutrition, and exercise and to take an active role in their care.

Somewhat like the traditional Chinese view of health, holistic medicine views optimal health as a state in which vital energy flows freely through the body, mind, and spirit.

Medical professionals who espouse a holistic approach may belong to the American Holistic Medical Association, which has a physician referral service, or the American Holistic Nurses Association. Information for the public on holistic health, as well as lists of professionals and institutions that use a holistic approach, are available through the American Holistic Health Association.

A new perspective

Learning about alternative medical systems can be worthwhile simply to get a different perspective. Even when the explanations of how the body works or why a person gets sick may sound outlandish, many alternative systems contain some valid insights into what it means to be human and what health is all about. For example, the idea that health requires a balance of body, mind, and spirit resonates with many Westerners, once they take the time to think about it. The idea that nutrition comes first in diagnosis and treatment, a key concept in ortho-molecular medicine, may sound familiar and make a lot of sense to people with diabetes.

Even if you never seek out an alternative medicine provider, there may be ideas you can take away from other medical systems that might make a difference in the way you manage your diabetes or other health-care needs. For example, how "balanced" do you feel, and what might you do differently to improve that balance? Do you need to "detoxify" your mind of negative thoughts? How could you better support your body's self-healing ability? Would being allowed to tell your story your way bring you relief, as Samuel Hahnemann, the inventor of homeopathy, believed? If so, how could you present that idea to your conventional health-care providers, so that they could serve you better?

Look for the concepts that have value for you, then think about or discuss with your health-care providers how to combine them with the best that Western medicine has to offer.

5. MIND-BASED TECHNIQUES

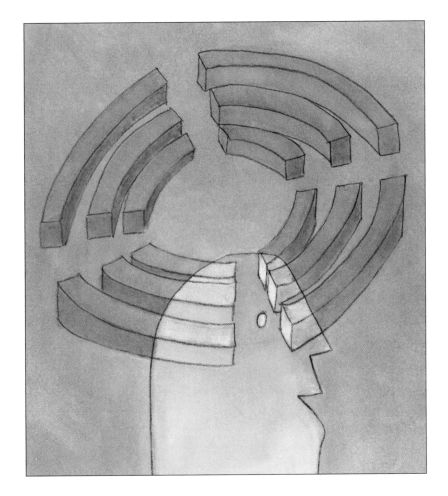

5.
MIND-BASED TECHNIQUES

Up until the 1960's or thereabouts, Western culture and medicine often treated the mind and the body as two completely separate entities. Yet everyone has experienced the mind–body connection. For example, just about everyone has blushed when embarrassed or anxious. Some people, when highly stressed, break out in acne, a rash, or even hives. People with chronic pain from conditions such as arthritis or neuropathy often report that their pain is worse when they feel depressed.

Many people with diabetes note that their blood glucose level is higher when they feel stressed, and it's not "all in their heads." When the body is mentally or physically stressed, it releases stress hormones, which prime the body to respond to a threat by raising heart rate, blood pressure, blood glucose, and sweating. In people who don't have diabetes, the pancreas secretes more insulin to deal with the increased glucose level in the blood. But people who have Type 2 diabetes may not be able to produce enough insulin to deal with the increased glucose level, and those with Type 1 are unlikely to have anticipated the stress and to have injected extra insulin to deal with it. The result, then, is high blood glucose. If the source of stress is acute and is dealt with promptly, there may be no long-term consequences. But if the source of stress becomes chronic, the elevated blood glucose levels can also become chronic and can contribute to the development of diabetes complications.

As more Western researchers have studied the connection between emotions and the body, particularly the immune system and blood pressure, the field of mind–body medicine has gained acceptance, and mind–body techniques are increasingly practiced at major medical centers. However, not all mind–body techniques require special training or the help of a therapist. Many can be learned and carried out on your own.

The following practices are those that start with the mind but that stimulate responses in the rest of the body. Their use is especially helpful in dealing with chronic stress. You may already use a number of these practices without even realizing the positive effects they can have on your body.

Positive thinking

Positive thinking, a term originated by clergyman Norman Vincent Peale, is the ability to change or reformulate your thinking so that you emphasize the upside rather than the downside in life. (Peale popularized the concept in his 1952 bestseller *The Power of Positive Thinking.*) In other words, it enables you to see the glass as half full rather than half empty.

Positive thinking looks for the good things that can come from bad things. For example, when asked what good can come of a diagnosis of diabetes, some common responses include "I'm learning to take better care of myself," "I have learned how to keep myself and my family healthier," and "I've found that exercise isn't so bad after all."

Similarly, a person who dislikes the task of monitoring his blood glucose levels could attempt to find a bright side, such as, "I could use a five-minute break a few times a day" or "All this hand-washing is probably protecting me against getting more colds."

Lest this sound Pollyanna-ish, researchers have found that people who use positive thinking have a higher level of immunoglobulin A in their saliva than negative thinkers. Immunoglobulin A is an antibody that protects the body against bacteria and viruses, so a higher level may mean fewer infections. That is worth the effort to think in a more positive manner.

Positive thinking is not about ignoring problems or making light of life's tragedies. People who think positively still experience anger, fear, sadness, and grief, but they are able to respond to these feelings with thoughts like "I can handle this" or "I'll get through this." Ultimately, positive thinking is about feeling in control of your life instead of feeling controlled by other people or outside events, but it doesn't always come naturally. Many people have to work at developing a more positive attitude. Some of the following suggestions may help you do that.

Affirmations

One way to think more positively about yourself is to use affirmations, or positive statements. An affirmation can be as broad as "I'm a good person" or much more specific, such as "I am losing weight now." While it may sound simplistic, repeating affirmations can influence your attitude. If you resent the idea of following a meal plan, try saying, "I choose to eat healthfully" rather than "I can't have the foods I like." Repeated often enough, this statement is likely to become the way you really feel.

Be aware that affirmations can be negative as well as positive, and if you say negative things about yourself often enough, you soon believe them. Learn to counter negative thoughts like "I'm a klutz" with positive ones like "Each time I exercise, I get stronger and more agile." When you make a positive affirmation, reinforce your words by visualizing a scene that embodies the affirmation. For example, you might imagine yourself eating a healthy meal, working out at the gym, gliding across a dance floor, or speaking confidently with your boss or doctor.

Positive affirmations can help in many areas of life, from sports, to business, to weight loss. Since repetition is key, some people choose to write down their affirmations and post them in places where they'll see them frequently, such as the bathroom mirror or the door of the refrigerator. You might also integrate one or more affirmations into your computer desktop or screensaver, or you could record affirmations on tape so you can hear them in your own voice.

Prayer

Prayer can have beneficial effects both for the person who prays and possibly for a person who is prayed for by others. When you pray, your heart rate slows, your blood pressure becomes lower, and your body uses oxygen more efficiently. Prayer is a quieting activity, much like meditation. In fact, some consider prayer a form of meditation.

Prayer is most effective if you are able to focus on your prayer without disruption from thoughts like "I need to go to a meeting" or "That neighbor is giving me trouble." According to Dr. Herbert Benson, a pioneer in the field of mind–body medicine and the physician who coined the term "relaxation response," prayers that include support words and peaceful intentions, especially if they are repetitive prayers, are most likely to elicit the biochemical and physical changes in the body that make up the relaxation response.

In his studies of meditation, Benson noted that all religious beliefs have some repeated phrase or process that appears to focus a person's mind away from the trials of the world, resulting in a state of calmness that more readily allows healing to occur. Among other health benefits, Benson and his colleagues found that a high percentage of people with sleep disorders were able to obtain quality sleep by using repetitive prayers or phrases.

Praying for others

Intercessory prayers are prayers spoken or thought by an individual or group of people concerned about the welfare of another.

Many religions have traditions of praying for the sick, and some research supports the belief that prayer has an impact on healing, even if the prayers are given at a distance. It certainly can't hurt, and it can have benefits for the people offering the prayers, so if you have the opportunity to be prayed for or to pray for others, give it a try.

Meditation

Meditation is well-known to calm and focus the mind. It has also been shown to benefit the body as well, by reducing such risk factors for cardiovascular disease as high blood pressure. There are numerous forms of meditation, none better than the others. The two described here are widely taught in the United States and also readily learned without formal instruction.

The Relaxation Response

The relaxation response was defined by Herbert Benson, M.D., author of the book *The Relaxation Response,* published in 1975. It is a physical state of deep rest that changes the physical and emotional responses to stress. Benson developed his technique for arriving at the relaxation response after studying practitioners of transcendental meditation who claimed they could lower their blood pressure with daily meditative practice. He found that they could, as well as slow their breathing and heart rate and reduce their oxygen consumption. In fact, if elicited regularly, the relaxation response has been proven to be an effective treatment for a wide range of stress-related disorders.

The following is the technique taught at the Mind/Body Medical Institute, a non-profit scientific and educational organization in the Boston area that was founded by Benson:

1. Pick a focus word, short phrase, or prayer, such as "one," "peace," "The Lord is my shepherd," "Hail Mary full of grace," or "shalom."

2. Sit quietly in a comfortable position.

3. Close your eyes.

4. Relax your muscles, starting with your feet and progressing to your calves, thighs, abdomen, shoulders, head, and neck.

5. Breathe slowly and naturally, and as you do, say your focus word, phrase, or prayer silently to yourself as you exhale.

6. Assume a passive attitude. Don't worry about how well you're doing. When other thoughts come to mind, simply say to yourself, "Oh well," and return to your repetition.

7. Continue for 10–20 minutes.

8. Do not stand immediately. Continue sitting quietly for a minute or so, allowing other thoughts to return. Then open your eyes and sit for another minute before rising.

9. Practice the technique once or twice daily. Good times to do so are before breakfast and before dinner.

Mindfulness meditation

Mindfulness meditation is a Buddhist way of meditating. It owes much of its current popularity in the United States and acceptance by mainstream medicine to Jon Kabat-Zinn, Ph.D., Professor of Medicine emeritus at the University of Massachusetts Medical School, where he was founding executive director of the Center for Mindfulness in Medicine, Health Care, and Society, and founder (in 1979) and former director of its Stress Reduction Clinic. Kabat-Zinn is the author of *Coming to Our Senses: Healing Ourselves and the World Through Mindfulness* and *Full Catastrophe Living: Using the Wisdom of Your Body and Mind to Face Stress, Pain, and Illness,* as well as CDs and tapes to help practice this form of meditation.

In mindfulness meditation, you focus on your breathing as a means of achieving moment-to-moment awareness. However, rather than being an end in itself, the goal of mindfulness meditation is to live each moment of your life fully. After all, there's only so long that you can focus on your breathing, but by learning to be anchored in the present moment, you can also learn to respond more thoughtfully when challenging situations arise.

The formal practice of mindfulness meditation is usually done sitting with your back straight, either in a chair or on the floor with a cushion for support. You begin the process of meditation by focusing on your breathing. Typically, however, as you try to focus, you become distracted by thoughts, sounds, or even odors. The idea is to treat these distractions as though you were an objective observer, without reacting emotionally. Once you have observed the distraction, you bring your thoughts back to your breathing.

Like the relaxation response, mindfulness meditation is most effective if practiced regularly, preferably every day. Mastering either form takes practice, however. It's not unusual to find your mind wandering or even to fall asleep when meditating. If you fall asleep, just try again another time. When you find yourself daydreaming, bring your mind back to your mantra or your breathing.

Meditation can improve diabetes control directly, by lowering blood pressure and lowering blood glucose levels by reducing the body's stress response. It can also help indirectly, by making you less likely to deal with stress by eating or by drinking alcohol.

Staying in the present also keeps you from focusing on what happened in the past—and possibly blaming yourself for it—or worrying about the future. It can put you in a calm frame of mind for learning from the past and planning for the future, both important for diabetes control.

Using a labyrinth

Using a labyrinth is another way to meditate. A labyrinth is a circular form with a path leading into and out of the center. Essentially, the user walks in and then walks out again. There are no blind alleys in a labyrinth as there are in a maze, so you can't get lost. In fact, the route in is also the route out. As you walk, you can pray, meditate, or let your mind wander while putting one foot in front of the other. There is no right or wrong way to walk the labyrinth. It's OK to go at your own pace, and if you meet someone on the path, you can step around him or step aside to let him pass.

Symbolically, the shape of the labyrinth relates to wholeness. The path can be a metaphor for life's journey. As you walk, you may choose to think about your life's journey—where you've been, where you are now, where you might be going.

Some traditions observe three phases of walking the labyrinth. The first phase is the inward walk, or the release; the second is standing in the center to receive; and the third phase is the return, or the time to integrate the experience. "Releasing" might include allowing yourself to fully experience feelings of grief, sadness, or anger brought on by your diagnosis of diabetes. "Receiving" might include saying a prayer or sitting quietly to see what comes to mind. And "returning" might include thinking about how you felt during the earlier stages, what you have learned, if anything, and what you take away from the experience. After you complete the labyrinth, you could also write down the thoughts and feelings you have experienced.

Labyrinths are found most frequently inside or outside churches but also in some medical centers, schools, and public parks. Some labyrinths are made with hedges while others are made of stone paths. Some include stations to pray for individual or world problems, to view beautiful scenery, to think about your relationships with others, or to watch a rock or flower or seed fall to the bottom of a vase. The best-known labyrinth is in the floor of the Chartres Cathedral near Paris.

The popularity of the use of the labyrinth is growing. If there's not one in your area, you can develop or purchase a floor mat with a design, or you can draw or use a hand-held labyrinth and follow the path with a pen or pencil or your finger.

Laughter

When you laugh, you release the same type of endorphins (chemicals similar to morphine) that you release when exercising. This may explain why you feel less pain, an increased sense of well-being, and less depression when laughing or exercising. Indeed, research indicates that laughing can have healthful effects ranging from lowering the level of stress hormones, stimulating the immune system, and decreasing pain perceptions to lowering blood pressure, increasing blood flow, and improving oxygenation in the body.

Writer and editor Norman Cousins was one of the first to write about the healing power of laughter in his book *Anatomy of an Illness as Perceived by the Patient: Reflections on Healing and Regeneration*, published in 1979. Diagnosed with ankylosing spondylitis, a connective tissue disease, Cousins found that laughter provoked by watching funny movies helped reduce the amount of pain he was feeling. While his is just one case study, humor has become a serious research topic, and any number of studies have confirmed that it not only feels good but is good for you.

Do you have a book of jokes to read or some funny videos to watch when things get "too heavy"? You might collect things that bring out a smile or a laugh, place them in an accessible box, and open the box when things seem the worst. If you could use some tips on using humor, try reading Loretta LaRoche's book *Relax! You May Only Have a Few Minutes Left: Using the Power of Humor to Overcome Stress in Your Life and Work*.

As you increase the laughs in your life, watch out for humor that is cruel. If it involves teasing or telling about someone else's embarrassing experiences, chances are it will hurt. As long as humor is not at someone else's expense, though, it can be just what the doctor ordered.

Guided imagery

According to Belleruth Naparstek, psychotherapist and creator of numerous guided imagery audio recordings, "Guided imagery is a process of deliberately using your imagination to help your mind and body heal, stay well, or perform well. It's a kind of directed, deliberate daydream, a purposeful creation of positive sensory images—sights, sounds, smells, tastes, and feelings—in your imagination."

Positron emission tomography (PET) scans show that the same parts of the brain are active whether a person performs an activity or imagines performing it. Athletes have long taken advantage of this phenomenon. When an athlete spends time imagining throwing a basketball through a hoop or clearing all the hurdles on a track (in addition to actually practicing doing it), in many cases, his performance on the court or track improves. Imagery can also be useful for people who are nervous about seeing the dentist. Instead of thinking about drills or other sharp metal instruments while sitting in the chair, a person might imagine lying on a beach, feeling warm, and listening to pleasant music. In many cases, the dental procedure seems to hurt a lot less.

A person with diabetes who feels nervous about giving himself insulin injections might use imagery to make it easier. For example, he might first imagine a very thin, sharp needle with a lubricated coating that allows the needle to slip through the skin cells without discomfort. He might imagine his body being relaxed, not "tightening up" to resist the needle. Or he might imagine the underlying nerves and blood vessels spreading apart as he pinches up skin on his abdomen for an injection, and the needle only going through skin and subcutaneous fat. He might then imagine himself giving several injections in a quick and matter-of-fact manner. By the time this person gives an actual insulin injection, it may be much less difficult than anticipated.

Imagery can be self-guided, or it can be guided by someone else, either in person or via an audio recording. If guided by a therapist or a recording, the technique usually begins with a relaxation exercise, followed by summoning up a mental image. The image would depend on the person's needs or situation. In some cases, a person would visualize a goal he wants to achieve, then imagine himself going through the process of achieving it. In others, a therapist might suggest starting with an image of a place where the person feels safe and comfortable before introducing other images. A person with a severe illness might then imagine tumors shrinking or invading microorganisms succumbing to aggressive immune cells. In some cases, a person might use metaphoric images, such as climbing a mountain and overcoming obstacles such as cliffs or being out of breath, rather than images of actual problems he is facing.

While the use of imagery has not been proven to cure serious illness, it may help psychologically, and it's possible that reducing the psychological stress of physical illness can have a real, physical effect. Even it doesn't, feeling better emotionally has great value.

Various types of practitioners offer guided imagery, including psychologists, nurses, and social workers, as well as people with no health-care background. While a number of organizations offer certification in guided imagery following a certain number of hours of training, there is no central licensing or certification required for practicing guided imagery.

Visualization

Visualization is related to imagery, but while imagery generally involves a narrative, visualization is more about focusing on one image or possibly color or sound. In some cases, a person chooses a particular image to focus on, such as a calm scene or an injured body part healing. In receptive visualization, a person allows his mind to flow freely and notices what images come in. Visualization can also be guided by a therapist or tape.

Here's a short visualization exercise to try (close your eyes or keep them open, as you prefer): Imagine a favorite place. Notice how peaceful it is. Think about the way it smells in your favorite place or, if it's an outdoor place, the color of the sky and trees nearby. Continue the visualization for several minutes. At the end of this period, note how you feel and whether you feel calmer than you did before your visualization.

Art as therapy

Art therapy has been used for more than 50 years to help with physical and mental healing. Art therapists work in hospitals, schools, prisons, and in private practice, among other places. Art therapy is often used to help people cope in the aftermath of natural disasters and other traumatic events. Research supports art therapy's ability to decrease distress, anxiety, and depression and to improve quality of life and feelings of vitality. It can be particularly well-suited to people who have trouble expressing themselves in words, such as children, but it's not for everyone. Some people find the emotions and memories stirred up by art therapy more distressing than cathartic.

Working with a registered art therapist is not necessarily required for art-making to be therapeutic. Creating art alone or with a group has also been shown to have health benefits. Any medium can be used to create art—clay, paint, fabric, collage, natural materials, etc. Drawing a picture with pencils or crayons can be an easy way to get started since it requires no special materials or equipment. Don't worry about having (or lacking) artistic talent or about being able to create representational images. Participating in the creative process is what's important.

Whether or not you "interpret" your artwork is up to you. You may decide that just creating it is enough, or you may try to put into words the emotions, events, or relationships depicted in the artwork. Sometimes explaining your work to others can help you see themes or symbols you hadn't noticed previously. In addition, other people may see things that you don't. However, if someone else's interpretation of your work doesn't feel right to you, you don't have to accept it.

Here are some ideas for exploring your feelings about diabetes through art:

■ Draw the first thing that comes to mind when you hear or think the word "diabetes."

■ Draw your experience of low blood glucose.

■ Draw your image of a syringe or lancet.

■ Draw a picture of yourself that shows your place in your family since being diagnosed with diabetes.

Over time, looking at the art you've created may clarify how your feelings have changed over the months and years.

Music as therapy

Music can have numerous, positive effects on the mind and body. It can be soothing, it can brighten your spirits, it can motivate you to exercise. Listening to slower music, especially with 60 beats or less per minute, can actually slow the heart rate. However, music can also have negative effects. Certain types of music may make you feel tense. Discordant, nonharmonious music has been shown to "shrivel" cells. Under a microscope, they can be seen getting smaller and out of shape. Pleasant music, on the other hand, can promote cell growth.

Many studies have been done on the health benefits of playing or listening to music. They have shown that music can reduce stress and pain, enhance immune function, alter brain-wave activity, reduce muscle tension, increase endorphin levels, and trigger feelings of inner peace. Music has also been shown to aid in neurological rehabilitation.

Music is called therapy when it is used to achieve therapeutic goals. In hospitals, music may be used to elevate patients' moods, induce sleep, reduce anxiety, and encourage relaxation. It may also be used along with anesthesia to alleviate pain. Music therapists who work with elderly people may use it to encourage physical movement and social interaction. For people with Alzheimer disease or other brain disorders, music may stimulate memories, improve mood, and increase orientation to the present. In children, music may be used to enhance communication skills and physical coordination. In people with mental illness, therapists may use music to help explore and express feelings or for imagery exercises.

Working with a qualified music therapist can be a rewarding experience, but you can also use music as self-therapy in any number of ways. Here are some ideas:

■ Listen to music and select works that perk you up, relax you, or influence your mood in the way you desire. Playing quiet music at bedtime may help you to get to sleep more easily.

■ Use music to inspire you to exercise. Faster music can help you keep up a brisk pace while walking or performing other aerobic activities. Dance music can get you dancing. Slower music may work best during resistance training, to prevent you from rushing through the exercises.

■ Play an instrument, alone or with others. Making music can enhance your ability to focus, temporarily take your mind off troubling thoughts, keep you involved socially, give you a sense of accomplishment, and just be plain fun.

■ Sing more often, whether or not you can carry a tune. Singing exercises the heart and lungs. It can improve mood. It can have spiritual benefits. Singing in an organized group has the added benefit of social interaction.

Dancing and drumming

Dancing as a healing art dates back to primitive times, when medicine men danced on behalf of their sick patients. Today, therapeutic dancing is generally done by the person seeking healing, not by the healer on his behalf.

Marian Chace, a modern dancer in the 1920's, is considered the founder of dance and movement therapy. After a career as a professional dancer, Chace taught dance classes in Washington, DC, beginning in the 1930's. She became interested in dance as more than a performance art when she noticed that some of her students were more engaged in the emotions they expressed in dancing than in the mechanics and technique of dance. Through working with psychiatric patients, Chace developed her theory that dance is a form of communication that fulfills a basic human need.

Today, dance and movement therapists work with diverse groups and individuals to improve self-esteem and body image, gain personal insight, and communicate more effectively. Dance therapy can have physical benefits, such as improved balance and greater muscle control, as well as psychological benefits, such as improved mood. The specifics of the movements done in a dance therapy session depend on the individual's or group's physical and mental abilities and needs. Therapists may choreograph movements for participants to follow, suggest certain movements or types of movements, ask participants to choreograph their own dances, or have participants improvise, or move freely, to music. While dance therapy is largely nonverbal, with the body expressing thoughts and feelings, some therapists and their clients also talk about the thoughts, feelings, and memories that arise during a session.

Registered dance therapists have a master's degree in dance/movement therapy or a related degree title and have completed many hours of supervised clinical work. The organization overseeing dance therapy credentialing is the American Dance Therapy Association.

Drumming is another mode of creative self-expression that can have similar benefits to dancing. Drumming allows a person to express his feelings, communicate with others in a drumming group, and feel connected with a group rather than socially isolated. Drumming can also be a form of exercise and of relaxation. It may offer an alternative for people who feel too self-conscious to dance or are unable to dance for some other reason.

Therapeutic drumming is currently used in numerous settings, from prisons to schools to psychiatric facilities to nursing homes. Some workplaces have introduced drumming sessions to enhance employee wellness. It is also becoming more popular as a recreational or therapeutic activity outside these settings, with drumming classes and workshops being offered around the country. In institutional settings, drumming classes or groups are often led by credentialed music therapists. In other settings, the leader may be a musician but not necessarily a registered or licensed mental health-care provider.

Eye Movement Desensitization and Reprocessing

Eye Movement Desensitization and Reprocessing, or EMDR, is a psychological treatment method that was "discovered" by psychologist Francine Shapiro in the late 1980's, after she became interested in psychoneuroimmunology—the study of how the mind affects the nervous system and the immune system. The intent of EMDR is to reduce the anxiety and distress associated with traumatic memories. It has been shown to be an effective treatment for post-traumatic stress disorder.

To use this technique, a person, with the help of his therapist, first decides on a distressing memory to focus on. He then identifies the most vivid visual image he can relate to that memory, a negative belief he carries about himself, and any related emotions or bodily sensations. He also identifies a positive belief. The person then focuses on the image, negative thought, and bodily sensations while simultaneously following the therapist's fingers with his eyes as they move back and forth across his field of vision for 20–30 seconds or more. Some therapists also use sounds, tapping, or other types of stimulation in addition to directing the eye movements. The person than lets his mind go blank and notices whatever thoughts, feelings, images, or sensations occur. This is repeated numerous times. When the person reports no distress related to the troubling memory, he is directed to focus on his positive belief.

The expectation is that the person will become desensitized to the memory, so it no longer causes distress. In addition, he will gain insight from this process, which will lead to behavioral change.

Exactly how or why EMDR works is not known. However, it should only be performed by properly trained, licensed psychotherapists. The EMDR International Association maintains a list of certified EMDR therapists.

Finding your mind–body connection

Some of the activities or types of therapies described in this chapter require the services of a professional therapist, while others can be tried on your own. Start with what feels comfortable to you. If working alone does not feel therapeutic or is boring or lonely, consider seeking outside help or the support of a group. In addition, give it time. Any new practice feels awkward at first. You may not see immediate results. In fact, you probably won't. But if you can find some pleasure or value in what you're doing and continue doing it for at least several weeks, you may start to feel some real benefits, such as feeling more relaxed more of the time, happier, or simply less stressed.

When you find a technique that works for you, keep tabs on your blood glucose control. You may be surprised to see that an activity that burns very few calories, when done regularly, helps to lower your blood glucose. It's not magic: It's the mind–body connection at work.

6. BODY-BASED THERAPIES

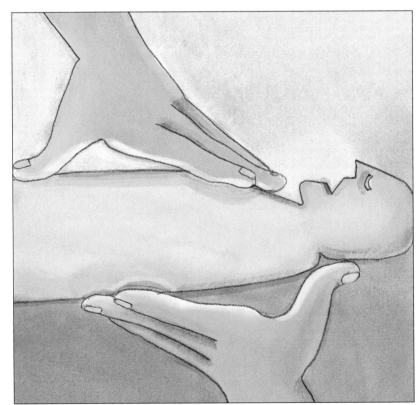

6.
BODY-BASED THERAPIES

Just as the mind influences the body, so does the body influence the mind. Pain from a backache or a headache can easily translate into a bad mood. Treating the body in ways that reduce pain and relax the muscles, therefore, can result in a happier, calmer state of mind.

This chapter looks at various techniques that focus on the systems of the body and its structures. These include the bones, the joints, the soft tissues, and the circulatory systems. While the goal of many of these methods is physical relaxation and pain relief, some have treatment goals that go beyond this. Providers of these techniques should be able to tell you what conditions can reasonably be helped by their mode of treatment.

Musculoskeletal manipulation

Musculoskeletal manipulations, or manual treatment of muscles and joints, can be helpful for certain conditions. Manipulations of various sorts may be performed by physiatrists (M.D.'s), osteopaths (D.O.'s), chiropractors, physical therapists, and sports trainers, depending on the nature of the problem and the training of the provider. The goal of musculoskeletal manipulation is to alleviate pain, restore a normal range of motion, and help the body function more efficiently.

Typical reasons to seek such treatment include back or neck pain and sports-related or work-related injuries affecting the limbs, spine, or neck. "Alternative" reasons to seek treatment would include conditions such as asthma, allergies, and ear infections, which have no obvious musculoskeletal connection.

Diabetes raises the risk of developing cer-

tain musculoskeletal problems, several of them involving the hands and shoulders, such as frozen shoulder, carpal tunnel syndrome, trigger finger, and limited joint mobility in the fingers. When seeking treatment for these problems, it's a good idea to start with your conventional health-care provider, who can educate you on what treatments may be effective for your condition and refer you to the appropriate specialist.

Massage

Massage is the systematic manipulation of the soft tissues of the body. It can help to relieve stress and muscular tension, reduce pain from injuries, and speed healing from certain acute and chronic conditions. A particular type of massage, called manual lymphatic drainage, can be useful in the treatment of lymphedema, a condition in which lymphatic fluid builds up in the tissues. Lymphedema in the arm is common following a mastectomy.

One of the primary benefits of all types of massage is relaxation. By sedating the nervous system, massage can bring a much-needed rest and a sense of well-being to the body. The caring touch of a massage therapist can also be a boost to self-esteem.

Massage increases the local circulation of blood and lymph, facilitating the transport of oxygen and other nutrients into the body's tissues. Improved circulation allows for more efficient uptake of insulin by the cells, so massaging an area where insulin has recently been injected could speed the insulin's entry into the bloodstream and cause low blood glucose.

Even in people who don't inject insulin, however, it's not unusual for blood glucose levels to fall during a massage, most likely because of its relaxing effects. This being the case, it's a good idea to bring a source of carbohydrate to treat hypoglycemia when receiving a massage.

Because massage works directly with the muscles and connective tissues (called *fasciae*), it may help to facilitate greater mobility. Deep-tissue massage can increase the range of motion of joints by releasing the connective tissue if there's contracture or scarring. This type of massage can be beneficial after surgery on a joint. Deep-tissue massage can also release chronic patterns of tension in the body.

No matter what type of massage you seek or why, communication between the massage therapist and the client is important. A massage therapist should ask you about your health history before proceeding with a massage treatment. If you have particular needs and concerns, share those with the therapist. Certain diabetic complications may make certain massage techniques more or less preferable. For example, if a person has peripheral neuropathy (damage to the nerves of the feet and sometimes hands) and is very sensitive to touch, a gentler touch may be needed. A skilled massage therapist should be able to adapt to your needs.

There are certain times when a massage is not recommended or precautions are in order:

■ Don't get a massage if you have a fever or are feeling unwell.

■ Don't get massaged near the site of an acute trauma such as an open wound, recent bruising, muscle tear, sprained ligament, contusion, chilblain, or burn, or over the site of a known tumor.

■ Don't get a massage when you have any kind of skin infection.

■ If you have blood vessel conditions such as varicose veins, phlebitis (inflammation of the veins), or thrombosis (blood clots), speak to your doctor before getting a massage.

■ If you have a chronic condition, such as cancer, heart disease, or advanced kidney or liver disease, speak to your doctor before getting a massage.

■ If you are pregnant, tell your massage therapist. Massaging certain areas of the body may induce labor.

Many states have passed legislation regarding the licensing of professional massage therapists and defining what level of education and/or national testing they need to practice legally. While the rules for certification and licensing vary widely from state to state, many require massage therapists to complete at least 600 hours of classroom instruction in massage therapy or be certified by passing an exam given by the National Certification Board for Therapeutic Massage and Bodywork.

To locate a properly qualified massage therapist in your area, call the American Massage Therapy Association's massage therapist locator service at (888) THE-AMTA (843-2682), or log onto www.amta-massage.org. You can also call the National Certification Board for Therapeutic Massage and Bodywork at (800) 296-0664, or look on their Web site, www.ncbtmb.com for certified practitioners.

In some cases, health insurance may cover part of the cost of a massage. If massage is prescribed by a physician, it increases your chances of receiving insurance coverage.

Swedish massage

Swedish massage is the most commonly used type of massage in the United States. Its main purpose is relaxation, and it is based on five specific techniques:

Effleurage. A massage generally begins and ends with long, gliding strokes called effleurage. At the beginning of a massage, this relaxes the muscles and prepares them for deeper treatment.

Petrissage. This kneading technique involves lifting the muscle away from the bone then rolling or squeezing it with gentle pressure. It can feel both soothing and stimulating. Petrissage loosens and

Body-Based Therapies

stretches muscle fibers and increases local circulation.

Friction. These are deep, circular or back-and-forth movements done with a fingertip or thumb, often near the spine or joints. Friction techniques can break up adhesions, or areas of thickening in the muscles and fascia, leading to greater mobility.

Vibration. This involves the therapist pressing his hands on a muscle and rapidly shaking for a few seconds to increase circulation.

Tapotement. This percussive, "beating" technique may be done using the outside edges of the hands, the fingertips, tight or loose fists, or cupped hands. It tends to be stimulating to the body.

Some additional techniques that a massage therapist might use include the following:

Trigger point therapy. Sometimes called neuromuscular massage, this therapy is used for the relief of soft-tissue pain and dysfunction. Similar to friction, it works on "trigger points," or small areas of tightness or tenderness within muscles. The tightness creates tight bands, or "knots," because of the contraction of the muscle fibers. A trigger point can be painful itself and also refer pain to other muscles. Massage helps the muscles to relax so the pain can dissipate.

Joint mobilization. This is a passive movement performed by the therapist, gently stretching or moving a joint to increase its range of motion and decrease pain. Joint mobilization is different from the type of joint manipulation performed by chiropractors.

Hydrotherapy. Moist heat packs may be used to relax a muscle or muscles before a massage begins. However, hot compresses should not be applied to the feet or lower legs in a person with peripheral diabetic neuropathy. Other hydrotherapy options, such as the use of a whirlpool, are more common in a spa setting or athletic facility.

Swedish massage is usually done on an unclothed body that is draped for warmth and modesty. Only the part of the body being worked on is uncovered. If you are uncomfortable undressing completely, however, discuss this with your therapist. Wearing underwear is generally acceptable.

Often a light oil, lotion, or powder is used to allow your muscles to be massaged without excessive friction on the skin. Let your therapist know about any preferences you may have regarding the use of oils or lotions on your skin. A typical Swedish massage lasts about an hour.

Sports massage

Sports massage therapy is specifically designed to meet the needs of athletes. It uses the techniques of Swedish massage as well as techniques from other styles of massage. In addition to simple relaxation, the goals of sports massage include calming an athlete's nerves before a competition, releasing muscular tension to improve sports performance and prevent injury, and speeding recovery after a hard workout or competition.

There are currently no legal guidelines for certification in sports massage in the United States. Ideally, however, a sports massage therapist should have a minimum of 50 hours of training in sports massage in addition to having the level of education and credentials recognized by the American Massage Therapy Association.

Craniosacral therapy

Craniosacral therapy is a technique practiced by some massage therapists (and others) that focuses on the bones of the head, spine, and pelvis. Its goal is to improve the functioning of the central nervous system by enhancing the circulation of cerebrospinal fluid. Supposedly, by placing his hands on the skull, the practitioner can feel rhythmic movements of the brain that are unrelated to heartbeat or breathing. Aberrations in this rhythm indicate ailments of various sorts, and a therapeutic effect can be had by applying slight pressure to the bones of the skull.

Proponents of craniosacral therapy suggest that it can have beneficial effects as a complementary treatment for a broad range of conditions, from brain disorders such as Alzheimer disease to ear infections to autoimmune diseases such as lupus.

Skeptics, on the other hand, express doubt that craniosacral therapy could have any effect on the body whatsoever. Indeed, most medical professionals believe that the bones of the skull are fused in adults and therefore not movable with gentle pressure. In addition, the concept of rhythmic brain movements has not been verified scientifically. However, craniosacral therapy appears to have a relaxing effect for some people.

Shiatsu

Shiatsu is a Japanese form of acupressure, in which pressure is applied along the meridians and acupuncture points through which vital energy, or ki, is believed to flow. The word shiatsu literally means finger (*shi*) pressure (*atsu*). Shiatsu practitioners may also incorporate palm pressure, assisted stretching, massage, and other manual techniques into their practice. Some common reasons to seek out shiatsu include neck, shoulder, and lower back problems; arthritis; depression; and anxiety.

There are many different schools of Shiatsu in Japan. There is the classic, or brusque, style; the more popular softer approach; and the barefoot style, in which the therapist may massage the meridians with his hands, elbows, knees, and feet. Regardless of style, the goal of shiatsu is to encourage the healthy flow of energy through the body.

The benefits of shiatsu may include relaxation, pain reduction, improved sleep, and improved mood. Unlike Swedish massage, shiatsu is usually done with clothes on.

Rosen Method

The Rosen Method combines gentle massage with a form of nondirective counseling. It was developed by Marion Rosen, a physical therapist who observed a strong association between emotional tension and muscular tension. She also noted that people who talked about their problems appeared to heal more quickly.

In the Rosen Method, practitioners feel for areas of chronic muscle tension in their clients as they perform their massage. They also pay attention to changes in muscle tension and shifts in the breathing. The practitioner responds to those changes with touch and words, observing aloud what is happening in the person's body. The idea is to allow the person to become more aware of his emotional state and possibly of information or memories held in the unconscious. However, while the goal of tapping into the unconscious is the same as that of psychotherapy, the Rosen practitioner does not attempt to interpret anything the person says in the way a psychotherapist would.

In some cases, simply becoming aware of emotions may be therapeutic and may allow a person to let go of chronically held muscle tension. In others, talking about the emotions may be beneficial. If awareness and talking are not enough, referral to a psychotherapist is recommended. In fact, the Rosen Method is considered by some to be a good adjunct to psychotherapy.

To find a Rosen Method practitioner, contact the Rosen Institute by calling (800) 893-2622, or use the links on the institute's Web site, www.rosenmethod.org.

Feldenkrais Method

The Feldenkrais Method is a way of changing habitual movement patterns so you can move, sit, and stand more comfortably. It was developed by Moshé Feldenkrais, a physicist who also practiced Judo. He was motivated by a knee injury to study physical self-rehabilitation techniques. He published his first book on his method in 1949 and subsequently taught his method and presented it to others through the early 1980's. Today the Feldenkrais Method is used by a broad spectrum of people, from those with physical limitations due to neurological or musculoskeletal problems, to athletes and performing artists.

Feldenkrais is taught either one-on-one or in a group. The one-on-one approach is called Functional Integration. In it, the practitioner guides the person's body or body part through new movement patterns, being attentive to any feelings of resistance in the joints or muscles. Through gentle exploration, the practitioner helps the person find less restrictive ways to move. The lessons are not learned intellectually, however, but rather through the nerves and muscles as they experience new ways of moving. Some people refer to the Feldenkrais method as a way of communicating with the unconscious through movement.

The group approach to Feldenkrais is called Awareness Through Movement. Students are guided verbally through sequences of easy, sometimes very small, movements. At times, they may be asked to visualize parts of their bodies or to focus on how a particular area of the body feels. The movements are not demonstrated by the instructor or presented as leading to a certain goal, so there is no expectation of what the movement "should" look like. Lessons generally last about 45–50 minutes and can evoke a state of deep relaxation. This approach to Feldenkrais can be done with audiotapes since a practitioner's touch is not required.

Because muscular patterns often have a psychological basis, Feldenkrais may affect a person on both the physical and psychological levels. A feeling of physical ease and freedom, for example, may be accompanied by a feeling of psychological ease and freedom, as well as an improved body image.

Certified practitioners and classes can be found through the Web site of the Feldenkrais Guild, www.feldenkrais.com, or by calling (800) 775-2118.

Alexander Technique

The Alexander Technique is a method of releasing habitually held muscle tension so the body can move, sit, and stand more comfortably. It was developed in the late 1800's by Frederick M. Alexander, an actor who was having trouble with his voice. By watching himself in mirrors, he traced his difficulty to a habit he'd developed of tensing certain muscles as he was about to speak. This discovery led to years of experimentation on how to lose this habit and use his body more naturally. Eventually, he developed his technique for reeducating the body and taught it to others.

Muscle tension can result from any number of things, such as sitting at a computer screen for long hours every day, wearing glasses that are the wrong prescription, and compensating for pain in one area of the body by overusing another area. Some people habitually clench certain muscles in response to emotions. Over time, the muscles may remain tight even when a person is not experiencing the emotion or sitting in front of the computer.

While the Alexander Technique can be explained in words and understood intellectually, it must be learned through the body to be effective. Just as the habitual tension has become automatic, or part of your "muscle memory," so must the feeling of released tension become part of your muscle memory.

Alexander Technique teachers observe students to see where they are holding tension. They then through words or touch suggest more "released" ways to stand, sit, or move. The Alexander Technique can be used for any type of movement or held position, from simple walking to playing a musical instrument to gardening or washing dishes at a sink. The Alexander Technique is generally taught one on one, and it usually takes at least 10 sessions to see lasting results.

Because holding muscular tension can be part of an emotional response, learning to release that tension can also have an emotional component. In some cases, the predominant emotion may be one of relief, but in some cases it can be one of vulnerability. A person who habitually maintains a crouched, protective stance, for example, may feel exposed when he releases the muscles that keep him crouched, thereby increasing the amount of chest and abdomen he shows the world.

An experienced Alexander Technique teacher will be familiar with the sorts of emotional responses students may have to this work and be able to respond in a professional manner. However, most Alexander Technique teachers are not psychotherapists, so if using the Alexander Technique is bringing up troubling memories or emotions, you might consider also seeing a licensed psychotherapist. Talking about the thoughts and feelings that cause you to hold tension may help you to change them or reduce their power over you, so you can take advantage of what the Alexander Technique has to offer.

Bowen Technique

The Bowen Technique is a form of gentle bodywork developed in Australia in the 1950's by Thomas Bowen. Although Bowen had no formal health-care or massage training, he was considered by many to be a gifted healer.

The Bowen Technique involves the practitioner manipulating points on the skin and muscle with light "rolling" movements. There are specific sets of movements that are performed on the neck, upper back, and lower back. These movements increase the circulation of blood and stimulate the nerves in the areas being manipulated. The autonomic nervous system is indirectly affected by the relaxing effect of the therapy. During a Bowen session, the practitioner occasionally leaves the treatment room for a few minutes to allow the person's body to absorb the effects of the work.

Bowen therapy can be done clothed or unclothed, and a person generally lies down to be worked on. The treatment lasts about 30–90 minutes. Afterward, the person is asked to drink plenty of water, take a walk, and not use any other forms of bodywork, such as massage, for the next week or so. This is to let the effects of the Bowen treatment linger as long as possible.

Bowen therapy has been reported to be relaxing and to be useful for a variety of conditions, including stress, headaches, fibromyalgia, chronic fatigue, and frozen shoulder. However, scientific studies of the Bowen Technique are limited, and it is not clear how the therapy exerts its effects. Some people believe that good responses are caused by vibrations set up in the body by the rolling motions. Others believe that the movements help to connect the body with the brain through the stimulation of the nervous system.

Bowen therapy should not be used by a person who has an infection or an infectious skin disorder, and certain aspects of treatment should not be done on pregnant women.

In the United States, the Bowen Technique is taught at the Bowen Research and Training Institute, Inc., in Florida (www.bowen.org) and at Bowen Therapy International in California (www.bowentherapy.com).

Reflexology

In reflexology, points on the feet and sometimes the hands and ears are believed to correspond to various organs and other parts of the body. Applying pressure to these points, particularly if the point feels tender when pressed, is believed to have beneficial effects on the corresponding body part. The theory for why this works is that pressing on particular points unblocks or encourages energy flow in the body. In that sense, the rationale for reflexology is similar to that for acupressure, in which energy is believed to flow along channels within the body, and blockages in the energy flow result in imbalances or disease symptoms.

The practice of reflexology in the United States started in the early 1900's with Dr. William Fitzgerald, an otolaryngologist (ear, nose, and throat specialist). Fitzgerald found that applying pressure to certain parts of the body had an anesthetic effect on other parts. Using this knowledge, he was able to perform minor operations on his patients without pain medicines. Fitzgerald named his method "zone therapy."

In the 1930's, a physiotherapist and nurse named Eunice Ingham expanded on Fitzgerald's work and mapped "reflex areas" in the body (similar to the meridians used in traditional Chinese medicine). She called her technique the "Ingham Reflex Method of Compression Massage." One of her students renamed it "reflexology." Ingham's theory was that pressure applied to specific locations on the body breaks up and moves crystals that interfere with blood circulation. The resulting improved blood circulation then stimulates the body's own self-healing mechanisms.

While the various theories behind reflexology are not supported by the Western understanding of how the body works, many people find a reflexology session relaxing, much the way a foot massage might be. In fact, many reflexologists start a session with a general foot massage before focusing on what are called "reflex points." Depending on how much pressure is applied to the reflex points, reflexology can be a little uncomfortable, but it should not cause lasting pain. Treatment sessions generally last 30–60 minutes.

Because reflexology involves pressing on the feet, people with diabetes should be cautious about its use. People who have any circulation problems, such as peripheral vascular disease or varicose veins, or any foot condition, such as neuropathy or arthritis in the feet, should speak with their health-care provider about the safety of reflexology before trying it. Do not use reflexology if you have a recent foot injury, active gout, or a communicable skin infection of the feet, or if you are in the first three months of pregnancy (there is some association with miscarriages). The relaxing effects of reflexology may lower your blood glucose level, so people susceptible to hypoglycemia should check their blood glucose after a session.

When you go for a treatment, the reflexologist should ask you about your health history, what if any medicines you are taking, and whether you use any medical devices such as a pacemaker. Depending on your answers, the therapist may avoid pressing on certain areas. He should also observe your feet for the type of arches you have, the condition of your toenails, as well as for the presence of any corns, calluses, and swelling (edema).

Various types of health-care providers and complementary care providers, including chiropractors, podiatrists, nurses, and massage therapists, offer reflexology. No licensing is required for reflexology itself (although the practitioners listed here would be required to have relevant licensing or certification in their respective fields). However, certification or training by the American Reflexology Certification Board and Information Service, International Institute of Reflexology, or Reflexology Association of America shows that a practitioner has achieved certain educational and skill standards.

Reflexology should not be relied on for any diagnostic purposes or for treatment of a specific ailment.

Trager Approach

The Trager Approach, also called Trager Psychophysical Integration, has been described as an intuitive and playful approach to movement reeducation. It was developed by Milton Trager, M.D., starting in the 1920's, when he was in his teens. He continued to practice, refine, and teach it over the next 50 years.

The goal of the Trager Approach is to help release patterns of tension in movement and posture. To do this, the therapist gently rocks, bounces, shakes, rotates, kneads, and pulls on the limbs and other areas of the body to release tense muscles and stiff joints. This work has an immediate relaxing effect, and proponents say it has lasting effects as well. Trager believed patterns of tightness are held in the mind and that his therapeutic manipulations were able to reach the unconscious mind, where those patterns are held.

The person receiving Trager therapy is generally clothed, and no oils or lotions are used. The number of sessions required depends on the person. For some, one is enough; for others, five or six sessions have the desired benefits.

In addition to the hands-on portion of the Trager Approach, often called table-work since the person lies on a padded table, therapists teach their clients Mentastics, a series of self-directed movements aimed at reinforcing and prolonging the benefits of the hands-on work. These exercises are sometimes taught in group classes as well as one-on-one.

While no large clinical trials have been done on the Trager Approach, anecdotally it appears to be beneficial for people with chronic neuromuscular pain such as sciatica or back pain. It also has been used to treat hypertension, migraine, and anxiety disorders. Some athletes say it has helped their performance. And some practitioners also report success in treating people with carpal tunnel syndrome, post-polio syndrome, muscular dystrophy, Parkinson disease, and other disorders that cause weakness or paralysis.

Certified practitioners of the Trager Approach can be located through the Web site of the United States Trager Association, www.trager-us.org. Certification is granted through Trager International (www.trager.com).

Rolfing

Formally called the Rolfing Method for Structural Integration, Rolfing is named for Ida Rolf, a biochemist who was influenced by osteopathic work, chiropractic work, and hatha yoga. Rolf developed the theory that injury, chronic stress, and emotional trauma could cause thickening and tensing in the body's connective tissue (fascia). Since fasciae virtually connect all the internal structures of the body, fascia that is thick and tense in one area can affect another area by pulling on it or restricting movement. Rolf developed a series of manipulations to stretch tight fasciae, increase freedom of movement, reduce chronic pain and tension, and improve body alignment.

Rolf died in 1979, but her 10-session basic Rolfing series is still used today. Each session generally lasts one to two hours and occurs a week or two apart. During these sessions, the Rolfer assesses the person's posture, alignment, and areas of tension and applies pressure to specific spots on the body to relax muscles and release tight fasciae. Manipulations are done while a person is sitting or lying down. A person may also be asked to stand and walk around occasionally to observe the effects of gravity on his balance and posture. One of the intended benefits of Rolfing is more erect posture, as the fascia holding the pelvis in place are made more flexible.

In addition to basic Rolfing, some Rolfers offer another sequence of sessions called Rolf Movement, which explore breathing and movement patterns. Once patterns that promote tension and asymmetry are identified, new patterns can be taught.

Rolfing has a reputation for being painful, because in its early days it often was. Today's certified Rolfers, however, are trained to be more in tune with their clients' comfort levels and to use techniques that cause less discomfort. However, the amount of pain caused by Rolfing manipulations varies from person to person.

Men generally wear underwear or swim trunks for Rolfing sessions. Women may wear underwear, a two-piece bathing suit, or loose-fitting shorts and a tank top.

While Rolfing is safe for most people, it should not be used by people with broken bones, severe osteoporosis, spinal disease, skin wounds, bleeding disorders, or blood clots in areas being manipulated. People using blood thinners should also not use Rolfing. It is generally not recommended for people with cancer. People with joint disease, inflammatory conditions, aortic aneurysm, or abdominal disease should consult their health-care provider before using Rolfing. Women in the first trimester of pregnancy should not use Rolfing.

Certification of structural integrators is provided by the International Association of Structural Integrators. Certified practitioners can be located through its Web site, www.theiasi.org, or call the association at (877) 843-4274.

Hellerwork

This form of bodywork was developed by Joseph Heller, an aerospace engineer who trained under Ida Rolf. It combines the deep-tissue work of Rolfing with movement reeducation and dialogue between therapist and client to foster a greater awareness of the mind–body connection.

A course of Hellerwork lasts for eleven 90-minute sessions, with part of each session devoted to bodywork and part to movement education. The dialogue can go on throughout the session. Before-and-after videotapes are sometimes made to observe a person's changed appearance.

The same precautions that apply to Rolfing apply to Hellerwork. It also may not be the right treatment for people with serious mental disorders. Although Hellerwork practitioners have some psychology and communication training, most are not licensed psychologists.

Certified Hellerwork practitioners can be found through the Web site of Hellerwork International, www.hellerwork.com.

Applied kinesiology

Kinesiology is the study of body movement. Many colleges and universities have departments of kinesiology that help prepare students for careers as athletic trainers, physical education teachers, exercise physiologists, and for other jobs related to sports and exercise. Many medical professionals, including occupational and physical therapists, also study kinesiology as part of their professional preparation.

While all of these people could be said to "apply" kinesiology in their work, the term "applied kinesiology" is used to refer to a specific system of muscle testing developed by a chiropractor named George Goodheart, Jr., in the 1960's. The theory behind applied kinesiology is that any number of health conditions are accompanied by specific muscle weaknesses. For example, a particular food allergy or organ dysfunction would have a corresponding muscle weakness. Through manual muscle testing, the practitioner identifies muscles that are not functioning well, then determines the cause and best treatment. According to this theory, the cause could be physical, emotional, or chemical in origin.

In addition to manual muscle testing, a practitioner would employ other diagnostic techniques, including taking a thorough history, performing a physical examination, and doing appropriate laboratory testing. Recommended treatments might include chiropractic adjustments (particularly if the practitioner is a chiropractor) as well as changes in diet, herbal remedies, or other conventional or complementary therapies. Follow-up muscle testing would be done to assess how well the treatment is working.

Although conventional doctors acknowledge that muscle weakness may accompany certain illnesses (both physical and emotional), most are skeptical of this system of linking specific muscle weaknesses to specific medical problems.

A certified practitioner of applied kinesiology must be a licensed health-care professional. There is no licensing for the practice of applied kinesiology itself, so anyone can call himself an applied kinesiologist with no legal repercussions. To find certified practitioners in your area, use the Web site of the U.S. chapter of the International College of Applied Kinesiology, www.icakusa.com.

Another organization that uses the word kinesiology in its name and teaches techniques of applied kinesiology is the Touch for Health Kinesiology Association. Touch for Health classes, which also include instruction on acupressure, are open to both licensed health-care or complementary care professionals and nonprofessionals. Some students are simply looking for a self-help method of health improvement, while others wish to go into practice as a touch healer or use Touch for Health techniques in their professional practice.

To learn more about Touch for Health, contact the Touch for Health Kinesiology Association by calling (800) 466 8342, or use their Web site, www.tfhka.org.

Yet another organization that uses the word kinesiology in its name is the Brain Gym International/Educational Kinesiology Foundation. Brain Gym is a program of 26 physical activities intended to enhance learning. Proponents say it can improve concentration, memory, reading, writing, organizing, listening, physical coordination, and more. Brain Gym is primarily used to help children develop their learning skills, although it can be used by people of all ages. For more information or to find classes in your area, call (800) 356-2109 or look on the Web site, www.braingym.org.

Colon therapy

Physicians have administered colon therapy, also known as colonic irrigation, as internal body baths since the time of the ancient Egyptians. Colon therapy was introduced to the United States in the 1890's by Dr. John Harvey Kellogg, who used colon therapy to avoid doing surgery on his patients who had gastrointestinal disease. (His treatments also included aerobic exercise and low-fat, vegetarian diets.) Colon therapy was also used to treat high blood pressure, infections, heart disease, arthritis, and even depression.

As antibiotics became available, the major use of colon therapy became "detoxification." One of the theories behind this practice is that fecal matter sometimes gets trapped in the lining of the colon and releases toxins into the body, causing symptoms ranging from gas and headaches to bad breath and digestive disorders. Direct observation of the colon during surgery and autopsies, however, has not revealed trapped fecal material.

Another theory is that certain types of foods leave a gluelike coating on the colon walls and that this substance needs to be removed. However, when medical doctors have perform colonoscopies to examine the large intestine for bowel cancer, no such coating or sticky residue is found.

While the use of an enema is sometimes appropriate to relieve constipation, there is no scientific evidence supporting the claims on which colon therapy is based. In addition, the frequent use of enemas carries some risks. Regular use of enemas can promote dependency on them for bowel evacuation. Other risks include changing the balance of the normal colonic bacteria, possibly leading to infection, and absorbing too much water through the colon, possibly leading to electrolyte imbalances and other problems. Enemas that include ingredients other than water can additionally irritate the colon. The use of contaminated equipment can lead to infection. And there is also the risk of perforating the colon wall, which is a very serious complication that can result in death.

Colonic therapy should never be used by anyone with intestinal disease, including diabetic diarrhea, or tumors of the rectum or colon. It should also not be used soon after bowel surgery, unless recommended by a conventional health-care provider. And it should not be used by people with heart disease or kidney disease because of the possibility of excessive fluid absorption.

If you choose to try colon therapy, find a practitioner who is certified by the International Association for Colon Hydrotherapy in San Antonio, Texas. You can contact this organization to find a certified practitioner in your area via their Web site, www.i-act.org, or by calling (210) 366-2888. Only the state of Florida requires colon therapy providers to be registered. Keep in mind that while the Food and Drug Administration has approved devices for medically needed colon cleansing, no colonic irrigation machine or system has been approved for routine use.

Although most "colon cleansing" is done by enema, some is carried out with laxative-type substances or herbs taken by mouth, which also have risks. Some of the herbs used may be habit-forming, while others can cause dehydration.

If you are concerned about constipation, try gradually increasing the amount of fiber in your diet, being sure to also drink more water as you eat more fiber. (However, if you have gastroparesis, or slowed stomach emptying associated with diabetic neuropathy, speak to your health-care provider about how much fiber to eat.) Keep in mind that many prescription drugs can have constipation as a side effect. If consuming more fiber doesn't help, or if constipation is accompanied by rectal bleeding, nausea and vomiting, or involuntary weight loss, see your doctor.

Chelation

Chelation is the use of intravenous infusions of a man-made amino acid called EDTA. In conventional medicine, chelation therapy is used to remove toxic metals, such as lead and mercury, from the blood.

Unproven uses include using it to prevent heart disease or treat atherosclerosis. At present, the risks of this practice outweigh any potential benefits.

Some practitioners offer "chelation enemas," which can be risky for the same reason that other forms of colonic irrigation are. Others offer "oral chelation," in which a person takes supplements such as garlic, vitamin C, zinc, and certain amino acids. The safety of this alternative depends on what supplements are taken and in what quantities. Similarly, the effectiveness would depend on the condition being addressed.

Hug therapy

It's well known that infants thrive on being held and cuddled. Children who are not touched as infants are known to not only develop emotional problems but have stunted physical growth as well. Most adults, too, enjoy human contact, though many get very little of it in their daily lives. Unlike infants, adults who have very little physical contact with others may overeat, because they confuse their yearning for touch with hunger, or they may seek sexual contact when what they really want is a reassuring, nonsexual touch. Similar to infants, however, adults who are rarely touched by others can develop emotional problems such as feeling lonely and depressed.

There are no easy answers to the problem of touch deprivation, but there are ways to touch and be touched more often. Having a massage or some other type of bodywork is one way to be touched in a safe, pleasurable, and nonsexual way. Even having your hair done at a salon or having a facial can provide a comforting type of physical human contact.

Another possible approach to the problem of touch deprivation is to make a point of giving and getting more hugs. This type of "therapy" may be easier to institute for people who already exchange at least a few hugs with an intimate partner, family members, or friends on occasion. It can be very difficult for people who feel embarrassed about asking for or needing a hug. If you're shy about asking for hugs or offering them to others, consider volunteering at a senior center or even at a cat or dog shelter. Remember, there are lots of people (and pets) out there who could use a hug. Nonetheless, care and sensitivity to yourself and others is needed when exploring this activity. If a full hug seems too intimate, placing a hand on someone's shoulder or hand may feel more comfortable, or even shaking someone's hand can connect two people in a nonthreatening, physical way.

If you decide you're ready to increase the number of hugs you give and receive, keep the following ground rules in mind:

■ Hugs are nonsexual.

■ Ask permission before you hug.

■ Give hugs only to willing recipients. If someone declines a hug, respect that person's desire not to be hugged.

To read more about therapeutic hugging, look for a copy of *The Hug Therapy Book* by Kathleen Keating.

Enjoying your body

Relief from pain and muscular tension are the primary reasons people seek out body-work and movement reeducation, and many of the techniques described in this chapter are effective for these purposes. But their benefits may go beyond the physical: Anything that makes your body feel better can also improve the way you feel about your body. Having a relaxing massage, for example, can remind you of what it's like to enjoy living in your body and taking pleasure in its sensations. Experiencing the nurturing touch of a bodywork practitioner as well as that person's ability to accept and respect your body as it is may help you to do the same. Bodywork and movement reeducation may also increase your body awareness, so you notice sooner when something doesn't feel right.

If you'd like to experience the benefits of body-based therapies but are not comfortable being undressed in front of a stranger, pick a therapy or method that doesn't require getting undressed. Have a shiatsu session rather than a Swedish-style massage, or sign up for a class in the Feldenkrais Method. Taking care of your body isn't all about eating right and exercising more. Sometimes it's just about loving and appreciating your body the way it is now.

7. Exercise: What It's Really Good For

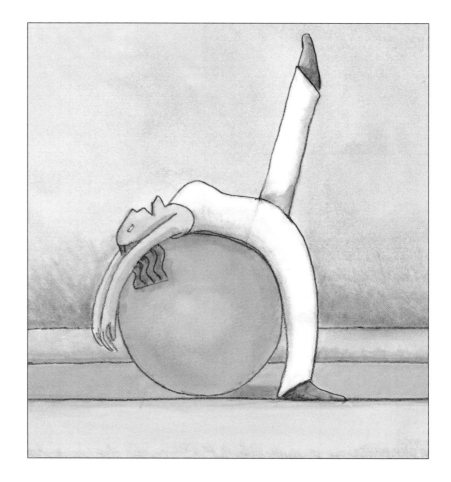

7.
EXERCISE:
WHAT IT'S REALLY GOOD FOR

Exercise is often viewed primarily as a weight-loss tool. This is unfortunate, because it is highly ineffective at producing weight loss on its own. If you consider that you must burn 3500 more calories than you consume to lose one pound, and it takes about 30 minutes of jogging to burn 250–300 calories, it becomes clear why it is unreasonable to try to lose weight solely by exercising.

Once the emphasis is off of weight loss, however, there is almost no end to the benefits of regular physical activity. Here are just some of them:

■ Reduces the risk of dying prematurely
■ Reverses and prevents heart disease
■ Lowers the risk of having a stroke
■ Reduces feelings of anxiety and depression
■ Improves self-esteem
■ Improves quality of sleep
■ Helps reduce blood pressure in people with high blood pressure
■ Improves balance, reducing the risk of falling
■ Helps maintain weight loss
■ Increases muscle and bone strength
■ Helps prevent osteoporosis
■ Helps control pain associated with arthritis
■ Reduces the risk of developing colon cancer
■ Promotes good mental and cognitive function
■ Delays the onset of Alzheimer disease.

Improved blood glucose control

One of the main benefits of regular exercise or physical activity for people with diabetes is improved blood glucose control.

Exercise has an insulin-like effect. It increases the sensitivity of the cell receptors to insulin, so that whatever insulin is available works more efficiently. Physical activity thus reduces insulin resistance and allows more glucose to enter the muscle cells. During a bout of activity, when the demand for fuel is high, receptors become hypersensitive to insulin, so that more glucose can enter the muscle cells and meet the demand.

Not only does blood glucose drop during activity, but it often continues to drop after activity. This is because your muscles continue to burn glucose at a higher rate as they cool down after activity and as they replenish the stored glucose (called *glycogen*) that was released and burned during activity.

Over the long term, regular physical activity can improve insulin sensitivity (or lower insulin resistance) by 20% to 30% by building muscle and reducing body fat.

Another important benefit of activity for people with diabetes is its ability to reduce the deeper abdominal fat known as *visceral fat*. Visceral fat is implicated in heart disease, insulin resistance, and other medical conditions. However, it is very sensitive to physical activity and readily releases fat for fuel in response to movement. Even when the amount of body weight lost is minimal, reducing visceral fat significantly improves insulin sensitivity.

Preventing highs and lows

Low blood glucose, or hypoglycemia, is the greatest risk of exercise for healthy people with diabetes. To prevent hypoglycemia during exercise, you need to both check your blood glucose level before exercise and know how the type of exercise you're doing affects your blood glucose. The only way to know how a particular type of exercise affects your blood glucose level is to monitor before and after the activity. If you're trying a new activity or you're active for a prolonged period, you may want to check your blood glucose level midway through the activity as well.

If your blood glucose level is below 100 mg/dl before exercise, the usual advice is to eat a carbohydrate-containing snack to raise it before starting to exercise. In addition, plan on eating enough carbohydrate before exercising so that your blood glucose level will be around 100 mg/dl afterward. You may also need to develop a plan with the help of your health-care provider to reduce your insulin or oral medicine before exercise. For more intense activity, a 50% or greater reduction may be necessary; for less intense activity, a 20% or 25% reduction may be sufficient.

If you inject insulin, don't inject, just before the activity, into a body part, such as a leg, that will be used intensively during an exercise or activity. Remember, too, that exercise causes increased blood flow to the skin, and this can cause injected insulin to enter the bloodstream earlier than it normally would, raising the circulating insulin level and possibly leading to hypoglycemia.

Always keep glucose in some form and an extra snack with you when you're exercising, participating in a sport, or increasing your activity. Wearing an identification bracelet or necklace is also useful, as is having some money on hand in case you need to buy some more food.

Don't forget to check your blood glucose more often than usual for up to 24 hours following heavy exercise. If you detect a pattern of delayed-onset hypoglycemia, you can prevent it by consuming extra carbohydrate or by lowering your insulin or oral medicine at the appropriate time.

High blood glucose

In some cases, your blood glucose level may go up with activity. The reason is that your liver always produces glucose when you are active. If you're not burning up as much glucose as your liver is producing, it's possible for the level of glucose in your bloodstream to be higher after activity than it was before. This doesn't mean that the activity didn't contribute to your fitness or that you didn't burn up glucose. It just means that during that particular activity session, you had more glucose in your bloodstream than your muscles could burn.

Blood glucose also rises during activity when you have a low level of insulin in your system at the time you're active. Although physical activity has an insulin-like effect, it can only lower your blood glucose when insulin is available. For this reason, people with Type 1 diabetes (whose pancreases do not produce any insulin) have a greater likelihood of blood glucose rising with activity.

In people with Type 1 diabetes, a blood glucose level above 300 mg/dl is dangerous because it raises the risk of *ketoacidosis*—a life-threatening complication. Whenever your blood glucose rises above this level, drink plenty of water and check your urine or blood for ketones. If you have any ketones, contact your doctor or diabetes educator for advice.

People with any type of diabetes are often told to restrict their physical activity when their blood glucose is above 240 mg/dl because of the risk of it going higher. In many cases, however, this is overly cautious advice that discourages people from activity and prevents them from realizing the benefits it offers. Most people can exercise safely when their blood glucose is above 240 mg/dl if they follow some simple rules: If your blood glucose is above 240 mg/dl, start your activity and, after 15 minutes, check your blood glucose level again. If it has decreased, continue your activity. If it is rising, stop your activity.

Pump precautions

Using an insulin pump has some advantages for exercise, particularly the ease of changing the basal insulin infusion rate to accommodate different schedules and levels of exertion. However, it is possible for an infusion set to get dislodged or for the insulin in a pump to get too hot or too cold during exercise.

Excessive sweating can cause your infusion set to dislodge, which may result in elevated blood glucose or even ketoacidosis if you fail to notice the displacement for some time. To prevent infusion set displacement due to sweating, try using a liquid skin adhesive, such as Skin-Tac-H, to anchor the set more firmly to your skin, or apply additional tape below the infusion set. You can also apply antiperspirant to your skin around the infusion site to minimize sweating beneath it. Or you can try wearing the infusion set in an area of the body that experiences less movement with activity, such as the buttocks.

When you exercise vigorously, you must adhere to the recommendation to replace your insulin infusion set every two to three days to prevent displacement or irritation at the insertion site. Metal needles are more likely to cause irritation than flexible plastic infusion sets. It is also recommended that you check the integrity of your infusion site following vigorous exercise, sweating, or water contact.

Another potential problem is that insulin is temperature-sensitive. Exercise in hot or cold environments can potentially cause insulin to degrade and lose effectiveness. When an insulin pump is placed close to your body during exercise in the heat, the insulin may become overheated; if the pump is placed outside your clothing in the cold, the insulin may freeze. If unexpected high blood glucose occurs under such conditions, replace both the infusion set and the insulin in the reservoir as a precaution.

Types of exercise

Exercise and physical activity are both good for you, but they're not exactly the same thing. Physical activity is any muscular activity that results in energy expenditure. Exercise is a particular kind of physical activity. Exercise is more vigorous (heart rate, breathing, and sweating all increase), sustained (it usually lasts 20 to 30 minutes), may require special clothing and a shower afterward, and usually involves a formal plan.

According to guidelines from the U.S. Surgeon General, you can be healthier and fitter if you accumulate 30 minutes of moderate-intensity physical activity on most, if not all, days of the week. "Moderate intensity" means walking at a speed of roughly three to four miles per hour, just fast enough to get a bit out of breath—but not gasping for breath—or engaging in any other activity that requires a similar level of exertion. Walking the dog, washing the car by hand, mowing the lawn, raking leaves, cleaning the house, and working in the garden can all qualify as moderate-intensity physical activity. It involves some effort, but not as much as you might think. Accumulating 30 minutes of activity means that you don't need to do it all at once. If you prefer, you can be active for, say, 10 minutes at a time, three times a day.

The benefits of vigorous exercise go beyond the health benefits of moderate-intensity activity. Vigorous exercise conditions the cardiovascular system, builds muscular strength and endurance, and increases flexibility. The American College of Sports Medicine (ACSM) guidelines for developing and maintaining health and fitness are 3–5 days per week of continuous aerobic activity for 20–60 minutes per session. In their latest position statement, the ACSM also recommends resistance training at least two days a week that includes one set of 8–12 repetitions of 8–10 exercises that condition the major muscle groups.

Aerobic exercise

Aerobic exercises include running, swimming, cross-country skiing, brisk walking, or any other activity that uses your large muscle groups, causes you to breathe a little harder, gets your heart pumping faster, and makes you a little warm and sweaty. Aerobic exercise is particularly good for your heart. If you follow a regular program of aerobic exercise, your heart will get stronger and will be able to meet your muscles' demands for oxygen-rich blood more easily.

Frequency, intensity, and time are all important to building aerobic fitness, but each must be tailored to your current level of fitness. The easiest way to measure how intensively you're working is to use a "perceived exertion" scale. On a scale of 1 to 10, with 1 being very light activity and 10 very hard, your exercise should feel like a 5, somewhat hard. Pay attention to your breathing to rate how hard you're working. You should be able to have at least short conversations while doing an aerobic workout.

Another way to measure the intensity of your exercise is to periodically take your pulse during exercise and calculate your heart rate. The goal is to work within your "target heart rate," which is usually 60% to 85% of your maximum heart rate. Your maximum heart rate is the upper limit of what your cardiovascular system can handle during physical activity, and it is usually calculated by subtracting your age from 220. Exercising within your target heart rate zone can help boost your fitness level.

To check your heart rate during exercise, stop your activity momentarily, take your pulse for 10 seconds, then multiply this number by 6 to calculate your beats per minute. (Some people prefer to use a heart rate monitor, which usually requires wearing a chest strap with a transmitter and a wrist monitor, although there are strapless models that take your finger pulse.)

If you're just starting an exercise program, keep your heart rate at the lower end of your target heart rate zone, and gradually work up to a higher intensity level. If you have heart disease or high blood pressure, discuss your target heart rate with your doc-

tor. Some high blood pressure medicines lower a person's maximum heart rate, so your doctor may recommend a lower target heart rate zone. Even at the lower limits, however, you'll gain cardiovascular benefits.

Strength training

Also known as resistance training, strength training involves working your muscles against a resistance, such as a dumbbell, elastic band, or your own body weight. Resistance training can make just about anyone's muscles and bones stronger. It can make carrying groceries or lifting children easier. You don't need to belong to a gym to use weights: Many people use household items like soup cans or detergent bottles, or they use the weight of their own body for resistance by doing push-ups and sit-ups. A nice bonus to weight lifting is that you can often see and feel impressive results relatively quickly.

With proper instruction, even elderly people can safely perform strength training exercises and achieve substantial improvements in strength, balance, and the ability to carry out activities of daily living.

Stretching

In fitness terms, flexibility is the ability to move your joints through a range of motion without straining the muscles. Stretching can help you maintain and possibly increase your flexibility. Although studies have shown that stretching does not prevent sports-related injuries, many people find that stretching before and after exercise feels good.

The easiest stretching technique to use on your own is called static stretching. To do it properly, stretch the muscle (or muscle group) until you feel the mildest bit of tension, hold that position until the muscle feels looser, then push just a bit farther. The amount of time it takes for muscles to feel looser is different for different people, so rather than counting to 20 or 30, focus on how your muscles feel, and stretch them until they feel looser.

For the most effective static stretch, do a brief warm-up (3–5 minutes) before stretching. At the gym, you might use an exercise bike or treadmill or other aerobic equipment at a light intensity to warm up your muscles before you stretch. At home, take an easy five-minute walk to get some blood in your legs, then do your stretches.

Cross-training

Cross-training simply means incorporating more than one sport or activity into your exercise program. Varying your activities not only prevents boredom but also causes you to exercise different sets of muscles, so you end up stronger overall, and it reduces the chance of injury from overusing a single muscle group. It also makes it easier to be flexible about your training plans: If it's too cold out to go for a bike ride, for example, you can work out at the gym or go swimming in a pool.

Before you start

Before you begin a new program of physical activity, make an appointment to see your doctor. While almost anyone with diabetes can benefit from moderate exercise, certain conditions and complications can be worsened by exercise or particular types of exercise. Your physician should evaluate your heart and circulatory system, eyes, kidney function, feet, and nervous system for evidence of complications. He may recommend delaying exercise until certain medical problems can be addressed, or he may have advice about the types of exercise you should or shouldn't do.

Heart and circulatory system

Exercise is part of the recommended treatment for many forms of heart disease, but overdoing it can be counterproductive. One way your physician can assess how well your heart handles work—and how much exercise is safe for you—is with a stress test (often called a treadmill test or an exercise test). During the test, a person is hooked up to a heart monitor and is asked to walk on a treadmill at varying speeds. The heart monitor generates an electrocardiogram, or a graphic representation of the electrical impulses in the heart. As the person walks, his heart rate, blood pressure, electrocardiogram, and how he feels are monitored.

Another test your doctor may administer is called a heart rate variability test. This test is used to diagnose *cardiac autonomic neuropathy,* which is an important factor for cardiovascular mortality in people with diabetes. Cardiac autonomic neuropathy may cause "silent" heart attacks, because people with this form of neuropathy don't feel cardiac pain.

Your doctor may also do tests to evaluate the blood flow in your legs. Decreased pulses or blood pressure in your feet and ankles, for example, can indicate that you may have peripheral vascular disease, or damage to the arteries that supply blood to your legs. This can cause *intermittent claudication,* or pain in your legs, when you exert yourself.

If you are diagnosed with heart disease or peripheral vascular disease, your doctor may refer you to a cardiac rehabilitation program for supervised exercise, or he may determine it's safe for you to exercise on your own, at a moderate pace.

Eyes

Having diabetes raises the risk of developing retinopathy, in which damage to the small blood vessels of the eye can lead to loss of vision. For people with nonproliferative diabetic retinopathy, the degree of severity dictates any exercise restrictions. Those with moderate to severe nonproliferative diabetic retinopathy are usually cautioned against activities that will raise blood pressure, such as power lifting or any movement that usually causes a person to hold his breath.

People with a diagnosis of proliferative retinopathy are advised to do low-impact cardiovascular conditioning exercises such as swimming, walking, and stationary cycling. They are cautioned against weight lifting, jogging, high-impact aerobics, racquet sports, doing exercises that require lowering the head below the heart, and anything else that involves bouncing, jarring, or holding one's breath.

People who have had laser photocoagulation treatments for retinopathy usually need to take some time off from exercise to allow for healing. Ask your eye doctor when it's safe for you to resume exercise.

Kidneys

Moderate-intensity exercise can be done by most people with kidney disease and may help them to have more energy. Good activity choices include swimming, dancing, walking, low-impact aerobics, light weight lifting, yoga, and tai chi. It's generally recommended that people with kidney disease avoid exercises that cause a significant rise in blood pressure, such as lifting heavy weights.

Feet

Everyone with diabetes should get in the habit of checking their feet after exercise for blisters or breaks in the skin. People with neuropathy in their feet may be advised to choose forms of exercise that don't put much pressure on the feet, such as using a stationary bicycle or rowing machine, swimming, or doing water aerobics.

When peripheral neuropathy in the feet causes numbness or loss of sensation, it can interfere with proprioception and balance. Proprioception is the reception of stimuli from receptors throughout your body that lets your brain know whether you are moving or standing still and where you are in relation to other things. Without good proprioception, it's easy to lose your balance, so doing non-weight-bearing exercises such as stationary cycling and rowing can reduce your risk of falling.

Nervous system

Neuropathy may be best known for affecting the feet, but in fact it can affect any nerve in the body. When neuropathy affects the nerves that control involuntary functions in your body such as digestion, heart rate, and sweating, it's called autonomic neuropathy.

If the nerves that help to regulate blood pressure are affected, the result can be *orthostatic hypotension,* or low blood pressure when you stand up or sit up from a lying-down position. If you have orthostatic hypotension, it's more important than ever to cool down after vigorous exercise. Stopping exercise abruptly can cause blood to pool in your feet and legs rather than circulate back to your heart, causing dizziness and even fainting.

If the nerves that regulate perspiration are affected, decreased sweating can lead to heat intolerance during exercise. If you don't sweat normally, it is extremely important to stay adequately hydrated and to not exercise in extreme temperatures. Loss of sweating in the lower body can cause dry, brittle skin on the feet, which can contribute to foot ulcer formation.

When the nerves that control the heart rate are affected, the result can be *exercise intolerance,* in which the heart rate remains unchanged instead of increasing and decreasing in response to your activity level. In people with cardiac autonomic neuropathy, heart rate is not a good indicator of intensity. (This is also true of people who take beta-blockers.) Instead, a person should pay careful attention to his level of perceived exertion and exercise in a moderate range.

Some cases of *hypoglycemia unawareness* may be related to autonomic neuropathy. People with hypoglycemia unawareness lack the usual warning signs of low blood glucose (hypoglycemia), such as shakiness, sweating, and palpitations. (These signs can also be obscured by exercise.) It is vital for people with hypoglycemia unawareness to frequently check their blood glucose level to prevent episodes of unconsciousness.

Autonomic neuropathy can also cause

gastroparesis, or slowed stomach emptying. Any effect of gastroparesis on exercise would be related to how quickly blood glucose rises after eating. If a person were to exercise too soon after eating—and before the carbohydrates in his meal were broken down to glucose—he could develop hypoglycemia. People with gastroparesis are advised to treat hypoglycemia with liquids that contain carbohydrate rather than solid food since liquids are absorbed more quickly.

In general, good activity choices for people with autonomic neuropathy include stationary cycling, recumbent cycling, and water exercises. Resistance exercises using light weights or elastic exercise bands may help maintain or increase muscle strength. Such exercises could be done while sitting, if necessary. Activities that should be avoided are those that cause rapid changes in body position (such as certain calisthenics) or that cause rapid and significant changes in heart rate and blood pressure (such as high-intensity running or lifting heavy weights).

Getting started

Once you've gotten your doctor's OK to proceed, along with any precautions for type of exercise, consider your current fitness level. One of the most common mistakes new exercisers make is doing too much too soon, which inevitably leads to feeling sore and discouraged the next day. So start with what you can do easily. Your first goal is to make exercise a habit. Once you are doing it regularly, you can concentrate on increasing the duration and intensity of your exercise sessions.

Consider also what you'd like to do and what's convenient. Walking is probably the most popular form of exercise. If you're just starting a walking program, try the technique of walking for five minutes in one direction then turning around and walking five minutes back to your starting point. When your ten-minute round-trip walk starts

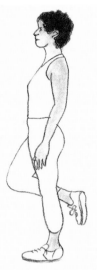

Stork

The stork is one of the simplest exercises to improve balance. Here's what to do:

■ Stand on one foot, arms at your sides, shoulders relaxed. Don't worry about how high you can hold your elevated foot in the air. An inch or two is fine.

■ Try to balance for 30 seconds. Repeat 2–3 times on each leg every day. Over the next few weeks, try to work up to 2 minutes.

Hint: Try not to "grab" the floor with your toes of the foot that's on the ground. It also helps to focus your eyes on one point while you try to balance.

To make the stork more challenging, try swinging your arms as if you were running. That will throw you slightly off balance, and you will need to make corrections to maintain your balance.

Another way to make the stork more challenging is to fold a bath towel over several times so it's four or six layers thick, then place it on the floor and stand in the center of it. It will be unstable because it's soft, but that's the idea because you want your proprioceptors—the sensory receptors that help you balance—to really work hard to improve your balance and strengthen your muscles.

feeling easy, increase it to six minutes out and six minutes back. Increase your distance by no more than 10% a week. Here are some more tips for a good walking workout:

■ Wear supportive shoes with cushioned socks. Synthetic "wicking" fabrics or wool will keep your feet drier than cotton socks.

■ Stand up straight as you walk, relax your shoulders, and look straight ahead.

■ Swing your arms with each stride, bending your elbows when you wish to increase your pace.

■ For more of a workout, include some hills in your route.

■ To pick up your pace (and burn more calories) use interval training: Walk faster for 30 seconds or so, then resume your regular pace for a minute or two. Alternate between faster and slower paces for several minutes or for as long as you can comfortably keep it up.

■ Another way to pick up the pace is to keep time to music as you walk.

■ Walk with a friend as a motivator.

■ Use a pedometer to count your steps for motivation.

■ Do some calf stretches before and after your walk to help prevent stiffness.

Swimming or water aerobics are good choices for people who have difficulty walking or standing. The water supports the body, so there's not as much pressure on the feet and ankles. Nonetheless, to protect the feet, wearing water shoes is recommended, both in the water and when walking around the pool or locker room.

When swimming, warm up for the first five to ten minutes with slow, easy strokes, and at the end of your workout, cool down in the same way. Increase the length of your swim gradually.

Low-impact aerobics is another good choice for exercise that's both safe and effective. (High-impact aerobics can be hard on the joints.) You can look for a low-impact class at your local gym or YMCA, or use an exercise video to get started. Some people also enjoy jogging, but be sure you

Using a Pedometer

Pedometers are pager-size devices that can be clipped onto a belt or waistband to count and record the number of steps you take. A pedometer can be a great motivator for increasing your activity level once you start monitoring how many steps you take in a day. The newer pedometers don't have to be calibrated to your stride length before use: You can just put one on and go.

Getting started. Wear your pedometer from morning until night every day for one week. Record your daily steps in a log, and at the end of the week, calculate your daily average. This is your baseline activity level. You don't have to start increasing your activity level during the first week; simply observe how many steps you take.

Setting goals. The current recommendation is to take 10,000 steps per day. Depending on your stride length, one mile is approximately 1900–2400 steps. Don't get discouraged if you currently take fewer than 10,000 steps. Any activity is better than none, and you can always work toward a goal of 10,000 steps a day.

Stepping it up. Try increasing your steps by 5% to 10% each week. For example, if you average 3,000 steps daily, try increasing your daily walk by 150 to 300 steps each week. In a few months, you'll be up to 10,000 steps per day.

Keep it simple. Purchase a device that measures steps only. Some pedometers can calculate distance walked or calories burned, but these devices must be calibrated and are more trouble to use. In general, the simpler the device, the better. Check your local sporting goods store for a simple pedometer.

have good running shoes to prevent injury. Also, if possible, run on a softer surface, such as dirt, a running track, or on asphalt rather than on the sidewalk.

Don't forget resistance training as a good place to start. If you choose to work with weights or dumbbells, one or two sessions with a qualified trainer (most gyms have them) will help you proceed correctly.

Overcoming barriers

Many people start exercising with great enthusiasm but quickly lose steam when the weather changes or an illness or business trip interrupts their routine. Here are some ideas to keep you going:

Chart your progress. Sometimes it helps to chart your progress in some way. Try keeping a calendar or journal where you write down what you've accomplished each day or each week. That way, you can easily look back and see how far you've come.

Find a friend. Some people find that having company makes it a lot easier to stick with exercise. Make sure your workout partner is reliable, and make sure you have a contingency plan for when he doesn't show up.

Take a class. Taking a class is a good way to learn something new, and it can add the structure to your regimen that you might need, especially in the beginning. Make sure that you sign up for a class at your level, and if it will make you feel more comfortable, tell the instructor that you are a beginner and would appreciate a little bit more attention in the beginning. Most instructors are more than willing to help.

Visualize success. If you just can't shake the feeling that you're out of your element in sneakers and sweatpants, try imagining your way out of the rut. Visualize yourself doing your activity, and "rehearse" it in your head. Just like a quarterback who reviews all the plays in his head over and over before the big game, you too can mentally prepare yourself for exercise.

Get some help. Schedule a session with an exercise specialist, such as an exercise physi-ologist or fitness trainer who can help you choose an exercise program that's right for you. (Check to see whether your health insurance provides for such visits. If it doesn't, try petitioning your insurance company with a request to pay for one consultation visit.) Many gyms and YMCAs offer a free or low-cost orientation session at the beginning of your membership, where you can have a staff member show you how to use the equipment and give you recommendations for an exercise program.

Try yoga or tai chi. Many Americans have come to appreciate the benefits of and enjoy doing yoga or tai chi. Both can build strength and stamina. Both also have a meditative aspect that tends to make people feel relaxed, even if their bodies are working or have worked hard.

Yoga

In its purest sense, yoga is a method by which a "union" with the divine or God is achieved. Most Westerners, however, practice it mainly to enhance physical and mental well-being. Practicing yoga regularly can increase flexibility, strength, stamina, and balance. It can also alleviate anxiety and depression, lower blood pressure and heart rate, and generally have a calming effect.

While popular images of yoga usually involve postures requiring great strength and flexibility, many basic poses can be done by just about anyone. In addition, poses can be modified to accommodate different abilities. While a typical yoga class includes postures that are done standing up, while seated on the floor, and from a lying-down position, "chair yoga" classes, for example, do all postures from a chair.

Even without formal modifications, however, yoga is not about holding postures "perfectly"; it's about paying attention to how your mind and body feel in the moment and doing the postures as best you can on any given day. In addition to performing postures, most yoga classes include a period of meditation, and some include chanting or breathing exercises. All of these serve as opportunities to tune in to your body and your mind.

There are many types and styles of yoga, some accentuating the physical component of yoga, others the spiritual or meditative aspects. *Hatha yoga* is considered a "basic" yoga style and is the root of several other variations. A basic hatha class is often a good introduction to yoga. Some of the other types of yoga commonly taught in the United States include the following:

Ananda. This style uses gentle poses to release tension and prepare the body for meditation and increased self-awareness. Students repeat silent affirmations while holding postures.

Ashtanga. Sometimes called "power yoga," this vigorous style uses rapid repetition of a series of postures in order of increasing difficulty. Ashtanga yoga provides more of an aerobic workout than some other styles.

Bikram. This style of yoga is done in a sauna-like room heated to at least 100°F. Bikram philosophy teaches that sweating helps the body release toxins. However, excessive sweating can also lead to heatstroke, so drinking lots of water before, during, and after doing Bikram yoga is a must. People who use insulin should also be aware that insulin can be absorbed into the bloodstream more quickly in high temperatures.

Integral. This spiritual practice uses gentle postures, chanting, and meditation to develop the individual as a whole.

Integrative yoga therapy. Often taught at hospitals or as part of a healthy lifestyle program, integrative yoga is usually combined with diet and exercise counseling to help people achieve better overall health or handle specific health problems.

Iyengar. In Iyengar yoga, props such as belts, benches, and blocks are used to help attain greater extension and better alignment in poses and breathing exercises. Poses are generally held longer than in other styles.

Kripalu. This style of yoga aims for a state of "meditation in motion," in which the body takes over and spontaneously performs movements to release mental and bodily tension. To attain this state, the intensity of meditation and the length of time poses are held are gradually increased.

Kundalini. This type of yoga blends postures and breathing exercises with Sanskrit chanting, meditation, and guided visualization.

Most yoga poses are done barefoot, which runs counter to the usual advice to people with diabetes to never go barefoot. One option is to wear nonslip socks (available through some yoga supply retailers) or yoga shoes, which have a flexible sole and are made by a number of major sneaker manufacturers. Another is to speak to your health-care provider about doing yoga barefoot, which may be acceptable if you're using a yoga mat and have no foot problems. People who have existing foot problems should consult their health-care provider before doing yoga since some poses can put pressure on the feet. It may be necessary to avoid those postures or make some modifications.

The presence of some other diabetes complications may also make it necessary to omit certain postures or modify them. People with retinopathy should consult their eye doctor about the safety of doing yoga and avoid any poses that put the head lower than the heart. People with certain forms of autonomic neuropathy may also need modifications.

All people with diabetes should be aware of how doing yoga affects their blood glucose and learn to make adjustments in their insulin or oral medicine doses, meals, or snacks. While doing yoga on a full stomach is not advisable, having a light snack is preferable to developing low blood glucose during class.

Tai chi

Tai chi is an excellent alternative (or addition) to walking or yoga. The slow, flowing movements may not look like they require a lot of energy, but in fact, tai chi has many of the same benefits as other forms of exercise, such as building strength, stamina, and agility. In addition, tai chi is known to reduce stress, improve mental focus, and improve balance. It has also been known to lower blood pressure and resting heart rate.

Tai chi originated as a type of martial art, but it is mainly used for exercise today and is considered an aspect of traditional Chinese medicine. The gentle movements are intended to cultivate and enhance qi, or "life energy," by stretching the *meridians,* or the channels along which energy is believed to travel in the body. In fact, because all living things are believed to have qi, tai chi is usually practiced outdoors so that those doing it can benefit from the qi in their surroundings. Sneakers and comfortable clothes are the preferred attire. If you practice indoors in a studio, however, you may be asked go barefoot or to wear shoes you don't wear outside.

As with yoga, there are several styles of tai chi. *Yang* style is widely practiced both in the United States and China. Other styles include *Wu, Hao, Chen,* and *Sun.* The style you learn is probably less important than finding classes that are convenient to you and an instructor that you like. Most tai chi movements are done standing, although they can be modified for people who can't stand. Deep breathing is always a part of doing tai chi. Advanced levels of practice can involve fast moves like jumping, kicking, and punching, or the use of swords, but it's not necessary to achieve these levels to reap the benefits of doing tai chi.

Many tai chi classes start with a relaxation exercise, followed by some warm-up exercises. Tai chi itself is done in choreographed sets of poses that flow together. Some instructors teach each movement of the set individually, and some perform the entire set while their students follow along. Learning each movement individually is sometimes easier, and it helps to practice it at home between classes. An entire tai chi set can last 10–20 minutes, and it can easily take months to learn an entire set.

Another aspect of tai chi that is similar to yoga is the idea that your best effort is good enough. Over time, you will develop more grace in your movements, but there is no wrong way to do tai chi.

If you have cardiovascular disease, joint problems, or other serious health issues, you should check with your doctor before practicing tai chi. However, in many cases, tai chi has been found to help people with chronic diseases due to its low intensity.

Qigong

Qigong (pronounced "chee-gong") is another Chinese form of exercise that includes breathing exercises, visualizations, meditation, and physical exercises. Like tai chi, qigong is considered both a form of martial art and a component of traditional Chinese medicine. Qigong exercises are often integrated into tai chi classes. Some qigong exercises are done standing, while others are done while sitting or lying down. Its purposes are similar to those of tai chi: physical health, mental relaxation, and the flow of qi throughout the body. While its main use is health maintenance, some people believe it can be used therapeutically by directing qi to a particular part of the body.

Learning the physical qigong exercises, sometimes called *moving qigong,* is like learning tai chi. Learning the meditative exercises, sometimes called *sitting qigong,* is similar to learning to meditate: A person allows his mind and body to relax, then focuses on his breathing and bodily sensations. He then intentionally thinks about energy flowing through the body and directs the energy to body parts that seem to need it.

There are a wide variety of qigong practices, ranging from the simple to the complex. While numerous qigong instructional videos and DVDs are available, learning from a live instructor has its benefits, such as being able to ask questions. Look for qigong classes at martial arts studios, places where tai chi is taught, or healing arts centers. The National Qigong Association directory is also a resource for finding instructors. Go to www.nqa.org or call (888) 815-1893.

Pilates

Pilates is a system of body conditioning known particularly for strengthening the core (abdominal) muscles. It was developed in the 1900's by Joseph Pilates, a one-time self-defense instructor. His original studio in New York City attracted many dancers as clients, and Pilates remains popular among dancers today. The results of practicing Pilates include not just stronger abdominal muscles but also better balance and posture, since a stronger abdomen means more support for the back.

Pilates exercises are taught in group classes and individually. Group classes, sometimes called "mat classes," may use no equipment or may use items such as rubber balls of various sizes and elastic bands for certain exercises. Studios devoted to the teaching of Pilates may have more elaborate pieces of equipment, including a table-like device called the Reformer. There are many, many exercises within the Pilates method, and different classes or instructors may favor different ones.

Many beginning Pilates exercises are performed lying down, either on one's back, front, or side. During a workout, attention is paid to the body's posture and alignment—particularly the position of the pelvis—and to one's breathing. Movements can be subtle but, when done correctly, powerful. In most cases, Pilates does not provide much of an aerobic workout, but the core strength it builds can make aerobic workouts such as walking or jogging more comfortable.

While Pilates exercises can be learned from books or videotapes, having a live instructor to observe your posture and answer questions is helpful. A good instructor can also suggest alternative movements or adaptations for people with injuries or physical disabilities.

What's stopping you?

There are lots of reasons people don't exercise regularly. Some people can't find the time. Others find it boring or hate the feeling of being out of breath and sweaty. Others are perfectionists and figure that if they can't do it perfectly, they won't bother to do it at all. And still others are in too much pain to get started or find that exercise causes them a lot of pain.

If you have a painful condition that prevents you from exercising or feel too depressed to move, it's important to have that issue addressed by a medical professional first. But if you aren't in pain or depressed, there's almost certainly a way to individualize a program of physical activity so that you can fit it into your life and stick with it. Examine your reasons for not exercising, and consider whether any of these tips can help get you started:

No time. Some people who make time for exercise find they have more time in their day, not less, because the exercise gives them more energy to accomplish daily tasks. In some cases, regular exercise can help you sleep better, which will also give you more energy. Examine your day to see whether there's an hour of television watching you could give up, a lunch hour you normally spend at your desk, or a commute that could be turned into an opportunity for a walk.

It's boring. Doing the same thing day in and day out is boring for many people. If that describes you, try varying your activities or, if that's not possible, try interval training, in which you alternate periods of intense exercise with more moderate periods. Exercising with a partner or group will also pass the time more quickly.

Don't like the feeling. Getting your heart rate up is good for your heart, but if you can't stand feeling out of breath or sweaty, try a slower activity such as tai chi or yoga, or try a water activity, in which the sweat is instantly washed off. In addition, only work out at an intensity that allows you to hold a conversation. If you're gasping for air, you may be working too hard.

Don't know how. Try walking, take a beginner-level exercise class, or arrange for a session or two with a personal trainer. There are lots of people out there who can help you get started.

It's embarrassing. If you feel self-conscious about your body or how you look when you exercise, first spend some time finding clothes you can wear comfortably in public. A T-shirt and loose-fitting sweatpants are acceptable for most activities. Next, look for an activity you feel confident doing or a facility where you feel comfortable. If there's no activity you can do with confidence, consider taking a class, finding a personal trainer, or even using a beginner-level video to get started.

Can't do it perfectly. There's no such thing as exercising perfectly. Stated another way, exercising regularly at a level you can handle is perfect. It's the best you can do. If you're worried about perfection, you may be setting unrealistic goals. There's no harm in challenging yourself, but practicing moderation and taking a break every now and then are important, too.

Even the most dedicated exercisers don't enjoy every single workout. But feeling better is a great motivator to get up and do a little activity even when you don't feel like it. Chances are, you'll feel better for having done it.

8. SUPPORTING THE MIND–BODY BALANCE

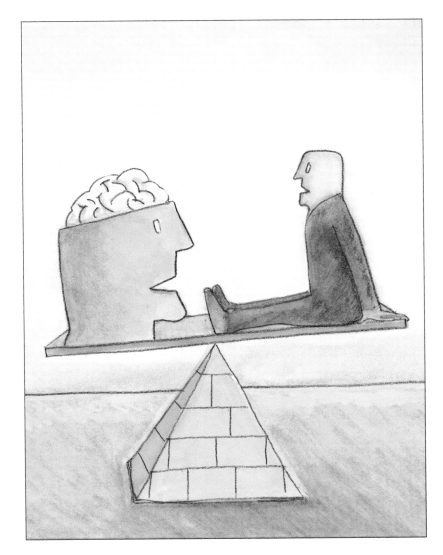

8.
SUPPORTING THE MIND–BODY BALANCE

Being in balance describes an ideal state of both mental and physical health, where the body functions well, and the mind is calm and peaceful. Life being what it is, however, that ideal state may exist for no more than minutes or even seconds at a time. The rest of the time is spent working toward that balance.

The good news is that people who work at balance feel calm and healthy more of the time, and they are able to get back in balance faster when new stresses arise. This chapter offers some more tools to work toward and maintain a balance of body and mind. Many of these tools help to access the subconscious mind, which is the part of the mind where attitudes, beliefs, and memories are held. Although you may be only vaguely aware or even completely unaware of the contents of your subconscious mind, it nonetheless directs much of your behavior. Learning more about your subconscious beliefs can help to explain why you think, feel, and behave the way you do, which is the first step toward changing thoughts, feelings, and behaviors that are no longer useful to you. As you bring your subconscious more in line with your conscious wishes and are able to increase the balance between your body and mind, you should see your blood glucose control improve.

Journaling

Keeping a journal can help you sort out your thoughts and feelings and make sense of your life. When you write in a journal (or speak into a tape recorder, if you prefer), you are writing only for yourself, so you can write any way you like, without having to worry about spelling, grammar, punctuation, or pronunciation.

Writing things down can have the immediate effect of unburdening your mind of intrusive thoughts. (This can help you to get to sleep if those thoughts are keeping you awake at bedtime.) It can also help you to get a new perspective on people or events. Often, situations don't look as bad or as unmanageable as they first seemed once you've written about them. On the other hand, writing about a situation could clarify just how bad things are, if your writing reveals a pattern of bad behavior, for example. Dating your journal entries can also help to put things into perspective if you later choose to review what you previously said or wrote.

If you're not sure how to get started journaling, try just writing down what happened over the course of your day. Then write down how you felt about the activities of your day while they were happening.

Another way to get started is to write down a chronology of your life. Once you've written down the basics, look for events or experiences you'd like to expand on. Rather than try to analyze why things happened the way they did, try to stick to what happened and how you felt about it. Keep in mind, however, that going over old memories can bring up sadness, anger, and other negative emotions. If writing about the past is too upsetting, it may be better to focus on issues you are currently living with.

Some people enjoy keeping a dream journal, in which they write down the dreams they've had. Dreams can provide an intriguing peek into the subconscious. However, when you analyze the possible meanings of your dreams, think about what the symbols in your dreams represent to you, not what they are said to represent in lists of dream imagery. Also, remember that dreams are often ambiguous; they don't reveal your thoughts, fears, or wishes with absolute clarity.

Yet another journaling technique is to write an "unsent" letter to someone. The purpose of an unsent letter is not to inform another person of how you feel but to give you the opportunity to fully express yourself. Again, write down what happened and how you felt. Don't try to guess why the other person behaved the way he did. Once you've written the letter, keep it for yourself.

If you're still having trouble getting started writing, you could simply describe the room or outdoor environment you're in, write down a conversation you had or overheard recently, or make a list of things that make you happy. Once some words are on the page, write down whatever thoughts pop into your head when you read those words.

While journaling can help you work through many types of problems, it's not a substitute for taking action. If you are able to do something to solve a problem, do it; don't just write about it. In addition, don't use writing as a way of complaining. Just complaining in your journal may make you feel worse, not better. Use journaling to discover how you feel and why you feel that way.

While journaling is generally used as an open-ended tool for self-discovery, it can also be used in specific ways for specific purposes. For example, a journal could be used to help you identify your unique symptoms of hypoglycemia. To use your journal for this purpose, make a point of writing down any feelings, thoughts, or bodily sensations you have just before episodes of low blood glucose. You might also ask the people who live or work with you whether they notice any particular signs or behavior when you have low blood glucose. Reviewing your notes may help you to identify signs of impending hypoglycemia that you hadn't noticed before.

This type of journaling might be particularly useful if you have hypoglycemia unawareness, a condition in which a person doesn't notice or doesn't experience early signs and symptoms of hypoglycemia. However, in many cases, hypoglycemia unawareness can be reversed by keeping your blood glucose level higher than normal for a number of weeks.

Journaling and grief

Journaling can be particularly helpful when you're grieving. Grief is a natural response to losing someone or something that is important to you. It's also a natural response to being diagnosed with diabetes or developing a complication of diabetes. Both are experienced as a loss—of good health, of the lifestyle you enjoy, of your freedom to live as you want, of your sense of who you are, or possibly of your hopes for the future. With time, you may realize you haven't lost all that you initially thought you had, but you must first grieve so that life can go on. Grieving can take a long time, but your journal doesn't mind how many times you repeat yourself or how long you stay on the same subject.

Here are some ways to use your journal when you're grieving over a diagnosis of diabetes or its complications:

■ Write down positive things about yourself, your health, and your body.
■ Write down your fears about your diagnosis. (Consider also discussing your fears with your health-care provider to get a realistic sense of the care your condition requires and how it may progress.)
■ If you are feeling guilty or blaming yourself in some way for having diabetes or a diabetes complication, acknowledge the need to forgive yourself (or your body, for failing you). Forgiveness can take time, but it starts with being aware of the negative blaming messages you're sending yourself and countering those messages with more compassionate ones, such as "I did the best I could at the time, and now that I have more infor-

mation, I'll act differently." Writing down both your negative thoughts and your statements countering those thoughts can help you work through this process.

Hypnosis

Hypnosis is a state of deep relaxation in which people are less critical and more susceptible to suggestion. Hypnotherapy is a therapeutic method that makes use of this state of relaxed, focused attention. Hypnotherapy has been used widely in smoking cessation and pain management programs, as well as to treat people with a history of substance abuse, headaches, anxiety, phobias, and many other health problems. Hypnotherapy has been shown to control nausea and vomiting from cancer medicines, reduce bleeding during surgery, steady heart rhythm, and bring down blood pressure. It has helped some people lose weight, controlled severe morning sickness, and given many people relief from muscle spasms.

It's possible to be in a hypnotic state during the course of everyday activities such as reading a book or watching a movie. Being hypnotized simply means you are awake but in a state of deep concentration. A person may also intentionally put himself in a hypnotic state using deep-breathing and concentration techniques.

A professional hypnotherapist might induce a hypnotic state by speaking in a soothing tone of voice, describing peaceful images, or playing soft music or recorded nature sounds. Once a person has entered the hypnotic state, the hypnotherapist might suggest methods for achieving specific goals, such as pain or stress relief, or he might use guided imagery to help a person envision himself achieving his goals.

Although a person is more susceptible to suggestion while hypnotized, he is not under the control of the hypnotherapist. Only if the suggestions given by the hypnotherapist are in accord with the wishes of the conscious mind do they pass into the unconscious. The value of hypnosis is to allow those suggestions in at all. The conscious mind has very strong defense mechanisms that protect a person's beliefs, whether or not those beliefs are helpful to him. When a person is hypnotized, his defense mechanisms relax, and new ideas can enter in.

While the use of hypnosis for the purposes of improved diabetes control has not been studied extensively, hypnosis can be useful for changing thoughts and beliefs that are counterproductive to good diabetes care. For example, thoughts such as "I will die early," "I'm bad," "I must be perfect," and "diabetes complications are inevitable" are inaccurate and can make taking care of your diabetes more difficult than it has to be. Subconscious fears, such as a fear of hypoglycemia, can also prevent you from taking steps to keep your blood glucose level in a near-normal range. Hypnotherapy can help to replace irrational fears with more realistic mental statements about the dangers of hypoglycemia.

At your first visit to a hypnotherapist, you would initially be evaluated in some way to test your ability to be hypnotized. If it appeared that you could be hypnotized (and most people can be), you and the therapist would then discuss your goals for treatment. During the therapy itself, you would most likely sit or lie on a reclining chair or couch, and the therapist would induce a trance. The therapist would then ask you to imagine a particular scene or make suggestions about your ability to control a habit or symptom. The therapist might ask you to recall a memory or emotion related to your treatment goals, but reputable hypnotherapists do not ask you to recall "past lives." At the end of the session the therapist will suggest how you will feel when you come out of your trance, then tell you to wake up. A hypnotherapist can also teach you to hypnotize yourself, which can be particularly useful for feeling more relaxed.

Many types of professionals, including physicians, psychologists, dentists, nurses, social workers, and marital or family therapists practice hypnotherapy. To find a health-care professional with training in hypnotherapy, ask your doctor for a reference, check the phone book for a local professional society, or contact one of the following organizations: American Society of Clinical Hypnosis, www.asch.net, (630) 980-4740; National Guild of Hypnotists, www.ngh.net, (603) 429-9438.

Hypnotherapy cannot cure any condition, nor can it make problems magically disappear, but it can alleviate a wide range of physical and psychological symptoms. The key to reaping the benefits of hypnotherapy is having the desire and willingness to change.

Relaxation techniques

Being relaxed is a very pleasant state, and it's also good for your body. When you're relaxed, your pulse rate is slower, your breathing is slower, your blood pressure is lower, and often, your blood glucose level becomes lower, too.

Learning to relax is a process that takes time and can't be forced. In fact, the harder you try to relax, it harder it is to relax. However, it is possible to "not try" and, as a result, learn to relax at will.

There are many ways to relax, including using the relaxation response, mindfulness meditation, and self-hypnosis. Progressive relaxation and autogenic therapy are two other options.

Progressive relaxation

Progressive relaxation is a method developed by Dr. Edmund Jacobson in the early 1900's. He noted that people often didn't know how to relax a muscle because they didn't know how a relaxed muscle felt. His method, therefore, involves progressively contracting and relaxing muscle groups to notice how they feel when tense and when relaxed. Jacobson observed that using this method relaxed not only the body but the mind as well. Many people find that practicing progressive relaxation helps them to fall asleep.

To use progressive relaxation, lie down in a quiet environment, close your eyes, and start by tensing your toes (or, if you prefer, your hands). Hold them in a contracted state for a few seconds, then release them. Continue up your body, tensing and releasing the major muscle groups in your calves, thighs, buttocks, abdomen, arms, chest, and shoulders. To tense your shoulders, squeeze your shoulder blades together in the back and release, then lift your shoulders toward your ears and release. Next, "scrunch up" then release the muscles in your face, raise your eyebrows as high as you can then release, and clench your jaw then release. When you've tensed and released all of the muscle groups you can isolate, notice how relaxed your body feels.

With enough practice, you may be able to relax a muscle or muscle group without contracting it first.

While most people can practice progressive muscle relaxation comfortably, it may not be a good technique for people who tend to get muscle spasms or who have certain types of chronic pain. For these people, autogenic relaxation may be a better choice.

Autogenic therapy

This method of relaxation, which uses visual imagery and body awareness, was developed in the early 1900's by German neurologist and psychiatrist Johannes Schultz. In the 1940's, Wolfgang Luthe, M.D., a student of Schultz, added repetitive therapeutic suggestions to the autogenic technique.

The general approach to using autogenic therapy is to imagine that the limbs feel heavy and warm, the abdomen feels warm, the heartbeat and breathing are slow and regular, and the forehead is cool. Simple statements, such as "my right arm feels heavy and warm," are repeated silently to gradually bring on a feeling of calmness and muscular relaxation.

One way to start using autogenic therapy is to sit or lie down in a quiet environment, breathe naturally, and repeat the following statements, while you visualize the body part or process:

- My arms and legs are heavy.
- My arms and legs are warm.
- My heartbeat is calm and regular.
- My breathing is deep and even.
- My abdomen is warm.
- My forehead is cool.

Autogenic therapy is believed to be safe for most people, but some people have been noted to have a sharp increase or decrease in blood pressure when using it. If you have abnormal blood pressure or heart disease, speak to your health-care provider before trying autogenic therapy.

Biofeedback

Biofeedback is a technique in which various monitoring devices are used to help a person learn to voluntarily alter normally involuntary body functions or reactions such as brain activity, blood pressure, muscle tension, or heart rate. Many people prefer biofeedback over medicine because of the lack of side effects.

Biofeedback has been shown to help people with a number of medical conditions, including asthma, Raynaud disease (intermittent episodes of decreased blood flow to the extremities), hot flashes, incontinence, and high blood pressure. It also seems to help people relax and enter a calmer state of mind, enhancing their overall health and well-being. The use of biofeedback therapy also enhances the body's use of glucose and can lower blood glucose levels for up to four hours after a session. Therefore, it is a good idea to check blood glucose levels frequently following biofeedback, particularly if you take insulin.

Biofeedback can be administered in a number of ways. An electromyogram (EMG) uses electrodes or other sensors to measure muscle tension. By showing people when their muscles are tensed, it can help them learn to relax these muscles, possibly alleviating such conditions as backaches, headaches, and neck pain, which are sometimes associated with muscle tension. It can also be helpful for medical conditions that are worsened by stress, such as asthma.

In temperature biofeedback, sensors are attached to the person's fingers or feet to measure skin temperature. A low skin temperature reading may indicate stress, so such a reading can serve as a prompt to begin relaxation techniques. This type of biofeedback may be useful in easing conditions related to circulation, including migraines and peripheral vascular disease.

In galvanic skin response training, sensors measure the activity of a person's sweat glands and the amount of perspiration on the skin, both of which are affected by anxiety. This type of biofeedback can be used to treat phobias and anxiety.

An electroencephalogram (EEG) monitors brain waves, which reflect different mental states, including sleep, wakefulness, and relaxation. Biofeedback using EEG may help people develop a calmer, more focused state of mind and may be useful in treating mood swings and conditions such as attention deficit disorder.

During a biofeedback session, a person is hooked up to various sensors, then taught mental or physical exercises that can help to affect the function that's causing a problem. For example, deep breathing, meditation, visualization, and muscle relaxation may aid in relieving stress-related symptoms. The sensors that are attached to the skin feed information to a monitoring device that translates physical responses into a tone that varies in pitch or a visual image of some sort. By controlling what's happening in the body, a person also controls the pitch of the tone or the appearance of the image. It may take 8–10 sessions to start seeing results, but it depends on the condition being treated. Most people who use biofeedback are also taught exercises and relaxation techniques to practice at home. Practicing for several minutes every day will speed improvement.

There is some evidence that biofeedback can improve blood flow to the feet in people with peripheral arterial disease or peripheral neuropathy. A study reported in the *Journal of the American Podiatric Medical Association* in 2001 was designed to determine the effects of biofeedback-assisted relaxation training on the healing of foot ulcers. While the control group received only traditional medical care, the experimental group received standard medical care combined with a biofeedback-assisted relaxation training program designed to increase blood circulation to the feet. In the experimental group, 14 of 16 ulcers (87.5%) healed, while in the control group, only 7 out of 16 (43.8%) healed.

Professionals who provide biofeedback training include psychiatrists, psychologists, nurses, dentists, physicians, and others. Certified biofeedback therapists can be found by contacting the Biofeedback Certification Institute of America, either via the Web site, www.bcia.org, or by calling (303) 420-2902.

Getting enough sleep

Anyone who's had trouble sleeping knows how unpleasant it can feel. But while one sleepless night will probably do no lasting harm (as long as you're careful about driving the next day), chronic sleep deprivation can be bad for your health.

Sleep gives the body time to relax and repair and also improves a person's ability to learn. Regularly getting at least two hours less sleep than you want can lead to insulin resistance, increases in appetite, and higher levels of stress hormones in the blood—all conditions that can contribute to the development of diabetes or make it harder to control diabetes. Some researchers believe there may also be a connection between sleep disorders and heart disease.

While lack of sleep can make it harder to control your diabetes, symptoms associated with high or low blood glucose can make it harder to sleep. Having high blood glucose can disrupt your sleep by causing you to wake up during the night to use the bathroom. Having low blood glucose, or hypoglycemia, during the night tends to lead to restless sleep. Hypoglycemia can cause nightmares, night sweats, or headaches; hunger that wakes you up to get food; or symptoms associated with daytime hypoglycemia such as rapid heartbeat, dizziness, or shaking.

Certain long-term diabetes complications can also make it difficult to sleep. Pain or restless legs from diabetic neuropathy can cause insomnia and consequently daytime fatigue. If pain is keeping you up at night, see your doctor for help with pain control. There are several approaches that can help with neuropathy pain, but it often takes trying several of them before you find what works best for you.

Type 2 diabetes also appears to be associated with a higher risk of sleep apnea, in which a person experiences interruptions of breathing during the night. Sleep apnea is more common among heavy snorers, who are usually, but not always, overweight. In sleep apnea, loud snoring is typically interrupted by about 10 seconds or more of silence, as breathing stops and then starts again—often with a loud snort or gasp. This pattern may repeat many times an hour throughout the night and may wake both the snorer and his bed partner. If you think you may have sleep apnea, it's worth checking out, because sleep apnea is associated with serious health problems, including heart disease.

Depression is a common cause of insomnia (and also of hypersomnia, or sleeping too much). Waking up too early is often a sign of depression. If you think you may be depressed, seek help from your health-care provider or a mental health professional.

Shift work commonly causes sleep problems and can also cause blood glucose control problems for people with diabetes. Shift work disrupts the body's internal clock, which regulates hormones depending on the time of day. At night, the body releases increased amounts of hormones that make the body more resistant to insulin. This may protect sleeping humans against low blood glucose during the night, but if you're up, working, and eating, it can increase the likelihood of high blood glucose. There's some evidence that the body may never fully adapt to shift work. Some people find that napping during their shift—in addition to making sleep a priority when they're not at work—is the best way to stay as alert as possible.

Tips for getting to sleep and staying asleep

Insomnia is frustrating, but it can be treated, often with self-help measures, including the following:

■ Get up at the same time every day.

■ Get some exercise during the day, but not too close to bedtime.

■ Learn to control your blood glucose levels. If you're not sure how, speak to your doctor or ask for a referral to a certified diabetes educator or a diabetes education program.

■ Cut back on caffeine, smoking, and alcohol. Although alcohol sometimes can help a person fall asleep, having a drink often leads to fragmented sleep and frequent awakenings during the night.

■ Have a bedtime routine, such as taking a warm bath or shower, having a light snack, listening to quiet music, or practicing a method of relaxation.

■ Do some gentle stretching before you go to bed.

■ Dim the lights in your home 20 minutes before bedtime.

■ If intrusive thoughts keep you awake, try writing them down on paper. Your mind has a tendency to let go of thoughts once they're written down.

■ Another way to deal with intrusive thoughts is to visualize putting them into a bubble, drawer, or box so they are separate from you.

■ If other efforts don't work, try "paradoxical intent," in which you instruct yourself not to sleep. As you try to stay awake, you will find yourself getting sleepier and sleepier.

Your sleep environment

Some people can sleep anywhere, but most sleep best in a dark, quiet, cool place. Here are some tips for turning your bedroom into a sleep room:

■ If possible, keep the room temperature around 60°F to 65°F.

■ Keep your bedroom as dark and as quiet as possible. However, if sounds from outside your room keep you awake, using a white noise machine may help.

■ Make sure your mattress is comfortable. Some studies have suggested that a medium-firm mattress is more comfortable than a very firm mattress for most people. If you ever sleep in a bed that is more comfortable than your own, don't miss the opportunity to find out the make or brand of that mattress. When buying a new mattress, spend 15–20 minutes trying it out before making a decision.

■ Be sure your pillow is comfortable and keeps your neck aligned with your spine.

Sleep aids

A few dietary supplements are promoted as treatments for insomnia, but none are recommended by major health organizations, either because they are unsafe or because they have not been shown to be effective. If your sleep problem is bad enough to consider taking supplements or other over-the-counter products, see your doctor to investigate underlying medical conditions that may be contributing to your lack of sleep.

Melatonin. Melatonin is a hormone secreted by the pineal gland that is believed to regulate the body's sleep and wake cycle. Normally, the pineal gland is inactive during the day and begins to secrete melatonin only when the sun goes down and darkness occurs. Melatonin levels rise sharply around 9 PM and stay elevated for about 12 hours.

Melatonin is also sold as a dietary supplement, either derived from the pineal glands of cattle or chemically synthesized. It may help some people initiate sleep, and it appears to be safe for short-term use. However, for melatonin to be helpful, the correct dose, method of delivery (oral or topical, for example), and time of day it is taken must be appropriate to the sleep problem, and in many cases, these specifics are unknown. Most commercial products are sold in doses that raise melatonin levels in the blood to much higher levels than are naturally produced in the body. Side effects of taking melatonin supplements can include fatigue and depression.

Valerian. Valerian is a botanical supplement derived from the root of the *Valeriana officinalis* or *Valerianae radix* plant. It is frequently used as a sedative to improve sleep. However, scientific studies have not shown it to be more effective than a placebo. It may have an additive effect when taken with barbiturates and benzodiazepines (drugs also used for insomnia), and it has been associated with liver toxicity when used long-term. Short-term side effects can include headache, morning drowsiness, and impaired alertness.

Kava. Kava is another botanical supplement sometimes used to treat insomnia. Kava is derived from the rhizome of the *Piper methysticum* plant. While it appears to have a sedating effect, it has also been shown to cause liver toxicity. In fact, the British, French, and Swiss governments have requested that kava be removed from the market, and the Canadian government has warned consumers not to use kava-containing products. It may have an additive effect when taken with barbiturates, benzodiazepines, alcohol, and sedatives. In the short term, kava can cause headache, impaired reflexes, visual disturbances, and restlessness.

Breathing techniques

Breathing is probably something you seldom think about until you can't do it naturally, because of a cold, for example. But perhaps you should think about it more often, because of what it can reveal about your state of mind: People who are relaxed tend to breathe slowly and deeply. People who are anxious tend to breathe quickly and shallowly. Quick, shallow breathing can actually make a person feel more anxious, because less oxygen is reaching his cells. The good news is that breathing slowly and deeply on purpose, or performing other regulated breathing exercises, can have the effect of calming your mind and body.

Breathing exercises, or at least attention to breath, are part of the practice of tai chi, qigong, and yoga. Many Pilates instructors also call attention to the right way to breath during Pilates exercises. And breathing correctly is even important for bodybuilding and strength training. (It's important to exhale with effort to prevent a sharp rise in blood pressure.)

There are lots of breathing exercises that can promote relaxation. Here are a few to try:
■ Breathe in to the count of four; hold your breath for the count of eight; breathe out to the count of four.
■ For 10 minutes, breathe in through your nose and out through your mouth.
■ Place a finger on one side of your nose to close that nostril, and breathe in through the other nostril for 10–12 breaths. Change sides every 10–12 breaths.

Learning breathing exercises like these can be especially helpful for people with asthma and people who get panic attacks. In some cases, an asthma or panic attack can be minimized with breathing techniques if the signs of an impending attack are noticed in time.

People with shortness of breath caused by chronic obstructive pulmonary disease are sometimes taught what is called "pursed lip" breathing, which is done as follows:

1. Relax your neck and shoulder muscles.
2. Breathe in (inhale) slowly through your nose for two counts, keeping your mouth closed. You don't have to take a deep breath; a normal breath will do. It may help to count to yourself as you inhale.
3. Pucker, or "purse," your lips as if you were going to whistle or blow gently on the flame of a candle to make it flicker.
4. Breathe out (exhale) slowly and gently through your pursed lips while counting to four.

To make sure air is going in and out the way you want it to, it helps to push your stomach out as you inhale and pull your stomach in as you exhale. Use the pursed-lip technique during the difficult part of any activity, such as bending, lifting, or climbing stairs. Practice it four to five times a day at first so you can get the correct breathing pattern.

Communication skills

Communication skills may sound unrelated to health care, but when you have a chronic condition like diabetes, they are necessary to staying healthy. Having good communication skills can help you get what you need from your doctor and from other health-care providers. It can help you get what you need from your family members and friends—and politely quell any tendencies on their parts to act like the "diabetes police." Learning to be assertive can also help in settings such as restaurants or when traveling. Here are some talking tips to keep in mind:

Be assertive. Let others know how you feel and what you need in clear, concise language. Keep in mind that your doctor may not realize you haven't fully understood his instructions, or your family members and friends may not know what kind of help you'd like with your diabetes care. The clearer you can be about what you need, the better able they are to provide it. If you have trouble articulating your needs, try writing them down before a doctor appointment or before you speak to the person you need to communicate with. Some people also find it helpful to bring a close friend or family member with them to doctor appointments, both to help ask questions and to hear and to remember the information given.

When you talk to others about difficult issues, try to state how you feel without accusing the other person of bad behavior. For example, rather than say, "You're not explaining it well," say, "I'm confused by what you're telling me."

Be honest. If you haven't been taking your diabetes medicines or haven't been exercising regularly, let your health-care provider know. Telling the truth can lead to a dialogue about why you haven't been taking the medicine (maybe you can't stand the side effects or can't afford it) or what a better approach to exercise might be. If your diabetes team doesn't know you're having problems, they can't help. Similarly, if they don't know that you're trying a form of complementary therapy, they can't tell you how it might interact with your conventional treatment.

Being honest can also help you deal with family members or friends who nag you about what you eat or otherwise police your behavior. If you lie to them, it's unlikely their behavior will change, and if they catch you in a lie, it will probably only reinforce it. On the other hand, if you admit to having trouble carrying out your meal plan or other parts of your diabetes regimen, they may be able to brainstorm solutions with you or offer constructive help.

Be sensitive. Other people have feelings, too, so pay attention to your word choice and tone of voice. Other people also have their own needs and priorities, which may sometimes conflict with yours. When you ask a favor, therefore, be prepared to hear the word "no" at times.

In addition, be aware that not everyone knows as much about diabetes as you do, and there may be times when you have to provide some education. Your boss, for example, may not understand why you would prefer to eat lunch at a particular time, but when you explain your medical needs, he may be willing to accommodate your schedule.

Listen. Communication is a two-way street. Once you have let your feelings and needs be known, listen carefully to what the other person has to say. Ask questions if you don't understand what is being said. Listening shows that you care about the other person and that you're willing to have a dialogue. When you listen, you may learn something you didn't know about the other person or hear something that either changes your opinion or points the way to a plan of action you can both agree to.

Be polite. Don't make nasty or snide comments in an effort to get your way or when you don't get your way. If the only thing you can think to say contains expletives, just keep your mouth shut until you've calmed down. Also, don't forget to thank a person who has performed a service for you, even if you paid that person for his service.

Pick your battles. There are some things worth fighting for and others that are not worth the effort. When a conflict arises, think about what's really important to you and whether the issue at hand is worth expending your energy.

Get help if you need it. Good communication skills are not innate; they're learned. If you're having trouble communicating, get some help. Participating in a diabetes support group is one way to get help. Chances are that others in the group have been in situations similar to yours and can let you know what has worked and what hasn't. A mental-health professional, such as a psychologist, can also help with communication difficulties. If your primary problems seem to be within the family, you might choose to see a family or marital therapist.

Building self-efficacy

Self-efficacy is the belief that you can carry out a certain action. It's an important concept for people with diabetes because they are often asked to carry out many actions to care for their diabetes. In some cases, these actions require changing old habits, such as eating habits, and adopting new ones, which is not an easy task for anyone.

Feeling confident about carrying out the actions necessary to control your diabetes requires education and training. If you don't know how to check your blood glucose or follow your meal plan, you won't feel—or be—able to do it. So getting the diabetes education and training you need from your doctor, diabetes educator, dietitian, or another health-care professional is the first step toward building your diabetes self-efficacy.

Here are some other tips for building your self-confidence:

Choose tools that help. Getting in the habit of checking your blood glucose is already a challenge, but if you have trouble using your meter, it may not seem worth the effort. Some blood glucose meters are easier to see than others, and some are easier to manipulate. If you're having difficulty using your meter, ask your health-care provider (or pharmacist) to show you some other models that may be easier for you to use. Similarly, some insulin delivery devices and lancing devices are easier to use than others. Make sure your tools are helping your efforts to control your diabetes, not hindering them.

Choose actions you want to take. There are many ways to improve your eating habits, increase the amount of physical activity you perform, and practice stress reduction. Choose methods or activities that appeal to you, not ones you think you "should" use or do. Or choose to work first on the barriers that are keeping you from making positive, health-related changes. If you really want something, you'll put energy into doing or getting what you want.

Set achievable goals. A goal should provide you with some challenge, but it must be realistically attainable. Rather than shoot for a huge goal and then fail, set smaller goals that will help you get closer to your larger goal. For example, rather than try to change your diet overnight, set a goal of eating a serving of vegetables every day. Once preparing vegetables has become routine, move on to another dietary goal.

Make an action plan. An action plan is a commitment to yourself to take one specific step toward your longer-term goal. The more specific and detailed the step, the better. Rather than say, for example, "I will exercise more," say something like, "I will take a 30-minute walk four days a week for the next four weeks."

Take stock of your progress. Once you have put your plan into action, periodically take a few minutes to assess your progress. Note what has been helpful and what hasn't, and give yourself credit where due. Revise your plan as needed, given your experience and increased self-knowledge. If your goal is health-related, write down any questions that may have come up to discuss with your health-care provider.

Expect setbacks. Habits take a long time to form and to break. If you've always coped with stress by sitting on the couch and watching TV for hours, you probably will find yourself doing it at some point, even if you've been religiously practicing the relaxation response. But just because you slip back into old habits sometimes doesn't mean you've failed permanently. The important thing is to get back on track and try to cope with stress in another way next time.

Reward yourself. The rewards of having a bowl of ice cream are obvious: It tastes good, and you enjoy it. The rewards of making the type of lifestyle changes that can lead to improved diabetes control are sometimes not so immediately obvious. It helps, then, to come up with rewards to yourself for successfully carrying out healthy behav-

Making an Action Plan

An action plan is a commitment to yourself to take one specific step toward your longer-term goals. An action plan can be made for anything you want to work on, from learning to ask for help to finding more time to exercise. Generally, the more specific the plan, the better. In addition, for a plan to be successful, it should meet the following criteria:

■ The action is something you want to do.

■ The action is something you can reasonably accomplish within the time frame specified.

■ The plan spells out, in as much detail as possible, when, where, for how long, and with whom you'll work toward your goal.

The following form can help you get started:

MY ACTION PLAN

This week I will _____
_____
_____ (state activity or behavior).

I will do this _____ times, for _____
(length of time or amount of activity).

I will do this activity _____
_____.
(when, where, with whom).

On a scale of 1 to 10, my confidence level that I will do this is _____. (Research shows that if your confidence level is 7 or higher, you will probably complete the plan. If it's lower than 7, you probably won't.)

The following barriers might get in my way: _____
_____
_____.

Here are some ways I might overcome those barriers: _____
_____.

iors. A reward would be something that is personally meaningful but doesn't undermine the new habits you are trying to form. **Get support.** Having a support group, or just one other person to encourage you, can provide an emotional boost when you're feeling discouraged. Your support network may also be able to help you brainstorm solutions when you come up against barriers to achieving your goal. They can also provide an outside perspective and probably point out how far you've already come.

The power of the mind

The conscious mind is the part of the mind a person is aware of. The subconscious mind (also called the unconscious mind) is the part a person is usually much less aware of. When a new idea pops into your head and you have no idea where it came from, it was your subconscious mind that put it there. When you drive to work without thinking about how to get there or how to drive a car, your subconscious mind did the work for you. When you automatically reach for a cigarette upon feeling stressed, your subconscious mind made the connection between stress and cigarettes.

In a sense, the subconscious mind is the sum of your experiences. Not everything in your subconscious mind is a bad habit or a painful repressed memory. But subconscious beliefs can be illogical and can lead to behavior that consciously doesn't make much sense.

If you're struggling with a bad habit, such as smoking, or can't seem to stick to a diabetes control regimen even though you know you should, or feel stuck in a life pattern you'd like to change, maybe it's time to use one or more of the tools described in this chapter to get in touch with your subconscious beliefs and attitudes to see what might be holding you back. Using a mind–body therapy won't necessarily lead to a quick fix, but it can be a way to bring your subconscious more in line with what you would consciously like for yourself in life.

9. NUTRITION: THE BASICS

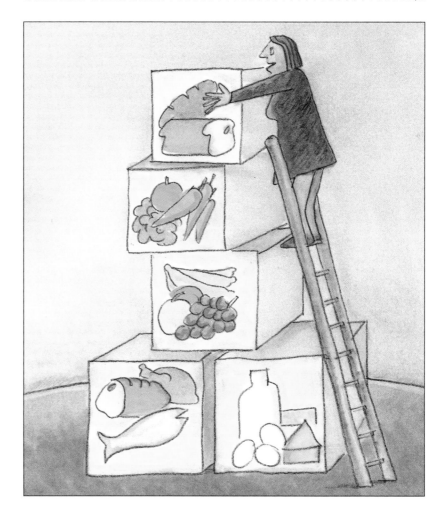

9.
NUTRITION:
THE BASICS

Following a meal plan tailored to your needs is one of the most important components of diabetes control. It's also one of the most difficult.

It's not that eating right is rocket science, but eating is about more than just survival. People eat not just to satisfy their physical hunger but for comfort and enjoyment. Food has a social role, so food choices may sometimes be influenced by the company you're in. Modern society surrounds us with cues to eat, from television ads to displays in grocery stores to carefully placed refreshment vendors in movie theaters and other places of recreation and entertainment. Even many schools and workplaces have vending machines these days. With food always present, it's easy to eat out of habit or on impulse rather than because you're hungry.

Eating right, then, requires both knowing what good nutrition is and paying attention to why and when you eat. This chapter reviews some of the basics of good nutrition as well as some guidelines developed specifically to help with diabetes control.

Dietary Guidelines for Americans

To function well, your body needs six essential nutrients: protein, carbohydrate, fat, vitamins, minerals, and water. Most people don't need absolutely precise amounts of any of these each day, but there are certain minimum requirements needed to stay healthy.

The Dietary Guidelines for Americans, published jointly by the Department of Health and Human Services (HHS) and the Department of Agriculture (USDA), are intended to make getting adequate amounts of these nutrients easier. If you eat the numbers of servings of food recommended by the guidelines, you will get enough of all the essential nutrients without having to count up every gram of protein and milligram of vitamin C. Last updated in 2005, the Dietary Guidelines for Americans describe a healthy diet as one that has the following characteristics:

■ It emphasizes fruits, vegetables, whole grains, and fat-free or low-fat milk and milk products
■ It includes lean meats, poultry, fish, beans, eggs, and nuts.
■ It is low in saturated fat, *trans* fat, cholesterol, salt (sodium), and added sugars.

The guidelines divide foods into six categories—grains, vegetables, fruits, oils, milk, and meat and beans—and offer guidance on how much of each to eat and more healthful choices within each group. Suggested numbers of servings are based on a person's age and sex. An individual would also need to take his size and level of physical activity into account. The more healthful food choices within each group are as follows:

Grains. Choose whole grains and whole-grain products over refined grains. Whole grains include brown rice, buckwheat, bulgur, oatmeal, popcorn, whole-grain barley, whole-grain cornmeal, whole rye, wild rice, amaranth, millet, quinoa, sorghum, and triticale.

Vegetables. Eat more dark-green and orange vegetables and more dry beans and peas. Dark-green vegetables include bok choy, broccoli, collard greens, dark-green leafy lettuce, kale, mesclun, mustard greens, romaine lettuce, spinach, turnip greens, and watercress. Orange vegetables include orange varieties of winter squash, carrots, and sweet potatoes.

Fruits. Eat a variety of fruit, and favor whole fruits over fruit juice.

Oils. Get most of your fat from fish, nuts, and vegetable oils. Limit intake of butter, stick margarine, shortening, and lard.

Milk. Choose low-fat or fat-free dairy products. If you don't eat dairy products, choose calcium-fortified foods or foods that naturally contain some calcium such as tofu made with calcium sulfate, tempeh, dried figs, dried beans, broccoli, bok choy, collard greens, kale, mustard greens, okra, and turnip greens.

Meat and beans. Choose low-fat or lean meats and poultry; use low-fat cooking methods; select fish rich in omega-3 fatty acids, such as salmon, trout, and herring; vary your protein sources by choosing more dry beans, nuts, and seeds in place of meat.

A person with diabetes can take away many good nutrition points from the Dietary Guidelines for Americans. However, the guidelines are intended for the general public and not intended as a therapeutic diet for any specific condition such as diabetes. For that, the American Diabetes Association (ADA) offers some guidance.

ADA Nutrition Recommendations

The American Diabetes Association's primary recommendation regarding diet is that each person with diabetes receive individualized nutrition guidance, preferably from a registered dietitian. Some of its other recommendations are as follows:

■ Monitoring the total grams of carbohydrate eaten remains a key strategy in achieving blood glucose control.

■ Using the glycemic index or the glycemic load to choose carbohydrate-containing foods may provide an additional benefit over just counting total carbohydrate.

■ Because the brain and nervous system require glucose as an energy source, restrict-ing total carbohydrate intake to less than 130 grams a day is not recommended in the management of diabetes.

■ A prudent approach to protein intake is to stick to the current recommended dietary allowance (RDA)—0.8 grams of protein per kilogram of body weight per day—particularly in people with any degree of chronic kidney disease.

■ Saturated fat intake should account for less than 7% of total calories.

■ Intake of *trans* fat should be minimized.

■ Weight loss is recommended for all adults with Type 2 diabetes (or prediabetes) and a body-mass index (BMI) of 25 or higher. The preferred method of weight loss is a reduction in food intake and an increase in physical activity.

■ For most people, weight-loss diets should supply at least 1,000–1,200 calories per day for women and 1,200–1,600 calories per day for men.

■ Routine supplementation with antioxidants such as vitamins C and E and beta-carotene is not recommended because of lack of evidence of benefits and because of long-term safety concerns.

■ Routine supplementation with chromium is not recommended because it has not been conclusively demonstrated to be beneficial.

Carbohydrate

Carbohydrate in food is what makes your blood glucose level rise, so reducing the amount of carbohydrate in your diet may help keep blood glucose levels lower. However, carbohydrate is an important source of water-soluble vitamins and minerals and fiber, which is why the ADA (in agreement with the National Academy of Sciences Food and Nutrition Board) recommends getting about 45% to 65% of calories from carbohydrate each day. For a person who consumes 2,000 calories daily, this works out to 225–325 grams of carbohydrate a day. For someone who eat 1500 calories a day, it works out to about 170–245 grams of carbohydrate.

As stated earlier, the ADA recommends an intake of no fewer than 130 grams of carbohydrate a day to provide the brain with adequate fuel.

Forms of carbohydrate include sugars, starches, and fiber, although fiber does not digest fully and hence does not raise blood glucose levels. Carbohydrate is found in most starchy foods (such as breads, cereals, potatoes, rice, pasta, and beans) as well as fruits, juices, milk, sweets, and to a lesser extent, nonstarchy vegetables.

Although all forms of carbohydrate (except fiber) are eventually broken down into simple sugars in the digestive system, some break down much more slowly and, as a result, raise blood glucose levels less. Highly refined carbohydrate foods tend to break down faster and raise blood glucose more than less-refined foods or whole grains. For example, regular cornflakes, which are made of refined grains, break down much faster than whole corn kernels. Foods that contain more soluble fiber, such as oats and oat bran, are also absorbed more slowly.

A tool for choosing sources of carbohydrate that digest more slowly is the glycemic index.

Glycemic index

The glycemic index (GI) ranks carbohydrate-containing foods on a scale from 0 to 100 according to how much they raise blood glucose levels after eating. Foods with a high GI are rapidly digested and tend to cause a marked rise in blood glucose level. Foods with a low GI are digested and absorbed more slowly and produce gradual rises in blood glucose level. Lists of foods and their glycemic index values are readily available on the Internet and in the book *The New Glucose Revolution,* which also explains how to use glycemic index values.

Even without consulting a list, however, it's possible to start putting the glycemic index to work by replacing the highly processed grains and cereals in your diet with whole-grain products. Choosing foods with a lower glycemic index may have benefits for weight control as well as blood glucose control since whole grains are higher in fiber and therefore more filling.

Glycemic index values can be helpful for meal planning, but they can vary from person to person. That's to say, one person may digest and absorb a given food faster than another person. That food, therefore, would have a higher glycemic index for the first person. Monitoring your blood glucose level 1½ to 2 hours after meals may help to determine how quickly you absorb certain foods or food combinations.

Because the glycemic index evaluates the quality of carbohydrate but not the quantity—and quantity is still the main determinant of how much a serving of food raises your blood glucose—nutritionists at the Harvard School of Public Health developed a way to take both quality and quantity into consideration. The result is the glycemic load.

Glycemic load

The glycemic load of a food is calculated by multiplying a food's glycemic index by the amount of carbohydrate (in grams) in a serving of food, then dividing that number by 100. The glycemic load may provide a more accurate indicator of how much a portion of food will raise your blood glucose level than just its glycemic index.

For example, say a particular type of fruit has a glycemic index value of 60, and a serving of that fruit contains 15 grams of carbohydrate. The calculation to determine the glycemic load of the serving of fruit is $60 \times 15 \div 100 = 9$. Some experts advise restricting the glycemic load of most meals to between 20 and 25, the glycemic load of most snacks to between 10 and 15, and the total glycemic load for the day to less than 100.

Calculating the glycemic load can help to compare foods or help you decide how much to eat of favorite foods that have a high glycemic index.

Fiber

The ADA encourages people with diabetes to choose fiber-rich foods but has not set specific recommendations for fiber intake.

There are two major types of fiber: insoluble fiber and soluble fiber. Insoluble fiber, which is found in whole wheat products, corn, and some other vegetables, aids in

Glycemic Index Values of Common Foods

The glycemic index of a food is a measure of how quickly it raises blood glucose after eating. The higher the number, the faster it raises blood glucose.

BREAD/CRACKERS

Bagel	72
Crispbread	81
Croissant	67
French baguette	95
Graham crackers	74
Kaiser roll	73
Pita bread	57
Pumpernickel	51
Rye, dark	76
Saltines	74
Sourdough bread	52
Stoned Wheat Thins	67
White bread	71
Whole wheat bread, high-fiber	68

CAKES/COOKIES/MUFFINS

Angel food cake	67
Banana bread	47
Blueberry muffin	59
Chocolate cake	38
Corn muffin	102
Cupcake with icing	73
Doughnut	76
Oat bran muffin	60
Oatmeal cookie	55
Pound cake	54
Shortbread cookie	64
Vanilla wafers	77

CANDY

Chocolate	49
Jelly beans	80
LifeSavers	70
M&M, peanut	33
Skittles	69
Snickers bar	40
Twix bar	43

CEREALS/BREAKFAST FOODS

All-Bran	42
Bran Chex	58
Cheerios	74
Cornflakes	83
Cream of Wheat	70
Crispix	87
Grape-Nuts	67
Oatmeal	49
Pancakes	67
Pop-Tarts	70
Puffed Wheat	67
Raisin Bran	73
Rice Krispies	82
Shredded Wheat	69
Special K	66
Total	76
Waffles	76

COMBINATION FOODS

Chicken nuggets	46
Fish fingers	38
Macaroni and cheese	64
Pizza (cheese)	60
Sausages	28
Stuffing	74
Taco shells	68

DAIRY

Chocolate milk	34
Custard	43
Ice cream	62
Milk, skim	32
Milk, whole	27
Pudding	43
Yogurt, low-fat	33

Nutrition: The Basics

preventing constipation. Soluble fiber, which is found in oats, oat bran, barley, apples, pears, dried beans and legumes, broccoli, and Brussels sprouts, can help to control cholesterol levels if eaten in adequate amounts.

The National Cholesterol Education Program's Therapeutic Lifestyle Changes rec-

FRUITS & JUICES

Apple	38
Apple juice	41
Banana	55
Cantaloupe	65
Cherries	22
Cranberry juice	68
Fruit cocktail	55
Grapefruit	25
Grapefruit juice	48
Grapes	46
Orange	44
Orange juice	52
Peach	42
Pear	37
Plum	39
Raisins	64
Watermelon	72

LEGUMES

Baked beans	48
Black beans	30
Black-eyed peas	42
Butter beans	30
Chickpeas	33
Lentils	25
Pinto beans	45
Red kidney beans	19

PASTA

Capellini	45
Couscous	65
Fettuccini	32
Macaroni	45
Spaghetti	41
Spaghetti, whole wheat	37
Tortellini	50

RICE

Brown rice	55
Instant rice	87
Long grain rice	56
Risotto	69

SNACK FOODS

Corn chips	74
Granola bars	61
Nutri-Grain bars	66
Peanuts	15
Popcorn	55
Potato chips	54
Pretzels	81
Rice cakes	77

SOUPS

Black bean	64
Green pea	66
Lentil	44
Minestrone	39
Split pea	60
Tomato	38

SPORTS BARS/DRINKS

Gatorade	78
PowerBar	58

SUGARS & SPREADS

Glucose tablets	102
High-fructose corn syrup (used to sweeten most regular sodas)	62
Honey	58
Pancake syrup	66
Strawberry jam	51
Table sugar (sucrose)	64

VEGETABLES

Carrots, boiled	49
Carrots raw	16
Corn	46
French fries	75
Potato, baked	85
Potato, boiled	88
Potato, instant	83
Potato, mashed	91
Sweet potato	44
Tomato	38

ommend that adults consume 20–30 grams of total fiber per day, or 10–25 grams of soluble fiber per day. However, people with any gastrointestinal problems such as gastroparesis, or slowed stomach emptying, should consult their health-care provider for individualized fiber intake advice. When increasing your fiber intake, it's a good idea to increase your fluid intake at the same time. Insoluble fiber can only help to prevent constipation if you consume adequate amounts of fluid.

Protein

Dietary protein is also a necessary part of the diet. Protein is used in the body to build and repair tissues and to regulate numerous bodily processes. It can also be used for energy if a person doesn't consume enough carbohydrate and fat. However, if you eat more protein than your body needs, it is stored as fat, not protein.

Sources of protein include meat, poultry, fish, dairy products, and eggs. However, it's not necessary to eat any animal products to get adequate protein: Grains, beans, nuts, seeds, and vegetables also contain varying amounts of protein, and there may be health benefits to getting more of your protein from plant sources. Recent research shows that people who get more of their protein from plant sources tend to have lower blood pressure.

The ADA currently takes the position that it is prudent for adults with diabetes to limit their protein intake to the RDA for protein, which is 0.8 grams of high-quality protein per kilogram of body weight per day. For a 150-pound person, that works out to about 54 grams of protein a day. For a 200-pound person, it's about 72 grams of protein a day. Depending on calorie intake, this level of protein intake is about 10% of total calories. This is less protein than a lot of Americans currently consume.

The ADA's rationale for its position is that a higher protein intake may be a risk factor for the development of diabetic kidney disease. However, there is much controversy over whether this is true and what a safe level of protein intake is in healthy people. Many authors of popular diet books advocate eating more protein to help with weight loss. Even the Joslin Diabetes Center's new nutrition guideline recommends getting 20% to 30% of total calories from protein based on studies showing a reduction in the risk for heart disease, a reduction in total body and abdominal fat mass, reduced insulin resistance, a preservation of lean body mass during weight loss, and an increased sense of satiety, or fullness, when higher amounts of lean protein are consumed.

However, the Joslin guideline cautions people with any signs of diabetic kidney disease, such as microalbuminuria, to check with a physician, preferably a nephrologist, before increasing their protein intake.

Fat

Fat is also necessary in the diet. Without fat, you could not fully absorb and use vitamins A, D, E, and K. Fat is also necessary to maintain healthy skin. And the body uses fat for energy to fuel physical activity and basic bodily functions.

Fat in the diet comes primarily from vegetable oils, animal products, such as meat and dairy products, and items made with oils and fat, such as baked goods. However, fat comes in different forms, some of which appear to have health benefits, and some of which have detrimental effects on the body. Here are the forms of fat you're most likely to hear about:

■ Saturated fatty acids tend to raise low-density lipoprotein (LDL, or "bad") cholesterol levels. Foods high in saturated fat include butter, coconut oil, and beef fat.

■ *Trans* fat raises LDL cholesterol and appears to lower high-density lipoprotein (HDL, or "good") cholesterol. Historically, fast foods, margarines, and commercial baked goods were high in *trans* fat, but that has started to change with mandatory inclusion of *trans* fat information on the Nutrition Facts panels of food labels.

■ Monounsaturated fatty acids may help lower LDL cholesterol levels if used in place of other fats. Foods high in monounsaturated fat include canola oil and olive oil.

■ Polyunsaturated fatty acids may help lower LDL cholesterol if used in place of saturated fat. Foods high in polyunsaturated fat include vegetable oils and seafood.

■ Omega-3 fatty acids are a type of polyunsaturated fat that appears to be particularly useful at lowering the risk of heart disease. These fats are found in high amounts in cold-water, fatty fish.

Confusing the matter is that all fats and oils contain a mixture of saturated, monounsaturated, and polyunsaturated fatty acids. That's to say, even canola oil contains a small percentage of saturated fat, and even beef fat contains a small percentage of polyunsaturated fat. The goal, then, is to choose foods that are "low in" saturated fat and *trans* fat and "high in" monounsaturated fat. This is made easier by reading food labels, which list grams of total fat, saturated fat, and *trans* fat separately. Labels on oils, margarines, and spreads may also list grams of monounsaturated and polyunsaturated fats.

While major health organizations generally agree that saturated and *trans* fat intake should be kept low, there is less consensus on the optimal percentage of total calories that should come from fat. The Dietary Guidelines for Americans suggest 20% to 35%; the National Cholesterol Education Program recommends 25% to 35%; and the Joslin nutrition guideline recommends 30% to 35%. According to the ADA, the best mix of carbohydrate, protein, and fat probably depends on the individual.

Water and sodium

Water is necessary for life. You can only go for a few days without water. Water helps regulate the body's temperature and keeps the body chemistry balanced. It also supports chemical metabolic reactions, such as those found in the stomach, the intestines, and the blood. Water also assists in the transportation of vitamins and minerals, gases, and waste products.

Any beverage is a source of water. Many foods are, too. Foods that contain a lot of water include vegetables, fruits, low-fat dairy products, and soups.

For years, people have been told they need a full eight cups of water a day. In the latest report of the Institute of Medicine of the National Academies of Science, however, researchers advise simply drinking when you're thirsty. However, since thirst sensations decrease with aging, elderly people may need to pay closer attention to their water intake. Some people may also avoid drinking water in an effort to control urinary incontinence. Although this tactic may help initially, it tends to work less well over time and is not recommended. Drinking too little water can lead to dehydration, heat exhaustion, and even heat stroke.

Certain people, such as those on kidney dialysis, have to limit their intake of fluids, including water, to prevent excessive weight gain between dialysis treatments. If your nephrologist has given you a fluid intake maximum, it is important to follow that advice.

It's rare for a healthy person to consume too much water, although some marathon runners have developed a condition called hyponatremia, in which excessive consumption of water dilutes the salt level in the body too much.

Sodium is also necessary for life, but only in small doses. According to the Food and Nutrition Board of the National Academies of Science, for healthy 19- to 50-year-old adults, 1500 milligrams of sodium a day is enough to replace the amount lost daily on average through sweat. For adults between the ages of 50 and 70, 1300 milligrams of sodium is adequate. And for adults over 70, 1200 milligrams is enough.

Having a high sodium intake can contribute to high blood pressure. The American Diabetes Association recommends limiting sodium intake to no more than 2400 milligrams per day, which is about the amount in one teaspoon of salt.

Alcohol

Moderate consumption of alcohol, particularly red wine, has been widely reported to reduce the risk for cardiovascular disease. Some researchers have attributed this cardioprotective quality to the significant amounts of the compound *resveratrol* naturally present in grape skins. Studies have shown resveratrol to be an effective antioxidant and to have anti-inflammatory properties. Other studies have attributed the lower risk of cardiovascular disease to the alcohol itself. However, drinking too much alcohol can raise the levels of triglycerides in the blood and lead to high blood pressure, heart failure, and weight gain through increased calorie intake. Even moderate consumption is not risk free, since even slight intoxication can contribute to traffic accidents and other sources of traumatic injury. For these reasons, major health organizations do not currently recommend starting to drink alcohol for its possible health benefits if you do not currently drink any alcohol.

Alcohol consumption poses the same risks for people with diabetes as it does for the rest of the population, and it also increases the risk of developing hypoglycemia (low blood glucose). This is because while the liver is busy metabolizing alcohol, it is not releasing glucose into the bloodstream. Drinking alcohol when you eat, such as during a meal, lowers the likelihood that you will develop hypoglycemia. To be sure of your response to the alcohol you drink, check your blood glucose level before and shortly after one drink to observe its effect. Be aware, however, that hypoglycemia can develop many hours after you finish drinking.

The ADA recommendations regarding the use of alcohol by adults with diabetes are that daily intake should be limited to a moderate amount. This is defined as one drink per day or less for women and two drinks per day or less for men. A drink equals 12 ounces of beer, 5 ounces of wine, or 1½ ounces of distilled spirits.

Vitamin and mineral supplements

Vitamins and minerals are chemical compounds required by the body to perform basic functions, such as energy production, carbohydrate metabolism, bone growth, oxygen transport, and heart contraction. Inadequate levels of certain vitamins and minerals in the diet can lead to serious diseases.

What constitutes adequate levels is established by the Food and Nutrition Board of the National Academy of Sciences. The recommended dietary allowance (RDA) is the amount found to be sufficient to meet the nutrient requirements of nearly all (98%) individuals in a group. In some cases, however, RDAs have not been established. The adequate intake (AI) is the amount believed to cover the needs of all individuals in a group, but lack of data prevents being able to state with confidence the percentage of individuals covered by this intake. The tolerable upper intake level (UL) is the maximum level of daily nutrient intake that is unlikely to pose a risk of adverse health effects in almost all individuals in a group.

Most major health organizations do not routinely recommend any vitamin or mineral supplements on the theory that following a balanced diet should provide all necessary vitamins and minerals. In addition, by eating whole foods, you may also get some nutrients that are not contained in supplements. Also, taking very large doses of some vitamins and minerals may be harmful.

However, there are instances in which a health-care provider may recommend supplements. A person who is unable or unwilling to eat a variety of fruits and vegetables, for example, might be advised to take a multivitamin and mineral supplement providing no more than 100% of his daily recommended intake. Some other instances in which supplements might be recommended include the following:

Very low calorie intake. If you are on a very-low-calorie diet, you may not get all of the essential vitamins and minerals you need, even if your selection of foods represents a balanced diet.

Very low calcium intake from food. A common consequence of a low calorie intake is a low calcium intake, which is believed to contribute to osteoporosis.

Chronic high blood glucose. High blood glucose can cause an increased loss of water-soluble vitamins and many minerals in the urine.

Food allergy or intolerance. People who cannot eat whole categories of food because of allergies or intolerances may come up short on certain vitamins and minerals.

Vegan diet. Those who follow a vegan diet, with absolutely no animal products, may be advised to take a vitamin B_{12} supplement, because vitamin B_{12} is present only in foods of animal origin.

Pregnancy. Many women are advised to take supplemental iron, folic acid, and calcium during pregnancy, both for their own health and that of the baby.

Older people. Some older people do not absorb certain nutrients efficiently and may need supplements. After age 50, the stomach lining produces less stomach acid, which is needed to process the vitamin B_{12} in food, so a deficiency may result. In the case of vitamin D, older people may not synthesize it readily in their skin and similarly, a deficiency may result.

Bariatric surgery. People who have had gastric bypass surgery or some other procedure for weight loss that severely limits their food intake are routinely advised to take certain vitamin and mineral supplements.

Certain vitamins and minerals often come up in the context of diabetes, including the following. It's a good idea to discuss these with your health-care provider before taking any of them regularly. If taking a supplement affects your blood glucose levels, you may need to lower the amount of blood-glucose-lowering medicines you take.

Alpha-lipoic acid

Also known as thioctic acid, alpha-lipoic acid is an antioxidant that is made in small amounts in the body but is not obtained from food. It appears to have some benefits of relevance to people with diabetes. In clinical studies, oral consumption or intravenous infusion of alpha-lipoic acid enhanced blood vessel relaxation and improved microcirculation. Some studies involving people with Type 2 diabetes have shown that treatment with alpha-lipoic acid improves blood glucose control. And in one study, people with diabetes who took 600 milligrams of alpha-lipoic acid per day had lower levels of protein in their urine than a control group. (Protein in the urine is a sign of kidney disease.) Perhaps most promising are studies showing that people with diabetes treated with 600 milligrams of alpha-lipoic acid per day for a matter of weeks or months had fewer symptoms of neuropathy, including heart rhythm abnormalities and pain, numbness, and burning in the feet.

While these study results are exciting, the long-term effects of taking high doses of alpha-lipoic acid are unknown.

Chromium

A trace mineral in the diet, chromium both enhances the action of insulin to help maintain normal blood glucose levels and appears to be directly involved in carbohydrate, fat, and protein metabolism. Chromium has been of interest as a possible aid to diabetes control ever since it was noted that people with a chromium deficiency develop diabetes-like symptoms.

However, determining who is deficient is difficult, because the levels of chromium in blood, urine, and hair do not necessarily reflect the body's stores. There is no evidence that all people with diabetes are deficient in chromium, nor that adding chromium to the diets of people who are not deficient has clear benefits.

The estimated safe and adequate dietary intake of chromium for adults is 50–200 micrograms. Many foods contain chromium, but most contain only small amounts. Meat and whole-grain products, as well as some fruits, vegetables, and spices are relatively good sources. In contrast, foods high in simple sugars are low in chromium. In addition, vitamin C and the B vitamin niacin enhance absorption of chromium, while diets high in simple sugars can increase chromium excretion in the urine.

Magnesium

A mineral needed by the body in very small amounts, magnesium serves important functions throughout the body and may play a role in how well cells respond to insulin.

Magnesium is a key component to over 300 enzymes in the body that regulate such functions as metabolizing food, making proteins, making muscles contract, and transmitting signals between cells. Magnesium deficiency may play a role in insulin resistance, the body's inability to use insulin effectively. However, the American Diabetes Association recommends screening for magnesium deficiency only in people at high risk for it, and magnesium supplementation only for people who are shown to be clearly magnesium deficient. While magnesium is a relatively nontoxic substance, taking supplements can lead to dangerously high levels in people with decreased kidney function.

Determining magnesium status can be difficult because only a very small percentage of the body's magnesium stores are in the blood. Magnesium deficiency is most commonly seen in people with impaired intestinal or kidney function, malnourishment, parathyroid disease, chronic alcohol abuse, or chronic diarrhea. Having chronically high blood glucose levels may promote magnesium loss through frequent urination.

The RDA for magnesium is 400 milligrams per day for men ages 19–30, 420 milligrams per day for men over 30, 310 milligrams per day for women ages 19–30, and 320 milligrams per day for women over 30. Good food sources of magnesium are legumes, nuts, whole grains, milk products, and green vegetables. Refined grains are generally low in magnesium.

Vanadium

A trace element for which there is no recommended level of intake, vanadium is believed to mimic the effects of insulin in some way. In studies, vanadium supplementation has been shown to decrease glucose release by the liver, increase the use of glucose for energy, and increase insulin sensitivity in people with Type 2 diabetes. However, some study subjects developed an upset stomach and other gastrointestinal side effects. Excess vanadium consumption is also associated with developing a green tongue. Long-term effects are unknown. Some researchers have recommended limiting vanadium intake to no more than 100 micrograms a day. The UL for vanadium is 1.8 milligrams per day. Food sources of vanadium include mushrooms, shellfish, black pepper, parsley, and dill seed.

A derivative of vanadium called vanadyl sulfate is heavily marketed to bodybuilders as a tool for increasing muscle mass. Suggested doses are often much larger than 1.8 milligrams. There is no evidence, however, that the supplement works as advertised.

Food combining and other theories

Food recommendations sometimes go beyond what to eat and also include when or how to eat. People with Type 2 diabetes, for example, are often told by mainstream registered dietitians to spread their carbohydrate intake out over the day. Each time a person consumes carbohydrate, the pancreas needs to release insulin to "cover" it. But in Type 2 diabetes, the pancreas may have trouble keeping up with demand. Eating small amounts of carbohydrate at each meal and one or two snacks lowers the demand at any one time.

People with diabetes may also be advised by mainstream health-care providers to eat "mixed meals," or meals containing carbohydrate, fat, and protein. Mixtures of these nutrients are generally digested more slowly than meals made up of mostly carbohydrate foods. Slower digestion generally means a lower rise in blood glucose level, and therefore less work for the pancreas.

Here are some other recommendations you may encounter as you explore the world of complementary medicine:

■ Some alternative medicine providers advocate specific rules for food combining. The theory is that certain foods are digested more easily when eaten alone or when eaten at the same time as certain other foods.

■ Others advocate food rotation schedules, in which each food is eaten only once every four days to minimize the allergic "stimulus" of each food.

■ Advocates of the alkaline diet theorize that it's better to eat foods with a pH level close to that of the human body. The pH scale is used to express level of acidity, with 7.0 being neutral, above 7.0 being alkaline (or basic), and below 7.0 being acid. Blood is normally slightly alkaline, with a pH range of 7.35 to 7.45.

■ Macrobiotics divide foods into yin and yang foods depending on how the food grows, where the food grows, the food's potassium and sodium content, and whether the food has a "hot" or "cold" effect on the body. It is believed that when the intake of yin and yang foods are not in balance, the person becomes ill.

While none of these approaches to diet is necessarily incompatible with getting adequate nutrients and maintaining blood glucose control, it would be wise to review any such food rules carefully. If a diet cuts out an entire food group such as dairy products, for example, note whether it includes other foods that supply calcium, magnesium, and vitamin D. Does the diet minimize saturated fat and sodium content? And most important, can you maintain blood glucose control while following this diet?

Fasting

Fasting is used for a variety of purposes. Some religions have ritual fasts, and some people believe fasting has a "cleansing" function. Fasting is also necessary for certain medical procedures and exams.

Because fasting can seriously disrupt blood glucose control, consult your health-care provider before participating in a fast. Even if you are not eating, your body still needs insulin to process the glucose that is released from the liver. If you take a long-acting insulin such as NPH, insulin glargine (brand name Lantus), or insulin detemir (Levemir), you may need to adjust your dose. If you use an insulin pump, you may need to adjust your basal rate.

People who take oral diabetes drugs may or may not be advised to stop taking them for the duration of a fast. If you usually take repaglinide (Prandin), nateglinide (Starlix), acarbose (Precose), or miglitol (Glyset) before meals, you probably won't need them since you won't be eating meals. People who take a sulfonylurea (glipizide, glimepiride, or glyburide) may be advised to stop taking it or to lower their dose since these drugs cause the pancreas to secrete insulin and can cause hypoglycemia. The drugs metformin (Glucophage), pioglitazone (Actos), and rosiglitazone (Avandia) should not cause hypoglycemia, but you should still consult your health-care provider about whether to continue using them during a fast.

It is generally recommended that people

with diabetes fast for no longer than a day. For any fast, it is recommended that you continue to drink water to prevent dehydration and reduce your level of physical activity. People with Type 1 diabetes may be advised to drink sweetened water or some other caloric liquid. This ensures that the body continues to use carbohydrate for energy rather than breaking down fat, which will create ketones and raise the risk of developing diabetic ketoacidosis.

If you choose to fast, do so with the cooperation of your diabetes health-care provider. Keep in mind that Western science has found no physical benefits to fasting and that many other practices can lead to spiritual growth without threatening your blood glucose control.

Weight loss

Many people with Type 2 diabetes are overweight when diagnosed and are told to lose weight. Learning about basic nutrition and working out an individualized meal plan is one step on the road to weight loss. But it usually isn't enough. Losing weight and keeping it off also usually involves behavioral changes and increased physical activity.

One proven technique for weight loss is to keep a food diary. By writing down absolutely everything you eat or drink, you're able to see how many calories you're really consuming and where the extra calories may be coming in. (Beverages often provide more calories than you'd think.) You can also see what happens when you skip breakfast, for example, and whether you're really eating all the servings of fruits and vegetables that you think you are.

Another way to change the way you behave around food is to pay attention to the types of things that cause you to overeat or to eat when you're not really hungry. Here are some common types of triggers:

Sensory triggers. You eat in response to the sight or smell of food.

Special occasion triggers. You tend to overeat on vacations, at parties, and during holidays.

Activity triggers. You associate eating with certain activities, such as going to the movies.

People triggers. You tend to make social plans that involve eating, or you eat in response to watching others eat.

Emotional triggers. You eat in response to your emotions. You may eat primarily in response to emotions such as sadness or anger, but you may also eat when you're happy.

Once you've identified your triggers, you may be able to figure out how to avoid them or respond to them differently. In many cases, common sense will do the trick. If the smell of fresh bread makes you want to eat it, stay out of the bakery. Bring an apple to the movie rather than buying popcorn. Buy only small portions of foods you tend to overeat (such as chocolate or potato chips) so you can have a taste but not have a big bag in the house tempting you.

In other cases, some of the strategies described in this book may help. Practicing meditation can help you learn to respond differently to negative emotions. Visualizing yourself eating less at holiday meals or on evenings out with friends may really help you eat less. Also, taking time to really enjoy your food can paradoxically lead to eating less of it.

Getting support is important, too. Attending a weight-loss support group can help you to feel less alone in your struggle. Finding health-care providers who give you the support you need is important, too. When it comes to getting support from friends or family members, it often helps to be specific about what kind of support you'd like. For example, you might ask that they join you in eating healthier meals. Or you might just ask them not to eat foods that you're trying to avoid in front of you.

The big picture

There are still many unknowns and controversies regarding food, but most health experts have agreed for many years that a healthful diet includes a variety of foods and emphasizes fruits, vegetables, and whole grains.

If you could use some help figuring out what to eat to stay healthy and keep your blood glucose in control, consider making an appointment with a registered dietitian who is knowledgeable about diabetes. Many insurance plans cover a certain number of hours of diabetes management education, including nutrition education (sometimes called medical nutrition therapy). You can also learn a lot about nutrition from resources published by authorities such as the American Dietetic Association and the American Heart Association.

Like any good habit, eating right takes attention and practice, but it can be done.

10. DIETS: HAVE YOU TRIED THIS ONE?

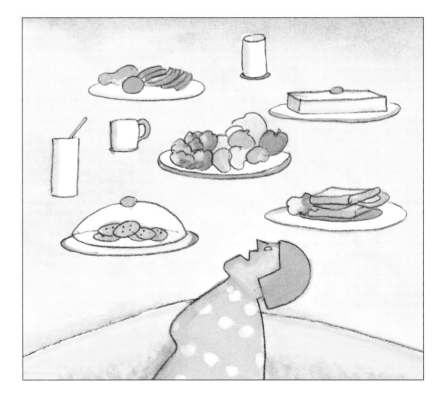

10.
DIETS:
HAVE YOU TRIED THIS ONE?

Americans—with and without diabetes—spend some $40 billion every year on dieting and diet-related products. Not a few of those dollars are spent at the bookstore, where diet books are perennial bestsellers. The sheer number of diet books for sale is a testament both to overweight Americans' great desire to lose weight and to the difficulty of losing weight and keeping it off. It's also a reminder that no one has found the single best diet for everyone.

This chapter describes some popular diets and the approaches they recommend for weight loss. Some have very precise instructions for what and how much to eat. Some have more general guidelines. And some approaches to weight loss are about not following a diet. Most will probably produce weight loss if followed to the letter, but for a diet (or nondieting approach to eating) to work, it's got to be one you can stick with for the long term.

In most cases, losing excess weight has the beneficial side effect of improving heart health and blood glucose control. However, switching to a meal plan that is much higher (or lower) in carbohydrate, protein, or fat than your current meal plan can disrupt your blood glucose control unless you plan for it. Before you start any new diet, review it with your health-care provider so that your medicine doses can be adjusted, if necessary. If your blood glucose levels come down, you may need less insulin or other diabetes medicines.

Pritikin Program

Nathan Pritikin was a 41-year-old inventor when he was diagnosed with cardiovascular disease in 1956. At the time, the recommended treatment was to take it easy, but Pritikin decided on another approach, based on his own reading about heart disease. He started jogging, adopted a low-fat vegetarian diet, and began his life's mission of teaching others how to reverse heart disease, high blood pressure, and diabetes with dietary and lifestyle changes. Pritikin died of leukemia in 1984, but his dietary approach lives on, both in books and in the Pritikin Longevity Center & Spa in Florida. For people who are able to stick with it, the Pritikin Program has been shown to lower low-density lipoprotein (LDL, or "bad") cholesterol, lower triglycerides, lower levels of C-reactive protein (a marker for heart disease), lower circulating insulin levels, lower blood pressure, and cause weight loss.

The Pritikin eating plan is low in fat and high in unprocessed, fiber-rich carbohydrates. It emphasizes whole grains, beans, peas, starchy vegetables, nonstarchy vegetables, and fruits. It is not a vegetarian diet, but it suggests eating no more than 3½ ounces of animal flesh per day and consuming only modest amounts of nonfat dairy products.

The basic approach to meal planning is to choose five servings of unrefined carbohydrate foods such as whole grains or beans per day, four servings of vegetables, three servings of fruit, two servings of calcium-rich foods, and one serving of animal protein. For those who prefer a vegetarian meal plan, the animal protein can be replaced with a serving of beans, peas, lentils, tofu, or other soy products. In addition, low-sodium, low-calorie beverages are encouraged, and the diet allows seven egg whites per week and 2 ounces of nuts, seeds, or avocado per day. Alcohol and caffeine intake should be limited. People who do not need to lose weight are encouraged to increase the amount of whole grains, vegetables, and fruits in their diet.

While all of these food choices could be simply cooked and eaten plain, most people prefer something a little fancier, at least occasionally. For that, the Pritikin Longevity Center & Spa Web site, www.pritikin.com, and many of the Pritikin books have recipes that use the low-fat, low-sodium ingredients recommended in the eating plan. In addition to books by Nathan Pritikin, several are also available by his son Robert, including *The Pritikin Weight Loss Breakthrough: 5 Easy Steps to Outsmart Your Fat Instinct.*

Ornish Lifestyle Program

The Ornish Lifestyle Program, developed by Dean Ornish, M.D., combines diet, exercise, and stress-reduction practices to prevent and reverse heart disease. The basic diet is low-fat and mostly plant-based. However, food choices for people with diagnosed heart disease are more restrictive than those for people who simply wish to lower their risk of heart and other types of disease. For stress management, Ornish recommends yoga, breathing techniques, meditation and imagery, and participation in support groups. And he advises that people get regular, moderate exercise. The Ornish Lifestyle Program has been shown to be highly effective in reversing even severe heart disease.

When it comes to food, Ornish recommends choosing primarily unprocessed fruits, vegetables, whole grains, and beans, including soy-based products. Moderate quantities of egg whites and nonfat dairy and soy milk products are also acceptable. People with heart disease are advised to avoid all high-fat plant-based foods, including all oils (other than 3 grams per day of flaxseed oil or fish oil to provide omega-3 fatty acids), nuts, and avocados. People who do not have heart disease may be more liberal in their food choices and may include moderate amounts of fish, skinless chicken, avocados, nuts, and seeds. However, everyone following the program is advised to limit high-fat animal-based foods, such as red meat and pork, and high-fat dairy products.

Ornish also advises taking a daily multivitamin that provides 100% of the recommended dietary allowance (RDA) of essential vitamins. It should include vitamin B_{12}, which is present only in animal-based foods, but exclude iron, except for women of childbearing age and people whose physicians have told them to take daily iron. In addition, Ornish recommends a daily fish oil capsule containing approximately 600 milligrams (mg) eicosapentaenoic acid (EPA) and 400 mg docosahexaenoic acid (DHA).

Certain hospitals in Pennsylvania and West Virginia have instituted programs to provide education and training in the various parts of the Ornish Lifestyle Program. For a list of these hospitals, look on the Web site of the Preventive Medicine Research Institute (of which Dean Ornish is the founder, president, and director), www.pmri.org. Medicare and some private insurance plans may cover the cost of such a program. You can also learn more about this program by reading the book *Dr. Dean Ornish's Program for Reversing Heart Disease.*

Volumetrics

The term "volumetrics" was coined by Barbara Rolls, Ph.D., a professor of nutritional sciences at Penn State University, who noticed in her research that people tend to eat the same weight or volume of food every day. Rolls subsequently showed that by choosing more foods with low energy density (or fewer calories per bite), you can eat the same volume of food that you're used to while consuming fewer calories.

Rolls divides foods into four categories according to energy density:

Very low energy density. Foods in this category have less than 0.6 calories per gram.

Examples include fruits, nonstarchy vegetables, nonfat milk, and broth-based soups.

Low energy density. Foods in this category have 0.6 to 1.5 calories per gram. Examples include starchy vegetables, grains, breakfast cereals served with low-fat milk, low-fat meats, beans and legumes, and low-fat mixed dishes, such as chili and spaghetti.

Medium energy density. Foods in this category have 1.5 to 4.0 calories per gram. Examples include meats, cheeses, pizza, French fries, salad dressings, bread, pretzels, ice cream, and cake.

High energy density. Foods in this category have 4.0 to 9.0 calories per gram. Examples include crackers, chips, chocolate candies, cookies, nuts, butter, oils.

In her books, Rolls offers helpful tips for putting theory into practice, with recipes, ideas for low-fat seasonings, and suggestions for eating out, such as taking home a portion of what you're served and sharing desserts. She includes formulas for calculating your calorie requirements and encourages exercise.

Dr. Rolls's books on volumetrics include *The Volumetrics Eating Plan* and *The Volumetrics Weight-Control Plan*.

Atkins Diet

The Atkins Diet was developed by cardiologist Robert Atkins, M.D., who first published *Dr. Atkins' Diet Revolution* in 1972 and updated it in *Dr. Atkins' New Diet Revolution* in 1992. The book *Atkins Diabetes Revolution* came out posthumously in 2004. Unlike the three diets previously described, the Atkins Diet is low in grains and other sources of carbohydrate. It also tends to be high in meat, although it could theoretically be followed by vegetarians who eat a lot of dairy products, eggs, soy products, and nuts.

The Atkins Diet is done in four phases: induction, ongoing weight loss, premaintenance, and lifetime maintenance. In the induction phase, a person is instructed to limit his carbohydrate intake to 20 grams per day. It is suggested that these 20 grams of carbohydrate come from either three cups of salad greens or two cups of salad greens and one cup of fresh, nonstarchy cooked vegetables. It is also permissible to eat 3–4 ounces aged cheese, a handful of olives, and half an avocado a day. All other calories come from protein and fat, which are not limited, but eating until full, not stuffed, is recommended.

The writers of *Atkins Diabetes Revolution* also recommend not charring meat (which can form carcinogens, or cancer-causing compounds), limiting cheese to 4 ounces a day, selecting full-fat dairy products and condiments (such as mayonnaise), avoiding *trans* fat, limiting intake of caffeine and diet soft drinks, and limiting use of artificial sweeteners to three packets a day.

The induction phase of the Atkins Diet is intended to be followed for at least two weeks and possibly much longer. It is intended to bring blood glucose levels into a more-normal range and to cause slow, steady weight loss. The second phase, ongoing weight loss, can be started when blood glucose and blood pressure levels are controlled in a normal range.

In the second phase, during which weight loss slows, 5 grams of carbohydrate are added to the diet each week until weight loss stops. At that point, 5 grams of carbohydrate should be subtracted from the diet to get the weight loss process started again. The new carbohydrate grams should come from vegetables, nuts, seeds, berries, and possibly legumes and fruits other than berries. (These last two are acceptable only if weight loss continues.) It is expected that as a person eats more carbohydrate, he will eat less protein and fat.

The third phase, premaintenance, is instituted when a person is within 5–10 pounds of his goal weight. He adds 10 additional grams of carbohydrate to his diet every day, which may come from starchy vegetables and unrefined whole grains. Again, grams of carbohydrate are added only as long as weight loss continues. If it stops, 5–10 grams of carbohydrate must be subtracted from daily intake.

Once a person has reached his goal weight, he should be very familiar with how much carbohydrate he can eat without gaining or losing weight. That is the amount to consume in phase four, lifetime maintenance. However, food choices remain important, and "junk food" is discouraged.

The Atkins Diet has been studied in clinical trials, and it has been shown to cause weight loss. However, when the effects of following the Atkins Diet were compared with the effects of following a low-fat, calorie-reduced diet, the people following the Atkins Diet had lost more weight than the other group after 6 months, but no more after 12 months.

Following the Atkins Diet may have some risks. While some people see their cholesterol levels decrease with the diet, others develop high cholesterol levels. There is also the possibility of developing high levels of homocysteine, a destructive amino acid created by the body as it breaks down protein. And consuming a high-protein diet is a risk factor for developing kidney stones.

South Beach Diet

The South Beach Diet was developed by cardiologist Arthur Agatston, M.D., to help his patients lose weight and lower their risk for heart disease. His basic recommendations include cutting back on processed carbohydrates, choosing carbohydrates with a low glycemic index, and keeping saturated fat intake low.

Like the Atkins Diet, the South Beach Diet is done in phases, with the first phase lasting two weeks, the second lasting until you've reached your ideal weight, and the third lasting forever—or at least until you gain weight and have to start over at phase one, which Dr. Agatston readily admits could happen. For each phase, menus, lists of acceptable foods, and recipes are provided. The food list for phase one is notable for having absolutely no fruits, grains, or legumes. According to Agatston, filling up on meats, low-fat or fat-free cheeses, nuts, eggs, tofu, low-fat or fat-free milk and yogurt, and nonstarchy vegetables for two weeks will reverse insulin resistance and end your cravings for carbohydrate-rich foods. Nonetheless, the food list for phase two includes fruit, whole-grain breads and cereals, legumes, and starchy vegetables.

Unlike the Atkins Diet, the South Beach Diet recommends avoiding foods high in saturated fat, such as full-fat dairy products and many cuts of red meat and chicken. Instead, it recommends choosing low-fat cuts of beef, pork, veal, turkey, and chicken. All types of fish and shellfish are encouraged.

The Zone

Barry Sears, Ph.D., author of *Enter the Zone* and *Mastering the Zone*, among other books, developed his diet out of a personal interest in preventing heart disease, which runs in his family. Through his research, he developed the theory that staying in good health depends on maintaining an ideal balance of *eicosanoids*, hormones, of which there are hundreds, which act as "master switches" that control virtually all human body functions. In his books, he says that eicosanoids are little known because they appear, do their job, and disappear "all in a flash." Their short life span, and the fact that they don't circulate in the bloodstream, make them difficult to measure.

According to Sears, by eating the right amount and types of protein, the right amount and types of carbohydrate, and the right amount and types of fat, you can achieve that ideal balance of eicosanoids and reach the metabolic state in which the body works at peak efficiency. He calls that state "the zone."

The first step to entering the zone is to determine your unique daily protein requirement. Here's how it's done:

■ Determine your lean body mass (using formulas in the book).

■ Assess your level of physical activity.

■ Based on your lean body mass and activity level, calculate your unique daily protein requirement (also using a formula in the book).

Once you know your protein requirement, it's time for meal-planning. Here's what Sears recommends:

■ Spread your protein requirement evenly over the day, in three meals and two snacks.

■ Add only enough carbohydrate to the meal or snack to maintain a protein-to-carbohydrate ratio of about 0.75. For example, if you eat 7 grams of protein, eat 9 grams of carbohydrate with it.

■ Choose sources of carbohydrate with a low glycemic index more often than those with a high glycemic index.

■ Add approximately 1.5 grams of fat for every 7 grams of protein in the meal or snack.

■ Avoid sources of arachidonic acid, which is found in egg yolks and organ meats, and saturated fat, which is found in high amounts in red meat and full-fat dairy products. Favor monounsaturated fat as much as possible.

■ Eat no more than 500 calories per meal and 100 calories per snack. If your daily protein needs are high, plan on having more than three meals a day, so that each contains no more than 500 calories.

■ Go no longer than five hours without a meal or snack.

To make things easier, Sears has provided lists of protein "blocks," or servings of recommended foods containing 7 grams of protein; lists of carbohydrate "blocks," or servings containing 9 grams of carbohydrate; and lists of fat "blocks" with 1.5 grams of fat.

Protein Power

Michael R. Eades and Mary Dan Eades, both physicians and authors of the book *Protein Power*, reason that since heart disease, high blood pressure, and diabetes are common diet-related diseases of modern man, modern man would be better off eating like Paleolithic man. While it would be impossible to know exactly what Paleolithic man ate, the theory they favor is that humans in that period had a diet composed of 65% foods of animal origin and 35% plant matter. The plant matter would be mainly wild vegetation and seasonal fruits, with very little to no cereal grains, since wild grains are virtually inedible, and widespread agriculture was not done in the Paleolithic period.

According to the Eadeses, Protein Power is not just a weight-loss plan but a nutritional program for treating diabetes and cholesterol and triglyceride disorders. In addition, they say they have seen reductions in symptoms from gastroesophageal reflux, ulcerative colitis, rheumatoid arthritis, and Crohn disease among their patients. However, they caution that people with diagnosed diabetes should consult their health-care provider before adopting this diet.

The six essential elements of the Protein Power plan can be summarized as follows:

■ Decrease your carbohydrate intake.

■ Decrease your calorie intake.

■ Exercise.

■ Alter your dietary fat profile.

■ Take supplements. (Specifics are given in the book for which and how much.)

■ Deplete the body of excess stored iron. (Specifics are given in the book for determining whether you have excess stored iron and what to do about it.)

The cornerstone of the program is to find your minimum protein requirement per meal using the tables in the book. The amounts work out to about 1.25–1.55 grams of protein per kilogram of body weight per day, which is somewhat higher than the RDA, 0.8 grams of protein per kilogram of body weight per day.

For fat intake, the Eadeses advise that if you're not trying to lose weight, you can eat as much fat as you want. If you are trying to lose weight, rein in your fat consumption.

Preferred fats are omega-3 fatty acids from cold-water fish, wild game, and flaxseed oil; monounsaturated fat from nuts, seeds, olives, and avocados; and naturally saturated fat from eggs, meat, poultry, and dairy products.

According to the Eadeses, carbohydrate is totally unessential to human health (because your liver can create glucose from amino acids and other substances). Nonetheless, they include some in their plan, with the advice to eat a wide variety of colorful fruits and vegetables, nuts, and green leafy vegetables. Their reasoning is that these foods supply needed antioxidants.

The Eadeses recommend starting with 7–10 grams of carbohydrate per meal (with an optional additional 10 grams per day in snacks). This "intervention" level should be maintained until cholesterol, blood glucose, and triglyceride levels are normal and you have approached your goal weight. At that point you can graduate to the "transition" phase, then to the "maintenance" phase, which includes more carbohydrate. Ideally, a person would find his unique ideal level of carbohydrate based on lab test results and weight gain or loss.

Sugar Busters

Like many diet books, *Sugar Busters! Cut Sugar to Trim Fat* devotes many words to explaining why this method works and why it is the best choice among diets. Essentially, however, their diet and lifestyle recommendations boil down to the following:

■ Cut out all refined sugar, corn syrup, molasses, and honey from your diet.

■ Choose whole-grain carbohydrate sources over refined grain products (such as white rice, white bread, cookies, and cakes).

■ Choose high-fiber vegetables, but avoid potatoes, corn, beets, and large helpings of carrots.

■ Choose low-fat dairy products.

■ Consume at least 1 gram of protein per kilogram of body weight per day (slightly more than the RDA, 0.8 grams of protein per kilogram of body weight per day).

■ Include both animal and plant sources of protein in your diet to get all of the amino acids you need. Choose lean meats and trim visible fat.

■ Eat small portions and regularly spaced meals and snacks.

■ Finish your evening meal by about 8 PM and don't eat after that.

■ Exercise for at least 20 minutes four days a week at an intensity that raises your resting heart rate.

According to the authors, all of these suggestions are aimed at lowering insulin secretion from the pancreas. The proposed benefits of this eating plan include weight loss, lower cholesterol levels, and reduced nighttime indigestion or heartburn.

Dr. Bernstein's Diet Solution

The author of *Dr. Bernstein's Diet Solution*, Richard Bernstein, M.D., was diagnosed with Type 1 diabetes in 1946, at age 12. He has had many years, therefore, to work on his approach to diabetes care and teach it to others.

Much of Dr. Bernstein's approach to diet is based on what he calls the "laws of small numbers." According to Bernstein, if you eat a small amount of carbohydrate, you can more accurately predict how it will affect your blood glucose level than if you eat a large amount of carbohydrate. Similarly, if you inject a small dose of insulin, you can more accurately predict how it will affect your blood glucose level than if you inject a large dose.

One of the reasons Bernstein gives for large amounts of carbohydrate having unpredictable effects is that the total carbohydrate listed on the Nutrition Facts panels of packaged foods may be inaccurate. If the total carbohydrate amount were off by 10% and you ate a serving you thought contained 20 grams of carbohydrate, you would be off by 2 grams of carbohydrate, which might not be a big deal. But if you ate a serving you thought contained 100 grams of carbohydrate, you would be off by 10 grams of carbohydrate, which could significantly affect your blood glucose level, particularly if you take premeal insulin doses to cover the carbohydrate in your meals.

The reasoning for small insulin doses having more predictable action is that injected insulin as a rule is absorbed unpredictably, and the larger the dose, the less predictability. Bernstein recommends that no insulin injection exceed 7 units; if more is needed, the dose should be broken up into several shots given to different areas of the body.

Because carbohydrate affects blood glucose level the most, Bernstein recommends a low-carbohydrate diet. The only carbohydrate-containing foods eaten should be slow-acting, such as salad greens; nonstarchy, nonsweet cooked or raw vegetables; heavy cream, unsweetened soy milk; hard cheese; cream cheese; plain, full-fat yogurt; tofu and meat substitutes made from soy; baked goods made with 100% soy flour; toasted nori (a type of seaweed); low-carbohydrate bran crackers; and nuts.

In general, Dr. Bernstein advises his patients to restrict their carbohydrate intake to about 6 grams at breakfast, 12 grams at lunch, and 12 grams at supper. Given these restrictions, the most calories in their diet come from meat, chicken, fish and other seafood, and eggs. The goal of this eating plan is for your blood glucose level to be the same after eating as it was before. If your blood glucose level increases by more than 20 mg/dl after a meal, either the meal content should be changed or your premeal dose of insulin or blood-glucose-lowering medicine should be changed.

Starting this meal plan without your physician's help is not recommended if you take insulin or oral medicines. Dramatically reducing your carbohydrate intake can rapidly lower your blood glucose level, so you may need to adjust your insulin or medicine doses.

Mediterranean Diet

The Mediterranean Basin includes parts of Greece, Italy, Spain, Portugal, southern France, Northern Africa (especially Morocco and Tunisia), Turkey and other parts of the Balkan region, and the Middle East (especially Lebanon and Syria). The Mediterranean diet usually refers more specifically to the dietary traditions of Crete, much of the rest of Greece, and southern Italy around the year 1960. Characteristics of the Mediterranean diet (and lifestyle) include the following:

Plenty of plants. Fruits, vegetables, potatoes, breads and grains, beans, nuts, and seeds are the backbone of the Mediterranean diet.

Not too much processed food. Minimally processed and, when possible, seasonally fresh and locally grown foods are emphasized.

Olive oil is the main fat. To fully reap the benefits of the high monounsaturated fat content of olive oil, it should replace other fats in the diet such as butter or margarine.

Low in saturated fat. The percent of calories from fat can range from 25% to 35% in the Mediterranean diet, but calories from saturated fat should account for no more than 7% to 8% of total calories.

Easy on dairy products. Daily consumption of cheese and yogurt is low to moderate.

Easy on animal protein. Weekly consumption of fish and chicken is low to moderate. Weekly intake of eggs ranges from none to four, including those used in cooking and baking.

Low in red meat. Red meat is eaten a few times a month, with total monthly consumption limited to 12–16 ounces.

Simple desserts. Typical desserts are fresh fruit. Desserts high in sugar are eaten only a few times per week.

Moderate wine consumption. No more than two glasses of wine per day for men and one glass for women may be consumed with meals.

Regular physical activity. Physical activity is done at a level that promotes a healthy weight, fitness, and well-being.

Another principle of Mediterranean eating is to savor every bite and relish the experience of eating.

People who follow a Mediterranean-style diet have been noted to have less chronic disease, including cancer and coronary heat disease, and a lower rate of recurrent heart attack. In fact, they have a lower mortality rate from all causes, even in old age. Perhaps not surprisingly, the guidelines for the Mediterranean diet are very close to the dietary guidelines of the American Heart Association.

There are numerous sources of information about the Mediterranean Diet. One is the book *The Mediterranean Diet* by Marissa Cloutier, M.S., R.D., and Eve Adamson. Another is the Oldways Preservation Trust, which maintains the Web site www.old-wayspt.org.

DASH eating plan

The DASH eating plan evolved from a clinical study entitled Dietary Approaches to Stop Hypertension. The study showed that elevated blood pressure levels can be reduced with an eating plan low in total fat, saturated fat, and cholesterol, and rich in fruits, vegetables, and low-fat dairy products. Reducing sodium intake as well as following this eating plan has been shown to lower blood pressure even more.

The DASH eating plan provides about 2,000 calories per day, and the recommended food choices and amounts are as follows:

■ 7–8 servings of grains per day, with a serving equaling 1 slice of bread, 1 ounce dry cereal, or ½ cup cooked rice, pasta, or other grain.

■ 4–5 servings of vegetables per day, with a serving equaling 1 cup raw leafy vegetables, ½ cup cooked vegetables, or 6 ounces vegetable juice.

■ 4–5 servings of fruit per day, with a serving equaling one medium fruit, ½ cup fresh, frozen, or canned fruit, ¼ cup dried fruit, or 6 ounces fruit juice.

■ 2–3 servings of low-fat or fat-free dairy products, with a serving equaling 1 cup milk, yogurt, or 1½ ounces cheese.

■ 2 or fewer servings of meat, poultry, or fish per day, with a serving equaling 3 ounces cooked meat, poultry, or fish.

■ 2–3 servings of fats and oils per day, with a serving equaling 1 teaspoon oil, 1 teaspoon soft margarine, 1 tablespoon low-fat mayonnaise, 1 tablespoon salad dressing, or 2 tablespoons low-fat salad dressing.

■ 4–5 servings of nuts, seeds, and dry beans per week, with a serving equaling ⅓ cup or 1½ ounces nuts, 2 tablespoons or ½ ounce seeds, or ½ cup cooked beans.

■ 5 or fewer servings of sweets per week, with a serving equaling 1 tablespoon sugar, 1 tablespoon jelly or jam, ½ ounce fat-free candy such as jelly beans, 1 cup lemonade, or ½ cup low-fat frozen yogurt.

More details on the DASH eating plan can be read online at www.nhlbi.nih.gov/health/public/heart/hbp/dash/index.htm. Updated paper copies can be ordered by calling (301) 592-8573.

Dr. Kushner's Personality Type Diet

Robert Kushner, M.D., is the medical director of the Wellness Institute at Northwestern Memorial Hospital in Chicago and coauthor, with his wife Nancy Kushner, M.S.N., R.N., of *Dr. Kushner's Personality Type Diet*. His approach to weight loss is based on his observations that different people have different barriers to weight loss. He asks the reader to identify his "diet personality," defined as the eating, exercise, and coping lifestyle patterns that have been preventing him from losing weight for good. To do this, he provides three quizzes, one on eating habits, one on exercise habits, and one on coping patterns.

Kushner has identified some common patterns, or "personalities," in each area. For example, some common eating patterns that lead to overconsumption include grazing all day on whatever food is convenient, sticking to a restrictive diet during the day then binging at night, and habitually taking large portions and finishing them. Some common barriers to exercise include hating the feeling of exercising, feeling self-conscious about exercising in front of others, sticking too closely to a routine and getting bored, and having no time to exercise. Common coping patterns that get in the way of weight loss include eating in response to emotions, having low self-esteem, having trouble saying no to others, and having unrealistic weight-loss goals.

Once a person has identified his main barriers, he can choose which to work on first. While Kushner offers some advice on healthful food choices and provides a selection of recipes, much of the advice in the book centers on behavior change.

One of the tools he recommends for everyone is keeping a diary or journal, in which you record what you eat (or drink), when you eat, how much you eat, where you eat, why you eat (including emotional triggers, such as loneliness, anxiety, or anger, activity-related triggers, such as a conflict at work, and environmental triggers, such as seeing a plate of doughnuts), and how hungry you are when you eat. He also advises writing down any physical activities you planned and any you carried out. Sometimes, simply the act of writing these things down can help to change behaviors.

Some of Kushner's other "prescriptions" for all diet personalities include the following:

■ Stop blaming yourself.
■ Know your lifestyle.
■ Make small changes.
■ Self-monitor to stay on track.
■ Identify recipes for success.
■ Be resourceful.

Intuitive Eating

As described in the book *Intuitive Eating: A Revolutionary Program That Works*, written by registered dietitians Evelyn Tribole and Elyse Resch, intuitive eating is based on trusting your body and listening to its signals. Intuitive eaters eat when hungry and stop eating when full. They do not follow weight-loss diets. They allow themselves to enjoy food, and they don't label foods "good" or "bad." Although their diets are not necessarily more nutritious than the diets of nonintuititve eaters, in general, they tend to have a healthy body weight and a low risk of heart disease since they don't overeat.

Becoming an intuitive eater, if you are not one now, takes time and effort, but it is possible and can improve your relationship to food, as well as help you lose weight. Here are some tips offered in the book for becoming an intuitive eater:

■ Reject the "diet mentality." Diets simply don't work.
■ Honor your hunger. Eat when you feel hungry. If you don't, you are more likely to overeat later.
■ Give yourself permission to enjoy food.
■ Discard the belief that some foods are "good" and some foods are "bad." While the authors don't encourage a diet of nothing but cookies and chips, they say that eating what you want when you want it tends to diminish the desire for "junk food," not increase it.
■ Pay attention to your stomach's feeling of fullness.
■ Savor every mouthful.
■ Learn to cope with your emotions without using food. Try doing something physical instead of eating.
■ Respect your body, and make sure your weight goals are realistic.
■ Learn to enjoy physical activity. Focus on how good it feels to move and be active.
■ Choose foods that are good for you and that you enjoy.

In addition to these tips, the authors suggest not going for more than four to five hours between meals and always keeping healthy snacks on hand, so that you can honor your hunger in a nutritious way rather than eating whatever is convenient.

Solution Method

Losing weight with the Solution Method, developed by Laurel Mellin, M.A., R.D., an associate clinical professor of family and community medicine and pediatrics at the University of California San Francisco's School of Medicine, requires mastering two developmental skills: self-nurturing and effective limit-setting. Instructions for learning these skills are included in the book *The 3-Day Solution Plan.* In part, learning and using these skills involves noticing whether you feel stressed or peaceful, being aware of your feelings and needs, and learning to get your needs met.

While results of the three-day plan are said to be immediate, more education and practice are encouraged to sustain them. This includes reading a second book, *The Pathway,* and purchasing various Solution Kits, which include a journal, CDs on various topics, and the opportunity to speak on the phone with a "Solution Provider." Those using the Solution Method are also encouraged to get support through individual coaching and groups set up by the program.

Getting started with the Solution Method can be done simply by purchasing books by Mellin at a bookstore, by visiting the Web site of the Institute for Health Solutions, www.thepathway.org, or by calling the institute at (415) 457-3331. The method is also taught at a few hospital wellness centers around the United States.

What they have in common

While the approaches to diet described here may seem diverse, there are a few points of agreement among most of them, including the following:

■ Listen to your body and only eat until satisfied, not stuffed.

■ Eat vegetables for needed antioxidants and other vitamins and phytochemicals. (Most of the diets also encourage fruits for the same reason.)

■ When choosing grain products, choose whole grains over refined grains.

■ Avoid *trans* fat.

■ Include physical activity in your weight-loss plan.

Many popular diets focus on achieving your "ideal" weight, but even a loss of 5% to 10% of your body weight can have significant health benefits if you are currently overweight. (That means 10–20 pounds if you weigh 200 pounds and 15–30 if you weigh 300.) If you can lose this much and keep it off, you haven't failed at weight loss. To the contrary, you've done your body a lot of good.

11. Herbal Remedies

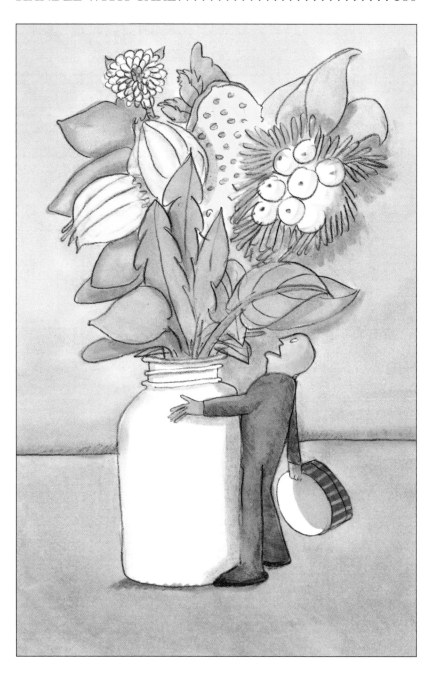

11.
HERBAL REMEDIES

Herbal supplements have become a multi-billion-dollar business in the United States. The reasons for their popularity include the desire to avoid taking prescription drugs, the hope that an herbal remedy will have fewer side effects than a prescription drug, the expectation that herbal remedies will cost less than prescription drugs, the appeal of having personal control over what is taken, the fact that no appointment with a medical professional is necessary to take herbal products nor is a prescription needed, the hope that an herbal remedy will help where pharmaceuticals or other conventional treatments have not, and the preference of some people to use a traditional remedy or "natural" product rather than something that was synthesized in a laboratory.

While some of these hopes and expectations have been realized some of the time, others have not. Some people have simply spent money on supplements that proved ineffective, while others have gotten seriously ill as a result of taking herbal supplements. And while having personal control is valued, many people would like more guidance from medical professionals on how to integrate herbal supplements into their health-care plan.

This chapter offers some guidance for the use of herbal and other botanical products, but it cannot take the place of a one-on-one consultation with a health-care professional.

How herbs are regulated

Herbal supplements are regulated under the Dietary Supplement Health and Education Act of 1994 (DSHEA). The DSHEA defines a dietary supplement as a product intended to supplement the diet that contains vitamins, minerals, herbs or other botanicals, amino acids, or a combination of these substances. To be considered a dietary supplement, it must be intended to be taken as a tablet, capsule, powder, softgel, gelcap, or liquid. It cannot be marketed as a meal replacement.

The DSHEA allows makers of supplements to market their products without first demonstrating to the Food and Drug Administration (FDA) that they are safe or effective. (In most cases, this information is unknown, since few dietary supplements have been subjected to large-scale studies of safety and efficacy.) However, in the case of some new dietary ingredients (ingredients that were not marketed in the United States before October 15, 1994), a premarket safety notification to the FDA is required by law.

Although the FDA does not evaluate dietary supplements before they reach the market, the DSHEA authorizes the FDA to remove products from the market that are later proven to be dangerous. In 2001, for example, the FDA issued a nationwide warning against products containing aristolochic acid (a compound found in the plants *Aristolochia fangchi* and *Asarum canadense*) and imposed a ban on further imports of such products. In 2004, the FDA banned products containing ephedra *(Ephedra sinica, Ephedra equisetina)* from the market. However, because banned products often remain available through the Internet, and other potentially dangerous supplements remain on the market, consumer advocates have called for stepped-up efforts to regulate the dietary supplement business.

Supplement labeling

Although not required to submit safety and efficacy studies to the FDA, supplement manufacturers are required to submit the language they intend to use on a supplement's label. Five statements are required on containers and packages of dietary supplements: the statement of identity (name of the dietary supplement), the net quantity of contents statement (amount of the dietary supplement), the nutrition labeling, the ingredients list, and the name and place of business of the manufacturer, packager, or distributor. The DSHEA allows manufacturers to include information on labels regarding the benefits of a supplement on the structure or the function of the body, but it does not allow manufacturers to label products with unproven claims that supplements will cure diseases.

Some herbal supplements have the word "standardized" on the label. This means the product contains a set amount of an active compound. Herbal products that are standardized are likely to have more predictable effects. However, standardization does not guarantee that a product is potent or effective. In many cases, it is not known exactly which compounds in an herb have beneficial effects. It's possible that some of the beneficial aspects of herbs may be lost when they are extracted and purified for the purpose of standardization. Herbs may be like food in the sense that whole foods have health benefits not provided by individual nutrient supplements.

Using supplements safely

Knowing the potential hazards associated with taking herbal supplements can help you to use them as safely as possible. Such hazards include allergic reactions to herbs, other side effects, interactions between herbs and prescription drugs, and contamination.

Almost any herb (or drug) can cause an allergic reaction. If you are sensitive or allergic to a particular herbal preparation, you could develop anything from a minor rash to an anaphylactic reaction, in which the upper airway may swell and breathing may become difficult. Anaphylactic reactions are

life-threatening. Herbs—as well as any substances used in manufacturing supplements such as dyes or fillers—may also have other side effects, just the way drugs do, but the labels of herbal supplements are not required to list potential side effects. It is prudent, therefore, to check sources of information besides a supplement's label before taking a given herb.

When herbs and drugs are taken simultaneously, the two can interact, usually in negative ways. If one substance interferes with the body's elimination of the other, the result can be too-high levels of either the drug or the herb (or both) in the bloodstream, causing, in effect, an overdose. On the other hand, an herb could also cause a drug to be metabolized more quickly than usual, making it less effective. Drugs and herbs can also interact when they have similar intended effects. For example, taking both a drug and an herb that prevent blood from clotting could raise the risk of excessive bleeding.

Contamination has been a recurrent problem with herbal supplements. Over the years, some supplements have been found to be contaminated with prescription drugs, lead, and arsenic, among other substances. While it's probably impossible to tell by looking whether a supplement is contaminated, the fact that it could be makes it that much more important to stick to brands that have a good reputation and to pay close attention to any side effects a supplement could be causing.

Mislabeling or misidentification is another possible problem with herbal supplements. It may be unintentional or deliberate, possibly an attempt to save on costs by using cheaper herbs. Choosing a reputable brand or manufacturer that has been evaluated by an outside organization should raise your chances of buying products that really contain what their labels promise. For example, the "USP-verified" label mark indicates that the U.S. Pharmacopeia, an independent, not-for-profit organization, has tested the supplement to assure that what's on the label is in the bottle, the supplement does not contain harmful levels of contaminants, the supplement will break down and release its ingredients in the body, and the supplement was made under good manufacturing practices. Similarly, ConsumerLab.com's "CL Seals" label mark identifies products that have met ConsumerLab.com's standards for quality, strength, purity, and availability, or the ability of the supplement to break down and release its ingredients in the body.

If you choose to try an herbal supplement to improve your diabetes control or any other health condition, here are some guidelines to follow for the sake of safety:

■ Discuss your plans with your primary health-care provider, and ask whether any of the supplements you'd like to try might interact with drugs you currently take or might have other negative side effects.

■ Do not use herbal preparations if you are pregnant or nursing. Some herbs are known to stimulate uterine contractions, which may increase the risk of miscarriage or premature labor. In addition, the effects of herbs on a fetus or baby are unknown.

■ Do not give children herbal supplements without first consulting their pediatrician.

■ If you get your doctor's OK to try herbal supplements, keep a log of all the supplements you are taking and the specific doses you are taking.

■ Try only one new supplement at a time so that you can more effectively gauge its effects.

■ Follow the dosage guidelines on the supplement label. Do not take more than the recommended dose.

■ Monitor your blood glucose levels more frequently, and keep careful records of your numbers. This is the only way to know what effect the supplement is having on your blood glucose levels.

■ Pay attention to any symptoms, such as headaches, nausea, rash, or changes in sleep patterns or mood, that may be side effects caused by a supplement. If symptoms persist, stop taking the supplement and see your doctor.

■ Store herbal supplements in their original containers with safety seals intact and out of the reach of children. Having the original container is important in case of accidental overdose or side effects.

■ Set a time limit for trying a supplement, usually three to six weeks. If it hasn't had any effect within that limit, stop using it.

■ If you are going to have any kind of surgery and have been taking one or more herbs, it would be wise to mention it to your anesthesiologist and surgeon and ask whether to stop the herb prior to the surgery (and also how long before surgery to stop taking it). Most herbs should be stopped at least one week before surgery. Only restart taking the herb when your health-care provider gives you the OK. Herbs that have anticoagulant or blood-thinning properties could cause bleeding if your surgical wounds haven't healed adequately.

■ If you are seriously ill, seek conventional medical care. Do not attempt to self-treat with herbal products.

Popular botanical remedies

Because of the laws regulating what may and may not be said on dietary supplement labels, it can be difficult to know what effect a product will really have. Here is what is known about some popular herbs and other botanicals:

Alfalfa

Tea, tablets, and capsules made of dried alfalfa (*Medicago sativa*) are reputed to have cholesterol-lowering and blood-glucose-lowering effects. However, scientific evidence supporting these claims is scanty. In addition, alfalfa plants contain phytoestrogens that may induce the growth of estrogen-dependent cancers, and alfalfa seeds may cause a relapse of lupus symptoms in people in remission from systemic lupus erythematosus. Fresh alfalfa sprouts have been linked to numerous cases of food poisoning, and people with diabetes are currently advised to avoid them for this reason.

Aloe

The thin, clear gel obtained from the inner portion of the leaves of the aloe vera plant *(Aloe barbadensis, Aloe vera)* is commonly used in skin and hair products for its alleged cleansing and moisturizing properties. Dabbing the gel from a freshly cut leaf is also a home remedy for minor burns and other minor wounds, a use supported by scientific studies. It may have a minimal blood-glucose-lowering effect when consumed, but there is not much evidence to support this use or other internal uses.

Aloe juice, or aloe latex, which is different from aloe gel and comes from a different part of the aloe leaf, has a potent laxative effect. In 2002, the FDA issued a rule stating that aloe juice was not recognized as safe for use in over-the-counter stimulant laxatives. Ingesting aloe juice is not recommended.

Artichokes

Whether eaten as a vegetable or taken as an extract in supplement form, artichokes *(Cynara scolymus)* are reputed to relieve indigestion and improve liver health. Scientific studies offer some support for these uses. Artichokes may also have a mild diuretic effect (meaning they increase urine output) and a blood-glucose-lowering effect.

Astragalus

Used mainly to protect the immune system, the root of the Astragalus *(Astragalus membranaceus)* may also protect the kidneys when used with the herb angelica, reduce fatigue in athletes, and protect against senility. It may have a positive effect on blood glucose control and act as a diuretic, but studies of these uses are limited.

Astragalus should not be taken by people who use immunosuppressant drugs because it may inhibit immune system suppression.

Banaba

A tea or extract made from the leaves of banaba *(Lagerstroemia speciosa)* has been used to lower blood glucose levels in people with Type 2 diabetes, as well as for weight loss. No significant side effects have been seen in short-term studies, but since few scientific studies have been done, the use of banaba is not recommended at this time.

Barley

Barley grain *(Hordeum vulgare)* is most commonly eaten as a food. In addition to the basic nutrition it provides, barley porridge may soothe a sore throat and help treat diarrhea. Barley is also a good source of soluble fiber, which can help lower blood cholesterol and possibly blood glucose levels if eaten in adequate amounts. Barley is also use as a poultice for skin ailments and as a facial mask.

Barley grass, which is grass harvested before the grain develops, is sold as a supplement, often with claims of numerous health benefits. Although barley grass is unlikely to cause any harm, it does not appear to live up to supplement makers' claims.

Bilberry

The fruits of the bilberry *(Vaccinium myrtillus)* are a rich source of antioxidants (compounds that may decrease the risk of heart disease, cancer, and other chronic diseases) and may improve blood circulation. They have been suggested as a treatment for diabetic retinopathy (eye disease), but so far only small studies have been done on this use. The dried berries, or a tea made from them, have traditionally been used in Europe as a treatment for diarrhea. A decoction of the dried fruit may also be used as a mouthwash or a gargle for inflammation in the mouth or throat. While generally safe, bilberry fruits or products made from them could theoretically interact with anticoagulant medicines such as aspirin or warfarin, potentially causing increased bleeding.

Less is known about the effects and the safety of the leaves of the bilberry. In animals, extracts from the leaf decreased blood glucose and blood triglyceride levels. However, chronic consumption of bilberry leaf tea or capsules is not recommended, because it can be toxic.

Bitter melon

Also called bitter gourd, bitter cucumber, balsam pear, karela, and charantin, bitter melon *(Momordica charantia)* is the most widely used traditional remedy for diabetes. It is commonly used in Asia, especially in India, and in Africa. Bitter melon is frequently eaten as a vegetable and looks like a misshapen, bumpy cucumber. As a treatment for diabetes, typically the juice or an extract of the unripe fruit is used. Dried or powdered forms of bitter melon are not believed to have the same activity. It is believed that bitter melon acts on both the pancreas and on nonpancreatic cells, such as muscle cells. Theoretically, consuming bitter melon while taking blood-glucose-lowering drugs could raise the risk of developing hypoglycemia (low blood glucose).

Black cohosh

The root and rhizome of black cohosh *(Actaea racemosa, Cimicifuga racemosa)* has become popular for treating symptoms of menopause, such as hot flashes, night sweats, mood swings, and vaginal dryness. It is also sometimes used to treat symptoms of premenstrual syndrome and pain associated with menstruation. So far, study results have been mixed on the effects of black cohosh on menopausal symptoms, but some have shown promise. It is not known how black cohosh works or whether it has an estrogenic (estrogen-like) effect, which could be a concern for women with a history of or a high risk for certain types of cancer. All women are advised to consult their physician before using it. Black cohosh can cause headache and stomach discomfort. It is not known to interact with any prescription

Finding Information on Herbs

These books offer information on hundreds of herbs and other dietary supplements, including their traditional uses and what modern scientific research has learned about their effects in the body.

THE AMERICAN PHARMACEUTICAL ASSOCIATION PRACTICAL GUIDE TO NATURAL MEDICINES
Andrea Peirce
William Morrow and Company, Inc.
New York, 1999

HERBAL MEDICINE
Expanded Commission E Monographs
Mark Blumenthal, Alicia Goldberg, Josef Brinckmann, Eds.
Integrative Medicine Communications
Newton, Massachusetts, 2000

PDR FOR HERBAL MEDICINES
Thomson Healthcare
Montvale, New Jersey, 2004

TYLER'S HERBS OF CHOICE
The Therapeutic Use of Phytomedicinals
James E. Robbers, Ph.D., and Varro E. Tyler, Ph.D. Sc.D.
The Haworth Herbal Press
New York, 1999

TYLER'S HONEST HERBAL
A Sensible Guide to the Use of Herbs and Related Remedies
Steven Foster, Varro E. Tyler, Ph.D.
The Haworth Herbal Press
New York, 1999

drugs, but this has not been studied extensively; it is thought to possibly interact with some drugs used to treat cancer.

Black cohosh should not be confused with blue cohosh *(Caulophyllum thalictroides)*, a plant that may have harmful side effects.

Boneset

The dried leaves and flowers of boneset *(Eupatorium perfoliatum)* were traditionally prepared as a tea to relieve the aches and pains of colds and flu, bring down fever, and treat loss of appetite and indigestion. The bitter taste of the tea can cause vomiting, particularly when served hot. Little is known about the long-term safety of boneset.

Buchu

Traditionally, buchu *(Barosma betulina, Barosma serratifolia, Barosma crenulata),* a plant native to South Africa, was used to treat urinary tract problems. It has also been used as a diuretic to treat high blood pressure and congestive heart failure as well as topically, to treat bruises. While buchu appears to be generally safe and is used in some commercial teas, it has not been shown to be particularly effective. However, because any herbal diuretic can irritate the kidneys, it is not recommended for people with kidney problems.

Burdock

The dried, ground roots of burdock *(Arctium lappa, Arctium minus)* have been promoted over the years as a diuretic, to stimulate hair growth, and as a treatment for skin problems such as psoriasis and eczema. None of these uses has been substantiated. In animals, the roots and leaves of burdock have shown some blood-glucose-lowering effects, but this has not been demonstrated in humans. Because burdock tends to grow in the same areas as belladonna (a poisonous plant), and the roots look very similar, the risk of contamination of burdock supplements is believed to be high. Fresh burdock root is also safely eaten as a vegetable and is high in fiber and nutrients. Some people also eat the young leaves and flower stalks.

Capsicum

Better known as red pepper, cayenne pepper, or chili pepper, the active ingredient in capsicum *(Capsicum frutescens, Capsicum annuum),* called capsaicin, is used in commercial, over-the-counter skin creams and ointments to treat painful neuropathy. While initial use may increase pain sensation, repeated application depletes the nerve fibers of the neurotransmitter substance P, leading to insensitivity to pain. Such creams or ointments must be applied four or five times daily for at least four weeks. Users must be sure to wash their hands after each application (or wear gloves to apply it) and not touch their eyes or mucous membranes with the cream.

Capsicum is also sometimes recommended to treat various gastrointestinal conditions, such as intestinal gas or diarrhea. However, because it can cause stomach irritation, caution is needed. Its utility in lowering blood cholesterol or decreasing the tendency of blood to clot has not been proven. Ingesting purified capsaicin is not recommended because of its potential to interact with a variety of prescription drugs. As a food flavoring, however, capsicum is considered safe.

Chamomile, German

In the United States, the flowers of chamomile *(Matricaria recutita)* are most often used to make tea, which is drunk for relaxation or to relieve heartburn or indigestion. It is also believed to have anti-inflammatory properties and is used in many commercial skin-care products as well as mouthwashes. Both internal and external uses of chamomile are believed to be safe. However, chamomile can cause allergic reactions in people who are allergic to ragweed, asters, chrysanthemums and should be avoided.

Cinnamon

Perhaps most familiar as a spice, cinnamon *(Cinnamomum verum, Cinnamomum cassia)* has been long used to treat loss of appetite, upset stomach, and intestinal gas. It is also commonly found as an ingredient in cough and cold remedies. More recently, studies have suggested that regular consumption of cinnamon can lower blood glucose levels in some people with diabetes, at least in the short term. Those who wish to try cinnamon as an aid to lowering blood glucose are advised to sprinkle moderate amounts of ground cinnamon—between ¼ to 2 teaspoons a day—on food and to monitor their blood glucose levels to assess its effect. Larger doses of ground cinnamon are not recommended: They can cause a fast heartbeat and accelerated breathing, followed by sedation. Consuming cinnamon oil is similarly not recommended because of its potential side effects, nor is putting the oil on your skin, where it can cause redness and burning.

Cranberry

A long-time home remedy for urinary tract infections, cranberry *(Vaccinium macrocarpon)* has been found to contain a substance that makes it difficult for bacteria to adhere to the bladder wall, which in turn makes it more difficult for the bacteria to grow. Some people drink cranberry juice daily to prevent urinary tract infections, while others drink larger amounts to treat them when necessary. Since most cranberry juices contain large amounts of sugar, artificially sweetened juice or capsules containing dried cranberry powder may be better choices for people with diabetes who wish to consume a cranberry product. It is also recommended that you see your doctor if you think you may have a urinary tract infection.

Dandelion

The roots and leaves of dandelion *(Taraxacum officinale)* have a long history of use in folk medicine in many parts of the world. Extracts of the leaves may have mild diuretic effects, while extracts of the root have mild laxative effects. Many other medicinal claims have been made for dandelion, particularly for stomach, liver, and kidney disorders, but

few clinical studies have investigated these uses. Some animal studies have suggested a moderate blood-glucose-lowering effect. Supplements containing dandelion roots or leaves should not be taken by anyone with bile duct obstruction, bowel obstruction, or gallstones.

Dandelion is also enjoyed as a food. The young, tender leaves can be eaten in salad, the more mature leaves steamed or sautéed, and the roots cooked and eaten as a vegetable. The roots are also sometimes roasted and used to make a coffee-like beverage.

Echinacea

Known to gardeners as purple coneflower, echinacea *(Echinacea purpurea, Echinacea angustifolia, Echinacea pallida)* has gotten a lot of attention in recent years as a treatment for the common cold. Some research suggests that if initiated within 24 hours of the onset of a cold, echinacea can decrease the duration of the cold but not the severity of symptoms. However, constantly taking echinacea has not been shown to prevent colds. In fact, it may be most effective when used sparingly. Current standard recommendations are not to take echinacea for longer than six to eight weeks at a time. It is unclear what sort of preparation of echinacea is most effective.

Because echinacea appears to stimulate the immune system, people with autoimmune diseases and people taking immunosuppressant drugs are advised not to take it. In addition, people with multiple sclerosis, tuberculosis, HIV, and AIDS are advised not to consume echinacea.

Elder

The flowers and fruits ("berries") of the elder plant *(Sambucus nigra)* are used to treat colds, flu, and fever. They may also have a diuretic, laxative, and anti-inflammatory effect. Elder flowers have traditionally been used in the treatment of diabetes, but few scientific studies have examined that use. While the flowers and fruits of the elder plant are safe (although the raw fruits may cause nausea and vomiting), the leaves and stems are toxic and should not be consumed.

Eucalyptus

The oil of the eucalyptus (*Eucalyptus globulus*) has both antiseptic and antibacterial qualities. It is used in many commercial products such as mouth rinses, cough syrups and lozenges, and inhalation vapors or topical ointments. Animal studies have shown eucalyptus oil to have a blood-glucose-lowering effect. However, caution is necessary when using dietary supplements or aromatherapy products containing eucalyptus oil. Even small amounts of oil taken by mouth have resulted in severe and deadly reactions. In addition, eucalyptus can enhance the sedating effects of drugs and other herbs, and it may weaken the effects of some prescription drugs taken simultaneously. Eucalyptus products should be kept out of the reach of children, and supplements should not be used by people with severe liver disease or inflammatory diseases of the gastrointestinal tract or bile ducts.

Herbal preparations made from the leaves of the eucalyptus plant are also sometimes used to treat respiratory tract ailments. Precautions regarding the leaves are similar to those for the oil.

Evening primrose oil

The oil derived from the seeds of the evening primrose plant (*Oenothera biennis*) contains about 9% gamma-linoleic acid, an essential fatty acid (one that is necessary for normal function). Other foods contain small amounts of gamma-linoleic acid, and the body produces some on its own from a number of dietary fats, but evening primrose oil is a concentrated source. Some studies have suggested that evening primrose oil may have a role in treating such diverse conditions as premenstrual syndrome, arthritis, multiple sclerosis, eczema, and painful neuropathy. However, more research needs to be done to confirm or refute the results of these studies and to establish therapeutic doses. Side effects from evening primrose oil may include headache and gastrointestinal symptoms. It can also precipitate seizures in people taking phenothiazines, a class of drugs used to treat schizophrenia and other mental disorders.

Fenugreek

Derived from the dried seeds of the plant, fenugreek (*Trigonella foenum-graecum*) has traditionally been used for numerous purposes, including as a laxative and treatment for gastrointestinal complaints and upper respiratory problems. Both the seeds and a defatted powder made from the seeds have been used as a treatment for diabetes. Fenugreek is one of the better researched botanical treatments for diabetes, with both human and animal studies suggesting it has blood-glucose-lowering activity. There is also research suggesting that fenugreek may improve blood cholesterol and triglyceride levels. Fenugreek seeds are very high in fiber, and it is believed that at least part of fenugreek's effects are achieved because the fiber slows the absorption of dietary carbohydrate.

Common side effects seen with high doses of fenugreek include diarrhea and upset stomach. It has also been reported that it may decrease blood coagulation, so people using anticoagulant medicines ("blood thinners") or aspirin should use fenugreek only under the supervision of their doctor. Because of its high fiber content, it may also alter absorption and effectiveness of other medicines taken at the same time. Fenugreek supplements should therefore not be taken at the same time as other medicines.

Feverfew

The leaves and extracts of the leaves of feverfew (*Tanacetum parathenium*) are most commonly used to prevent and treat migraine headaches. A few studies have found that feverfew is safe for this use, although its effectiveness has yet to be conclusively demonstrated. Taking feverfew may also reduce the painful symptoms of arthritis, but again, evidence for this use is inconclusive. Because chewing fresh feverfew leaves and drinking tea made from the leaves have been reported to cause mouth ulcers, capsules or tablets may be a better choice for those who wish to try it. People who are allergic to ragweed, chrysanthemums, or marigolds may also be sensitive to feverfew. Feverfew should not be used by people taking aspirin or anticoagulants ("blood thinners").

Fo-ti

Also called he-shou-wu, fo-ti (*Polygonum multiflorum*) is the root of a plant native to Asia. It is used as a folk remedy in Chinese medicine and appears to have a laxative effect. While Chinese medicine distinguishes between the effects of "raw" and "cured" fo-ti, Western studies usually have not, and when purchasing fo-ti in the United States, it is often impossible to tell which type it is. Fo-ti has been recommended as a treatment for diabetes, heart disease, and tumors, but there is no conclusive evidence for any of these uses.

Garlic

One of the top-selling herbal supplements in the United States, garlic (*Allium sativum*) is best known for its potential protective effects against cardiovascular disease. It has been claimed that garlic can decrease blood cholesterol levels, decrease high blood pressure, and decrease the likelihood of blood clots forming. Studies suggest that it may indeed have these properties, at least to a modest extent. Garlic may also have a mild blood-glucose-lowering effect. However, fairly large doses of tablets, capsules, or fresh garlic are needed for therapeutic effects. Topically, garlic may have an antifungal effect, but it is also known to cause skin irritation.

Garlic appears to be generally safe when taken as a supplement. Common side effects include mild stomach discomfort and an unusual body odor, although deodorized garlic tablets, which should not cause a body odor, are available. However, because of garlic's possible ability to decrease blood clotting, it may increase the risk of bleeding in people who take aspirin or anticoagulant medicines. People who take such drugs, therefore, should consult a health-care professional before taking garlic supplements. Use of garlic should be discontinued at least seven days before surgery or dental procedures that may cause bleeding. Garlic may also reduce the effectiveness of certain immunosuppressant drugs and drugs used to treat HIV and AIDS. For those who wish to try garlic as a supplement (and for whom it is safe), either fresh garlic cloves or enteric-coated dry garlic preparations appear to be most effective.

Ginger

Derived from the rhizome of the plant, ginger (*Zingiber officinale*) is most commonly used to prevent or treat nausea and other gastrointestinal complaints. Some say that it prevents motion sickness when taken half an hour before a trip. It is also commonly used as a tea to soothe sore throats and other cold symptoms. As a food, ginger is on the FDA's GRAS (generally regarded as safe) list. Possible side effects of taking ginger as a supplement include heartburn, and very large doses may cause heart arrhythmias and central nervous system depression. Ginger supplements should not be taken by people taking anticoagulants. It may also enhance the effects of blood-pressure-lowering and blood-glucose-lowering drugs. People with gallstones should consult a physician before taking ginger.

Ginkgo

The concentrated leaf extract of ginkgo (*Ginkgo biloba*) appears to have numerous beneficial effects on the circulatory system.

It is used to treat peripheral vascular disease, which can cause intermittent claudication, or leg cramping during walking. It is also used for ailments related to reduced cerebral blood flow, such as dizziness, tinnitus, and problems with memory and concentration. It may be of some use for improving functioning in people who have Alzheimer disease. Ginkgo has also been studied for the treatment of sexual dysfunction in men and women and may be effective in the treatment of some cases of erectile dysfunction.

Only standardized ginkgo products should be used. Possible side effects of taking gingko include stomach upset, diarrhea, flatulence, headache, dizziness, and palpitations. Since ginkgo reduces the rate at which blood clots, people taking aspirin or anticoagulants should not also take products containing gingko. Ginkgo should generally be stopped prior to surgical or dental procedures. Ginkgo may theoretically affect insulin secretion and blood glucose levels, so regular monitoring should be done when taking ginkgo.

Ginseng

The root of the ginseng plant *(Panax ginseng, Panax quinquefolius)* has long been used to bolster mood, immunity, and ability to deal with stress. It is also believed by some to be an aphrodisiac. Several human studies have reported that ginseng may lower blood glucose levels in people with Type 2 diabetes. It may also increase the blood-glucose-lowering effect of insulin and drugs in the sulfonylurea class (glyburide, glipizide, and glimepiride). However, more and larger studies are needed to establish its possible therapeutic doses and long-term safety and effectiveness as a treatment for diabetes. Ginseng is generally well-tolerated, but long-term use has been associated with skin rash, diarrhea, sore throat, increased blood pressure, excitability, anxiety, depression, and insomnia. It may also have some mild, estrogen-like properties, possibly caus-

ing breast tenderness, loss of menstrual periods, and postmenopausal vaginal bleeding. And it may increase the risk of bleeding when taken with aspirin or anticoagulants.

The term "ginseng" is also used for Siberian ginseng *(Eleutherococcus senticosus),* a plant native to Siberia, Korea, and some parts of China. In spite of the name, Siberian ginseng is not believed to have the same effects as plants of the *Panax* genus.

Glucosamine

Not a botanical product, glucosamine is a natural substance found in and around the cells of cartilage. Glucosamine supplements are often taken by people with osteoarthritis along with chondroitin (also a natural substance found in and around cartilage cells) for pain relief. Some researchers believe these substance may aid in the repair and maintenance of the cartilage cells that line the joints. Some also believe that glucosamine inhibits inflammation and stimulates new cartilage cell growth, while chondroitin enhances the cartilage's strength and resilience.

Studies suggest that these substances do have a painkilling effect for some people with osteoarthritis. A three-month trial should establish whether they have any beneficial effects for an individual. However, it's worth keeping both a pain diary and careful blood glucose monitoring records if trying glucosamine. It has been shown to raise blood glucose levels in some people with diabetes. In addition, people with shellfish allergies should avoid glucosamine and chondroitin supplements because they are often made from crustacean shells.

Goldenseal

A popular ingredient often promoted along with echinacea to treat upper respiratory infections, goldenseal *(Hydrastis canadensis)* has not been found effective for any medicinal uses. In addition, the myth that taking goldenseal prevents detection of illegal drugs in urine is untrue. Public demand for

Plants With Blood-Glucose-Lowering Potential

Some 400 plant products have been reported to have blood-glucose-lowering effects, including those listed here. However, in most cases, not enough research has been done to establish that these plants are consistently effective at lowering blood glucose or safe at doses required to lower blood glucose.

COMMON NAME	BOTANICAL NAME
Bitter melon (also known as balsam pear)	Momordica charantia
Aloe	Aloe vera, Aloe barbadensis
Barley	Hordeum vulgare
Burdock	Arctium lappa
Cashew	Anacardium occidentale
Churchsteeples	Agrimonia eupatoria
Cinnamon	Cinnamomum verum
Dandelion	Taraxacum officinale
Common maidenhair	Adiantum capillus-veneris
Corn	Zea mays
Cumin	Cuminum cyminum
Damiana	Turnera diffusa
Devilsclub	Oplopanax horridus
Devil's tongue	Amorphophallus konjac
Eucalyptus (also known as Tasmanian bluegum)	Eucalyptus globulus
Fenugreek	Trigonella foenum-graecum
Fo-ti (tuber fleeceflower)	Polygonum multiflorum
French plaintain	Musa paradisiaca
Gale of the wind	Phyllanthus niruri
Garden cucumber	Cucumis sativus
Garlic	Allium sativum
Ginseng, American	Panax quinqeufolius
Ginseng, Chinese	Panax ginseng
Guar	Cyamopsis tetragonoloba
Gymnema (also called miracle fruit)	Gymnema sylvestre
Hairy beggarticks	Bidens pilosa
Holy basil	Ocimum tenuiflorum
Horse chestnut	Aesculus hippocastanum

COMMON NAME	BOTANICAL NAME
Indian banyan	Ficus benghalensis
Ivy gourd	Coccinia grandis
Java plum	Syzygium cumini
Juniper	Juniperus communis
Kidney bean	Phaseolus vulgaris
Licorice weed	Scoparia dulcis
Madagascar periwinkle	Catharanthus roseus
Maitake mushroom	Grifola frondosa
Matrimony vine	Lycium barbarum
Nalta jute	Corchorus olitorius
Olive	Olea europaea
Onion	Allium cepa
Pride of India	Lagerstroemia speciosa
Professor-weed	Galega officinalis
Psyllium (also known as sand plantain)	Plantago psyllium
Purple loosestrife	Lythrum salicaria
Reishi mushroom	Ganoderma lucidum
Saltbush	Atriplex halimus
Siberian ginseng	Eleutherococcus senticosus
Spinach	Spinacia oleracea
St. John's bread	Ceratonia siliqua
Staghorn sumac	Rhus typhina
Trumpet tree	Cecropia obtusifolia
Virginia water horehound	Lycopus virginicus
Wheat	Triticum sativum
White Egyptian lotus	Nymphaea lotus
White lupine	Lupinus albus
White mulberry	Morus alba
Whortleberry	Vaccinium myrtillus
Yellow trumpetbush	Tecoma stans

goldenseal has been so high in recent years, though, that the plant is in short supply, raising the possibility that other, similar herbs may be substituted for goldenseal in dietary supplements.

Gosha-jinki-gan

A blend of 10 herbs used in traditional Chinese medicine, gosha-jinki-gan has been tested in mice and rats for its possible uses as a treatment for diabetes. Studies suggest that it increases blood flow to the extremities, may decrease insulin resistance, and may be useful in the treatment of painful diabetic neuropathy. Time will tell whether this blend catches on as a complementary diabetes treatment in the West.

Grape seed extract

Best known for its antioxidant properties, grape seed extract (Vitis vinifera) may lower blood pressure, prevent atherosclerosis, and improve cholesterol levels. It may also help prevent varicose veins and fight some forms of cancer. Small studies suggest that grape seed extract may help slow retinopathy, but more research is needed. Grape seed extract is associated with few side effects, although it may enhance the effects of anticoagulants and lead to increased bruising or bleeding.

Green tea

Made from the same plant as black tea, green tea (Camellia sinensis) is produced by lightly steaming the freshly cut tea leaves. All tea contains antioxidants called polyphenols. Because green tea is less processed than black or oolong tea, it is believed to contain more polyphenols. The benefits of regularly drinking green tea may include a lower risk of heart disease, lower blood glucose levels, better dental health, and stronger bones. Some studies suggest that people who drink tea or take supplements containing green tea extract burn more calories, but it is unclear that consuming tea products leads to significant weight loss.

The role of green tea consumption in the prevention of various types of cancer has also been studied, sometimes with positive results. However, in 2005, the FDA, in evaluating a petition for a qualified health claim for green tea, concluded that it is highly unlikely that green tea prevents either breast or prostate cancer and that there is no evidence that it reduces the risk of gastric, lung, colorectal, esophageal, pancreatic, ovarian, and combined cancers.

Green tea contains caffeine, so it can cause jitteriness or sleeplessness, just like other sources of caffeine. It may also enhance the effects of other herbal products or drugs with a stimulant effect.

Guar gum

A type of viscous fiber derived from the guar bean (Cyamopsis tetragonoloba), guar gum has been shown to lower blood cholesterol, blood pressure, and, in people with diabetes, postmeal blood glucose levels and fasting blood glucose levels. Guar gum is used in small amounts in commercial food products, cosmetics, and pharmaceuticals and is sold as a fiber supplement. However, it is banned in over-the-counter weight control products because of numerous cases of esophageal, gastric, and intestinal obstruction.

Possible side effects of taking guar gum supplements include abdominal cramping, bloating, gas, and diarrhea. If taken without adequate fluids, it can cause esophageal, gastric, and intestinal obstruction. It should not be used by people with gastrointestinal problems. Guar gum may slow the absorption of some drugs, including some used to treat Type 2 diabetes, if taken at the same time. It may also reduce absorption of some carotenoids when taken with a meal.

Gymnema

A traditional diabetes treatment in India, gymnema (Gymnema sylvestre) is believed to act by improving the function of the pancreatic beta cells (the cells in the body that produce insulin). Gymnema may also decrease glucose absorption from food and improve the ability of the body to use glucose for energy. In some studies it has also been shown to reduce cholesterol levels. Gymnema is also known as gurmar, which means "sugar destroyer," because chewing the leaf of the plant decreases the sensitivity of taste buds to sweet tastes. In some studies, this has led to a short-term decrease in food consumption. While gymnema has no known toxic side effects, most experts believe that more studies are needed before it can be widely recommended as a complementary treatment for diabetes.

Hawthorn

The dried leaves, berries, and blossoms of hawthorn *(Crataegus laevigata, Crataegus oxycantha, and Crataegus monogyna)* are sometimes used for treating early stages of congestive heart failure and minor heart arrhythmias. It lowers blood pressure and may also be useful in the treatment of angina, although not for acute attacks since the effects of the herb work slowly. However, self-treatment of serious heart problems, such as these, is not recommended, and finding supplements containing standardized doses may be difficult. Hawthorn may also interact with prescription drugs taken for heart conditions.

Holy basil

An herb native to India, where it is called tulsi, holy basil *(Ocimum sanctum)* has historically been used for many medical conditions, including heart problems, asthma, bronchitis, and arthritis. Evidence from animal studies suggests that it may help control blood glucose levels and blood cholesterol levels. So far, its use has no known side effects.

Hoodia

A botanical product widely promoted as an appetite suppressant, hoodia *(Hoodia gordinii)* is a cactus extract said to keep South African tribesmen from feeling hungry during long hunts. While a compound isolated from hoodia reduced food intake in rats, similar effects have not been seen in humans. Very few studies have been done on hoodia, and the FDA has warned manufacturers and distributors of hoodia products against making unsubstantiated and misleading claims about weight loss.

Horsetail

In Europe, horsetail *(Equisetum arvense)* is used as a diuretic, for kidney stones, and for urinary tract infections. It is occasionally used for osteoporosis and wound healing. However, there are few scientific studies to support these uses. Horsetail appears safe when used in moderate amounts, but large amounts can have toxic effects. Horsetail contains an ingredient that destroys thiamine (vitamin B_1), which could lead to deficiency with long-term use. People with kidney disorders or edema due to heart problems should avoid horsetail.

Licorice

The roots and rhizomes of the licorice plant *(Glycyrrhiza glabra, Glycyrrhiza uralensis)* are used extensively in traditional Chinese medicine and also in some European countries. Licorice appears to have some effectiveness as a cough remedy, for treating stomach ulcers, and as an anti-inflammatory. However, the active ingredient in licorice, glycyrrhizin, has well-known toxic effects, including headache, sodium and water retention, excessive excretion of potassium, high blood pressure, heart failure, and cardiac arrest. Deglycyrrhizinated licorice products should not produce these side effects, but they may have no therapeutic benefits either. In the United States, licorice is used mostly to flavor tobacco products and as an ingredient in some pharmaceutical products. Licorice candy sold in the United States is usually flavored with anise oil. Anyone should use caution when consuming licorice, and people with high blood pressure, heart disease, or kidney or liver disease should avoid it.

Milk thistle

The fruit of the milk thistle (*Silybum marianum*), also called silymarin, has been traditionally used for liver complaints or to protect the liver from toxins. It is used in Germany as a supportive treatment for inflammatory liver conditions and cirrhosis. Possible side effects include gastrointestinal problems such as upset stomach or diarrhea and allergic reactions in people allergic to ragweed. The leaves of the milk thistle plant have no known therapeutic effects.

Nettle

An extract of the root of the nettle plant (*Urtica dioica*) is used to treat benign prostatic hypertrophy (noncancerous, enlarged prostate), while the leaves are known to have a diuretic effect. Some evidence suggests that taking nettle leaf may reduce hay fever symptoms. In folk medicine, nettle was used to treat arthritis or to stimulate hair growth on the scalp, but no scientific evidence supports these uses. While nettle tea has been tested for its blood-glucose-lowering potential, it is not recommended for people with diabetes; studies suggest that it may raise, not lower, blood glucose levels. In addition to being used as an herbal remedy, the tops of young nettle plants are sometimes cooked and eaten for food; they provide about the same amounts of beta-carotene and vitamin C as other green, leafy vegetables.

Possible side effects of consuming nettle include stomach upset, sweating, and skin irritation. Indeed, the leaves and stalk of the plant, which is also known as stinging nettle, are known for their painful sting when touched. Because it acts as a diuretic, nettle should not be taken by people with kidney problems, and it is not an effective treatment for edema caused by congestive heart failure.

Nopal

The stem or leaf of nopal cactus (*Opuntia streptacantha*) is a traditional Mexican treatment for Type 2 diabetes. Usually, cooked or fresh nopal is used for this purpose, but extracts from the fresh plant have been used as well. In studies where about 500 grams of fresh or cooked nopal were eaten before or with a meal, decreases in blood glucose, cholesterol, and triglycerides were seen. It is thought that the high fiber content of nopal may be at least partly responsible for these effects. There are no known side effects of eating nopal, other than those you would expect from increasing your fiber intake.

Passionflower

The aerial parts of the passionflower (*Passiflora incarnata*) are popularly used in Europe as a sedative, tranquilizer, or treatment for insomnia. However, its effectiveness is unproven, and its mechanism of action unknown. The FDA does not recognize passionflower as safe and has prohibited its use in over-the-counter sleep aids, although there are few reports of serious side effects.

Peppermint

Peppermint (*Mentha x piperita*) and its active ingredient, menthol, are widely used in over-the-counter cold remedies, cough and throat lozenges, topical nasal decongestants, ointments, and other products. Tea made from peppermint leaf is prized for its stomach-settling properties. However, the FDA does not allow peppermint oil to be used as an ingredient in over-the-counter digestive aids, saying it is ineffective for this purpose. As a dietary supplement, peppermint oil has shown some effectiveness for the treatment of heartburn and irritable bowel syndrome, but caution is in order when consuming peppermint oil as a dietary supplement. Consuming too much can cause heartburn and irritate the skin. Even a little can aggravate symptoms of hiatal hernia. It should not be used at all by infants and small children. Pure menthol should never be ingested by anyone; it is toxic and can be fatal.

Psyllium

The seeds or seed husks of psyllium *(Plantago ovata, Plantago isphagula)* are high in soluble fiber and are commonly used in bulk laxatives as well as in some breakfast cereals. Adequate consumption of soluble fiber can not only help prevent constipation but also lower blood cholesterol levels. It is important to consume adequate amounts of fluid when taking high-fiber products such as psyllium. Psyllium supplements should not be taken by people with bowel obstructions. People with delayed stomach emptying should consult their physician before increasing their fiber intake. While side effects are generally mild, severe allergic reactions to psyllium have occurred, mostly in pharmaceutical workers repeatedly exposed to large quantities of psyllium.

Raspberry

Raspberry leaves *(Rubus idaeus* and *Rubus strigosus)* have a long history of use for the treatment of diarrhea, menstrual pain, and numerous complaints related to pregnancy. They have also been used to treat diabetes. However, no reliable studies support any of these uses. Raspberry may have some use as a mouthwash or gargle, and it is believed to be generally safe.

St. John's wort

The leaves and flowering tops of St. John's wort *(Hypericum perforatum)* have shown promise in studies as a treatment for mild to moderate depression. The evidence does not support using it for severe depression. Because St. John's wort interacts with numerous prescription drugs, herbs, and supplements, people are advised to consult a physician or pharmacist before taking it. (It's a good idea to see a physician anyway, if you think you're depressed, for proper diagnosis and treatment.)

St. John's wort should generally not be taken along with prescription antidepressants. It may take four or more weeks of taking St. John's wort to get to "therapeutic" levels. Side effects include fatigue, dizziness, mild stomach upset. It can also cause photosensitivity (sensitivity to light), causing a skin rash, so it is recommended that people avoid direct sunlight after taking St. John's wort. Internal use of St. John's wort should be discontinued one week before surgery. St. John's wort is also used externally as an ointment to treat wounds and skin infections, a use also supported by research.

Saw palmetto

The berries of saw palmetto *(Serenoa repens)* are used primarily to relieve symptoms associated with benign prostatic hypertrophy, such as difficulty initiating urination and frequent nighttime urination. Although saw palmetto is widely used in some European countries, studies are mixed on its effectiveness. However, few serious side effects are associated with its use; the most common complaints are gastrointestinal upset. Nonetheless, because the symptoms of benign prostatic hypertrophy are similar to those of other prostate and urinary tract disorders, it is advisable to see a doctor for a diagnosis of the problem before self-prescribing saw palmetto.

Shiitake mushroom

Generally eaten as a food rather than taken for medicinal purposes, shiitake mushrooms *(Lentinula edodes)* may nonetheless have health benefits beyond basic nutrition. They may help to prevent cancer, and they may have a blood-cholesterol-lowering effect. Maitake mushrooms *(Grifola frondosa)* may have similar effects. In addition, extracts of maitake mushrooms are reported to lower blood glucose levels in animals. Since few studies have been done in humans, however, consuming these mushrooms as foods, not supplements, is currently recommended.

Soy

Both foods and supplements made from soy *(Glycine max)* have been studied for their effects on cholesterol, hot flashes associated with menopause, prevention of breast and other forms of cancer, treatment of cancer, osteoporosis, and prevention of cardiovascular disease. Many of soy's benefits are believed to come from its isoflavones (including genistein and daidzein), compounds believed to have estrogen-like effects in the body and for this reason often called phytoestrogens. For the most part, scientific evidence is mixed on soy's medicinal uses. In addition, there is concern that soy could encourage the growth of estrogen-dependent cancers or interfere with drugs used to treat such cancers. However, the moderate intake of soy foods, such as soy milk, tofu, and soy "burgers," is believed to be safe and nutritious for most people. Soy is a vegetarian source of "complete" protein that contains no cholesterol and virtually no saturated fat.

Stevia

Derived from the leaves of a South American shrub, stevia *(Stevia rebaudiana)* has gained popularity in the United States for its sweet taste. In the amounts usually consumed, stevia has negligible calories and carbohydrate, so it does not raise blood glucose levels. However, because the FDA has not given it GRAS (generally recognized as safe) status, it can only be sold as a dietary supplement, not a sweetener. Nonetheless, when consumed in moderate amounts, it is believed to be safe. A few studies, most of them using lab animals and not humans, have examined stevia's potential use as a diabetes treatment. Research results have been mixed, but some suggest that stevia may have a blood-glucose-lowering effect.

Valerian

Derived from the root of the plant, valerian *(Valeriana officinalis* or *Valerianae radix)* is frequently used as a sedative to improve sleep. However, scientific studies have not shown it to be more effective than a placebo. It may have an additive effect when taken with barbiturates and benzodiazepines (drugs also used for insomnia), and it has been associated with liver toxicity when used long-term. Short-term side effects can include headache, morning drowsiness, and impaired alertness.

Dangerous botanicals

Any herb can be dangerous under certain circumstances—if taken in megadoses, for example, or by someone who is allergic to it. As herbal use has become more popular in the United States, however, some herbal products have been shown to be dangerous under any circumstances, and others should be used only under the supervision of a qualified herbal therapist. The following herbs and supplements should not be self-prescribed:

Akee

Unripe akee fruit *(Blighia sapida)* has a hypoglycemic (blood-glucose-lowering) effect, but it is toxic, as are akee seeds. Ingesting unripe akee fruit causes vomiting and sometimes death.

Chaparral

Leaves of the chapparal plant *(Larrea tridentata),* also known as creosote bush, were once thought to have anticancer effects but have been linked to cases of liver and kidney injury. The FDA removed chaparral from its GRAS (generally recognized as safe) list long before passage of the DSHEA. The agency issued another warning in 1992 regarding consumption of chaparral and one of its components called nordihydroguaiaretic acid (NDGA).

Coltsfoot

Traditionally used for coughs and bronchial congestion, the leaves, flowers, and roots of the coltsfoot plant *(Tussilago farfara)* have been shown to be toxic to the liver.

Comfrey

Traditionally used for wound healing, the leaves, roots, and rhizomes of comfrey *(Sym-*

phytum officinale) are known to be toxic to the liver when taken orally. In 2001, the FDA asked all manufacturers to remove products containing comfrey from the market.

Ephedra

Also called ma huang, ephedra *(Ephedra sinica, Ephedra equisetina)*, derived from the root and rhizome of the plant, was widely promoted in the United States as an aid to weight loss. However, it can increase heart rate, raise blood pressure, cause nausea and vomiting, and also cause insomnia and feelings of anxiety. Use of ephedra has also been linked to some deaths. The FDA banned dietary supplements containing ephedra in 2004, after it determined that ephedra posed an unreasonable risk to those who used it.

Germander

At one time a popular weight-loss remedy, germander *(Teucrium chamaedrys)* has been linked to numerous cases of hepatitis and shown conclusively in the laboratory to be toxic to the liver.

Kava

Derived from the rhizome or rootstock of the *Piper methysticum* plant, kava beverages have a long history of ritual use in various cultures of the Pacific Islands. In Europe and North American, kava supplements have been used mainly for anxiety, stress, and insomnia. However, kava is believed to cause liver toxicity. In fact, the British, French, and Swiss governments have requested that kava be removed from the market, and the Canadian government has warned consumers not to use kava-containing products.

Lobelia

Traditionally used to treat asthma and chronic bronchitis, the dried leaves and tops of the lobelia plant *(Lobelia inflata)* have more recently been used to help with smoking cessation. In large doses, it can cause vomiting, as well as difficulty breathing, rapid heart rate, low blood pressure, and even death.

Sassafras

The root bark of sassafras *(Sassafras officinalis)* has no medicinal properties but does contain safrole, a substance known to be carcinogenic. The FDA banned the use of sassafras volatile oil and safrole as food additives or flavors in 1960.

Ma huang

See ephedra.

Yohimbe

Derived from the bark of the West African *Pausinystalia yohimbe* Pierre tree, yohimbe has long had a reputation as an aphrodisiac and as a treatment for erectile dysfunction. It works by dilating blood vessels in the skin and mucous membranes. However, it also raises blood pressure, making it unsafe for some people. In addition, it acts similarly to a monoamine oxidase inhibitor (a type of drug used, rarely, to treat depression), which means it interacts with numerous foods and drugs. Serious side effects reported with its use include kidney failure, seizures, and death.

Knowledge about herbs and other botanical supplements continues to grow as scientific studies are done and adverse effects are reported to the FDA. If you self-prescribe herbs, it is important to stay up to date on reports of side effects. Regularly checking the Web site of the FDA, www.fda.gov, is one way to stay abreast of developments in this area.

Aromatherapy

Aromatherapy is the use of essential oils from plants for the purpose of healing the body, mind, and spirit. Essential oils are concentrated extracts taken from the roots, leaves, or blossoms of plants. The word "aroma" in aromatherapy suggests that this form of therapy involves mainly the scent of the oils, and indeed, odor is a big part of it.

The most popular use of aromatherapy today is probably just smelling essential oils for relaxation, stimulation, or a reduction in pain perception. However, essential oils may also be applied to the skin through massage or by adding a few drops of oil to bathwater. In these cases, the oils may have an effect on the body by being absorbed through the skin. Less commonly, essential oils are ingested. However, swallowing essential oils should not be done without the guidance of a knowledgeable healthcare provider. In addition, it's important to keep essential oils out of reach of children. They may smell good enough to taste, but many are toxic when ingested.

Proponents of aromatherapy believe that essential oils work both emotionally and physically. (Synthetic oils, while they may smell nice, are not believed to have the same physiological effects as essential oils.) Emotionally, they may make you feel better by evoking pleasant memories. Physically, they may help to relieve certain conditions by stimulating the immune, circulatory, or nervous systems. While there are no established uses for aromatherapy in the treatment of diabetes, anything that reduces stress can be of benefit for diabetes control. There has also been some research on the use of essential oils to accelerate wound healing and reduce skin infections.

When choosing an essential oil for the purpose of mood elevation or relaxation, what matters most is your personal response to the aroma—and using it in a safe manner, of course. Here are some popular essentials oils and medicinal properties they are commonly believed to have:

Clary sage

(*Salvia sclarea*) is a natural pain killer that is helpful in treating muscular aches and pains. It is also relaxing and can help with insomnia.

Eucalyptus

(*Eucalyptus globulus* or *Eucalyptus radiata*) is traditionally used to treat respiratory prob-lems, such as coughs and colds, by relieving congestion. It is also believed to boost the immune system and relieve muscle tension.

Geranium

(*Pelargonium graveolens*) can be both relaxing and uplifting; it may be an effective antidepressant. It is also sometimes used for skin care.

Jasmine

(*Jasminum officinalis*) is an effective antidepressant and may improve quality of sleep.

Lavender

(*Lavandula angustifolia*) is relaxing. It reduces anxiety and may improve sleep. It is also used for treating wounds and burns and for skin care.

Lemon

(*Citrus limon*) is uplifting yet relaxing. It may improve mood and increase mental alertness, and it's also used to treat wounds and infections as well as for house cleaning and deodorizing.

Peppermint

(*Mentha x piperita*) may be used to treat headaches, muscle aches, and digestive disorders such as slow digestion, indigestion, nausea, and flatulence.

Roman chamomile

(*Chamaemelum nobile* or *Anthemis nobilis*) is relaxing and can help with sleeplessness and anxiety. It's also used for relieving muscle aches and tension and for treating wounds and infection.

Rosemary

(*Rosmarinus officinalis*) is mentally stimulating and uplifting and may also stimulate the immune system and the digestive system. It is sometimes used to ease muscle aches and tension.

Tea tree

(*Melaleuca alternifolia*) is a natural antifungal that is used for treating infections such as athlete's foot and ringworm. It is also believed to help boost the immune system.

Ylang ylang

(Cananga odorata) is relaxing, can reduce muscle tension, and is a good antidepressant.

While many health and beauty aids are scented with these and other herbs, most aromatherapists contend that only pure, natural, unadulterated essential oils have true medicinal properties. Essential oils should be stored in a cool, dark place to prevent oxidation.

Methods of use

There are a number of safe ways to use essential oils at home, including the following:

On a handkerchief. Put 2–4 drops of an essential oil on a tissue or cloth handkerchief. Holding the tissue in your hand, bring it close to your nose and inhale deeply several times. Close your eyes to avoid irritation. Depending on the oil you use, this method can help keep nasal passages open or promote relaxation or sleep.

Massage. Mix 10–20 drops of an essential oil into 1 ounce of a base, or "carrier," oil, such as almond, olive, safflower, or sesame oil. Use the mixture to massage sore or tense muscles. Diluting essential oils in this way reduces the risk of their causing a skin irritation or allergic reaction. However, it's a good idea to try the oil on a small area first, before doing a whole-body massage, to make sure you don't have a reaction to it. In addition, keep the oil mixture away from your eyes, genitals, and any breaks in the skin.

Bathwater. Add 5–10 drops of an essential oil to a tub filled with warm water. Swish the water around a little to disperse the oil, then enjoy a relaxing bath. If you don't want a full bath, place 5–7 drops of essential oil in a basin of warm water and soak your hands or feet for 10–15 minutes.

Steam inhalation. Boil 2 cups of water, then pour the water into a sturdy bowl. Add 2–7 drops of an essential oil. Position your face about a foot from the bowl and inhale the scented vapors for several minutes. Close your eyes to avoid irritation. You may also drape a towel over your head to concentrate the vapors. Inhaling steam may relieve nasal or chest congestion.

Room freshening. Prepare a bowl of hot water as if for steam inhalation, but instead of inhaling it, simply place it in a room to allow the scent to fill the air. Since you won't be directly inhaling it, you can add up to 10 drops of essential oil.

Another option for room freshening is to put 10–15 drops of an essential oil in a 4-ounce spray bottle filled with water. Shake the bottle then spritz the air around you. Shake again before each use. (Avoid spraying oils onto light bulbs.)

A device called a diffuser can help to disperse oil into the air so the aroma is distributed throughout the room. Several types of diffusers are sold, including candles, clay pots, electric heaters, and heaters with fans. Another option is a nebulizer, a device that breaks down an essential oil into a fine spray before dispersing it into the air.

Compresses. Moist warm or cool compresses are sometimes used to relieve certain types of pain. Cool compresses can reduce pain, swelling, and bruising after an injury. Warm compresses may relieve menstrual cramps or may be used to bring boils to a head. To make a compress, add 5–7 drops of an essential oil to 2 cups of warm or cool water. Swish the water around to disburse the oil, then dip a small towel in the water. Wring it out and place on the body area to be treated. Allow compress to come to body temperature, then remove.

Gargling. Add 1–2 drops of tea tree, caraway, or fennel oil to 1 cup of water and mix well. (Alternatively, use 5 parts water to 1 part apple cider vinegar.) Use mixture to gargle, then spit out; do not swallow. Gargling can be useful for sore throats and canker sores.

Precautions

While most external aromatherapies are usually safe to self-administer, some precautions are in order:

■ People who are allergic to nuts should not use oils derived from nuts, such as almond or peanut oil.

■ Pregnant women should not use aromatherapy without the guidance of a knowledgeable practitioner. Some essential oils can be harmful to the fetus or induce miscarriage if taken internally and possibly if used externally. These include the essential oils of basil, thyme, clary sage, calamus, mugwort, pennyroyal, sage, rosemary, juniper, and wintergreen.

■ People with asthma should consult a knowledgeable practitioner before using essential oils. Certain aromatherapy oils can trigger bronchial spasms.

■ People with epilepsy should use caution when using aromatherapy. It's possible that oils that tend to have a stimulating effect, such as camphor, peppermint, and rosemary, may provoke more frequent seizures. On the other hand, the use of relaxing oils may reduce the frequency of seizures.

■ When using essential oils in any application, care must be taken not to inhale the actual oil. Doing so can lead to a type of pneumonia called lipid pneumonia.

■ It's possible to become sensitized to an oil after one or more uses. If an oil causes any skin irritation or other allergic-type reactions, even if it didn't on previous uses, stop using it.

■ Essential oils are highly volatile and flammable so they should never be used near an open flame. Anything used to clean up a spilled oil is also highly flammable.

While many people use essential oils on their own, some prefer to consult an aromatherapist for individualized guidance. However, there is no licensure for the practice of aromatherapy; anyone may call himself an aromatherapist. At this time, "certification" in aromatherapy simply means a person has completed some coursework in the subject. However, some licensed massage therapists, chiropractors, and other health-care providers have training in aromatherapy. If you'd like to explore aromatherapy in depth, making an appointment with one of these professionals is probably a good place to start.

Handle with care

Herbal remedies don't require a prescription for purchase, but they can have effects as powerful as drugs that do. Also like drugs, they can have serious side effects, but unlike drugs, they don't come with a package insert that lists common or possible side effects. Nor do herbs come with information on possible drug interactions, even though many of them can interact with prescription or over-the-counter drugs and other herbal supplements. Because it is still largely up to the user to research what is known about the safety and effectiveness of herbal remedies, they should be approached with care and caution.

Even when you've done your research on the uses, safety, and effectiveness of a dietary supplement, keep in mind that self-diagnosis and self-treatment are risky. If you think you have a medical problem serious enough to need treatment, see a health-care professional for a proper diagnosis. Most medical problems are more treatable when caught and treated early. Once you know what you're up against, ask your health-care provider whether herbal products could complement your other treatments.

Certain botanical remedies have been found to help control diabetes and its complications, and more will no doubt be discovered in the future. It is unlikely, however, that they will take the place of insulin in the treatment of Type 1 diabetes or be a substitute for diet and exercise in the treatment of Type 2 diabetes. But they may be valuable tools in the toolbox for achieving the best diabetes control possible.

12. BIOFIELD THERAPIES

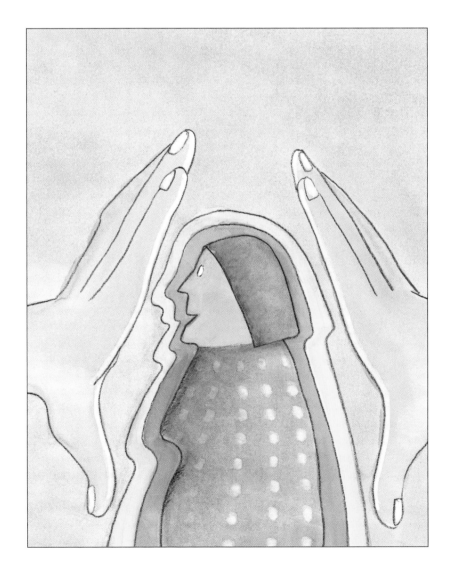

12.
BIOFIELD THERAPIES

Biofield therapies are based on the belief that energy fields exist in and around the human body. Some traditional healing methods such as acupuncture are based on this premise, and some newer ones such as therapeutic touch, healing touch, and polarity therapy are, as well. (There has been no scientific detection of such a human energy field, however.) Some biofield therapies use fine needles or light physical touch to affect a person's energy field. In others, practitioners do not touch the person at all but rather place their hands near the body and use hand motions or their own energy to "unblock" or "smooth" a person's energy field. The purpose of all biofield therapies is healing, whether physical, emotional, or spiritual.

While the use of biofield therapies does not necessarily depend on holding any particular spiritual beliefs, some have more of a spiritual flavor than others. For example, some practitioners call upon "higher powers" or "spirits" to guide them in their work. This practice goes against the belief systems of some people and can cause distress if they're not prepared for it. If you feel that this is a potential area of concern for you, find out as much as possible about the background and basic beliefs associated with a specific energy therapy before you start. In addition, check out your potential practitioner and ask questions about his beliefs, training, and practices to avoid conflicts.

Therapeutic touch

Therapeutic touch is a derivative of "laying on of hands" healing. Its underlying premise is that healing is promoted when the human energy field is in balance, while disease is manifested when this energy is out of balance. In spite of the name, therapeutic touch generally involves no direct physical touch between practitioner and recipient. Those trained in this method believe that by passing their hands in the air several inches above a person's body, they can feel energy imbalances, often as a sensation of heat, cold, tingling, pulsation, pulling, or tightness.

The technique of therapeutic touch was developed in the 1970's by Delores Krieger, R.N., a professor of nursing at New York University School of Nursing, and Dora Kunz, a clairvoyant and a healer who served as a mentor to Krieger. The basic steps involved in performing therapeutic touch are as follows:

1. The healer becomes centered in a meditative state and focuses his intent on helping the person in need of healing.

2. The healer moves his hands over the person's energy field to assess where on the body healing is needed.

3. With rhythmic hand motions, the healer begins to move or redistribute the energy around the body to clear, or "unruffle," areas of congestion or add energy to areas that are lacking in it. The healer also visualizes transmitting life energy to specific areas of the body, also to correct imbalances.

4. The healer reassesses the energy field to determine if further intervention is needed.

Therapeutic touch is most commonly practiced by nurses to elicit relaxation, help heal wounds, and help reduce pain. It may be performed while a person is sitting or standing. Clothes are usually worn, and a person might even be covered with a blanket if the room is chilly or he so desires. Most of the time, the healer's hands are held about 2–6 inches above the person's body, with the palms facing down. However, the healer might massage a particular area of the body if he senses the need and the recipient is comfortable with physical contact. The average treatment lasts about 20 minutes.

While most therapeutic touch practitioners are in the nursing profession, some massage therapists, physical therapists, chiropractors, acupuncturists, and others practice therapeutic touch as well. Proponents of therapeutic touch believe that anyone can be taught to sensitize himself to feel human energy fields.

Although therapeutic touch is taught at more than 100 hospitals and health centers worldwide, there is no formal certification program in the United States. To find a qualified therapeutic touch practitioner, the Nurse Healers–Professional Associates International, whose mission is to advance the practice of therapeutic touch, maintains a list of practitioners on their Web site, www.therapeutic-touch.org, and it has a toll-free phone number, (877) 326-4724. The organization recommends looking for a practitioner who performs therapeutic touch on an average of two times per week, has at least five years of experience doing it, and has completed at least 12 hours of therapeutic touch workshops.

Healing touch

Like therapeutic touch, healing touch is an approach to rebalancing and restoring the energy system of the body to enhance the body's natural healing abilities. Also like therapeutic touch, healing touch was developed by a nurse, in this case Janet Mentgen, R.N., in the 1980's. Healing touch is most often used to reduce pain and promote relaxation.

Healing touch uses a variety of techniques to assess both the energy field surrounding the body and the flow of energy within the body. For example, to assess energy flow within the body, a pendulum might be held over the chakras, or centers of physical or spiritual energy identified by some Eastern philosophies, to identify weaknesses. There are seven main chakras, located approximately on the crown of the head, forehead, throat, heart, solar plexus (behind the stomach), pelvic floor, and base of the spine, or coccyx. If the pendulum swings very little, the chakra is closed, or blocked. If the pendulum has a wide, circular swing, the chakra is open (or has been opened by the treatment). When a practitioner detects a closed chakra, he uses various hand movements to unblock it so that energy may flow freely through it.

Other healing touch techniques have names, such as hand scanning, magnetic unruffling, chakra connection, headache techniques, ultrasound, chakra spread, and the Scudder technique. Depending on the technique used and the recipient's comfort level, the practitioner's hands may or may not touch the person receiving treatment.

Healing touch is usually done with the person receiving treatment lying clothed on a massage table, although he could also sit in a chair or lie on a bed, if that were more comfortable. Normally, the practitioner starts by asking the person why he has come for healing touch before moving on to assessment techniques. Treatment sessions may last anywhere from 10 to 60 minutes.

Certification in healing touch is administered by Healing Touch International. Training toward certification includes five progressive levels of education and practice and a mentored apprenticeship. While many healing touch practitioners are licensed health-care professionals, anyone may take healing touch classes and be certified in its practice. For listings of certified healing touch practitioners as well as healing touch clinics that are open to the public, visit the Web site www.healingtouchinternational.org. The organization can also be contacted by phone, at (303) 989-7982.

Reiki

Reiki (pronounced ray-key) is an energy healing system believed to have ancient Tibetan roots. It was introduced in Japan in the early 1900's by an educated Japanese businessman named Mikao Usui. In Reiki, energy is believed to flow from the universal to the practitioner to the person needing it for emotional, physical, or spiritual healing. In this way, the practitioner can give energy to a person who needs it without depleting his own supply.

In a Reiki treatment, the practitioner lightly places his hands on the recipient's body. The recipient remains fully clothed and usually lies down to receive the treatment. The position of the practitioner's hands is changed about every five minutes, and a treatment lasts about an hour. Some people report a gentle tingling warmth coming from the practitioner's hands.

During the placement of hands, the Reiki practitioner may meditate on certain symbols that relate to his intent as a healer. For example, meditating on one particular symbol may increase the power of the energy flow, while meditating on another may help to provide emotional healing.

Proponents of Reiki believe it can also be given from a distance, with no physical touch between healer and recipient. The healer uses a picture of the person he would like to send Reiki to, writes the person's name on a piece of paper, or simply thinks of the person and also meditates on the distance-healing symbol. The healer need not know the person; he could choose to send energy to a world leader, a celebrity, or a complete stranger.

There are no prerequisites or qualifications to becoming a Reiki healer. It is taught through a series of "attunement" rituals, in which the student learns to experience increased energy flowing through his hands. The energy can then be used to heal himself and others. Students are also taught a number of formalized hand positions for healing various parts of the body, as well as the Reiki symbols used to enhance treatment.

Numerous hospitals in the United States offer Reiki to patients to reduce anxiety and depression, speed healing, and counteract side effects of treatments, such as chemotherapy and radiation therapy for cancer. Reiki may also be used for treating chronic pain resulting from conditions such as arthritis. However, Reiki is considered a complementary therapy, not a cure for any particular condition.

While there is no national or statewide licensing of Reiki practitioners, some may be licensed as nurses, physical therapists, or massage therapists. One resource for finding a Reiki practitioner is the Web site of the International Center for Reiki Training, www.reiki.org, which can also be contacted by phone at (800) 332-8112.

Polarity therapy

Polarity therapy is a four-part approach to balancing the flow of energy in the body. It combines bodywork, stretching postures, nutrition, and psychological counseling to open energy blockages and encourage natural healing. It was developed in the 1940's by Randolf Stone, an osteopath, chiropractor, and naturopath. Stone was looking for a unifying thread that would link together all of the healing arts. Through his travels to China and India and his studies of traditional therapies, he concluded that the unifying thread is the vital energy of nature, which flows in and around the body.

The name polarity therapy is based on Stone's belief that various parts of the body have positive electromagnetic energy and various parts have negative electromagnetic energy. For example, the right hand carries a positive charge, and the left hand, a negative charge. The center of the body is neutral. Stone also identified a number of energetic patterns in the body; some flow vertically, some horizontally, and some spiral from the top of the body downward or from the center outward.

In polarity bodywork, the therapist makes use of these energy patterns by simultaneously stimulating a positive and a negative area to improve energy flow. Bodywork techniques include "scanning" the body with the hands (similar to therapeutic touch), and gentle rocking, stretching, and manual pressure. It is not necessary to undress to receive this type of bodywork.

The stretching postures developed by Stone are similar to yoga postures, except that a person gently rocks once he has assumed the posture. Vocal expression is sometimes added to the postures to further stimulate energy flow. Stretching postures are to be done for a few minutes, several times a day.

Stone believed that foods also have different types of energy, so that diet can either enhance or unbalance energy flow in the body. A typical polarity diet is vegetarian, although specific suggestions for food choices would be based on a person's health problems.

To open energy blockages caused by negative feelings, polarity therapists may ask a person questions about possible sources of conflict or may allow a person to speak spontaneously if he wishes. The therapist offers support as the person talks about emotional issues. The object is to promote self-awareness. While the training for polarity therapists includes classes to develop listening and communication skills, most polarity therapists are not licensed psychotherapists.

Common reasons to seek polarity therapy include back pain, chronic headaches, chronic fatigue, digestive complaints, fibromyalgia, arthritis pain, respiratory problems, and stress-related illnesses. Polarity therapy has also been used to promote postsurgical wound healing and to regain range of motion in muscles and joints after surgery. A typical polarity therapy session lasts 60–90 minutes.

There is no licensing of polarity therapists in the United States. However, the American Polarity Therapy Association has set standards of training for practitioners. Some people practice only polarity therapy, while others practice it in addition to massage therapy, chiropractic, osteopathy, and mental health care. To find a qualified practitioner, check the listings on the association's Web site, www.polaritytherapy.org, or call the association at (303) 545-2080.

Acupuncture

Acupuncture, which is discussed at more length in Chapter 4, is an ancient Chinese therapy that uses carefully placed fine needles to balance the flow of qi (energy) along the body's meridians (the channels along which qi is believed to flow). When there are blockages in the energy flow, the body's yin–yang balance may be disrupted, and health problems can result. (Yin and yang are the opposing but complementary forces that exist everywhere in the universe, including in the human body.) While numerous studies have found acupuncture to be therapeutic for certain health conditions, its mechanism of action remains unexplained in Western terms.

Auriculotherapy

Auriculotherapy could be thought of as acupuncture or reflexology for the ears. However, while the earliest uses of ear acupuncture date back to ancient China, auriculotherapy as it is practiced today was developed in the 1950's in France by a physician named Paul Nogier. After becoming aware of an acupuncture point on the ear that, when stimulated, relieved sciatica, Nogier developed a system of reflex points on the external ear that he believed corresponded to all other parts of the body. Stimulation of these points—with acupuncture needles, electricity, manual pressure, lasers, magnets, or "ear pellets" (hard objects attached to parts of the ear with adhesive tape for specified periods of times)—can theoretically bring about healing in distant areas of the body.

Auriculotherapy is often used to control pain or alleviate substance abuse. Side effects can include ear soreness during and after the treatment.

Certification in auriculotherapy is granted by the Auriculotherapy Certification Institute to people who have completed the required coursework and hold a national or state health-care license. The institute maintains a list of certified practitioners, which can be accessed through its Web site, www.auriculotherapy.org.

Acupressure

Acupressure uses the same principles as acupuncture but uses pressure to stimulate points along the meridians rather than needles. Like acupuncture, acupressure was developed in China, and its use is believed to predate acupuncture by a couple of thousand years. However, there are several varieties of Chinese acupressure, such as tui na and qigong massage, and other cultures have developed their own versions, as well. Shiatsu, for example, is a Japanese form of acupressure. Reflexology, developed in the United States, could also be considered a form of acupressure.

Acupressure may be applied using fingers, knuckles, palms, and even elbows and feet. In the United States, acupressure is generally used to relieve pain, reduce stress, and improve overall well-being. It can be done by a trained professional or self-administered, which can be useful in countering headaches or nausea, for example, or chronic pain or sinus problems. If you wish to use acupressure on yourself, it helps to have a trained therapist show you where and how to apply pressure. Sometimes self-applied acupressure is combined with meditation or visualization to enhance the effects.

A professional acupressure session could last from 15 minutes to an hour, depending on the problem. The person receiving acupressure generally sits or lies on a massage table. The therapist may work through clothing or ask the person to remove his clothing.

While acupressure is generally safe, there are some precautions, many of which are the same as for any kind of massage or soft-tissue manipulation:

- Never press on an open wound, swollen or inflamed skin, or a bruise, surgery scar, varicose vein, or broken bone.
- Do not apply pressure over the site of a known tumor.
- If you have phlebitis (inflammation of the veins), or thrombosis (blood clots), speak to your doctor before having acupressure therapy.
- Certain acupressure points must be avoided during pregnancy. Be sure to tell your practitioner if you are or may be pregnant.

There is no licensing procedure for acupressure practitioners. However, you can find practitioners certified in Asian bodywork therapy by searching the online directory of the Web site of the National Certification Commission for Acupuncture and Oriental Medicine, www.nccaom.org. Another way to find trained acupressure practitioners is via the Web site of the Acupressure Institute, www.acupressure. com. The Web site of the American Organization for Bodywork Therapies of Asia, www.aobta. org, also has a member listing.

Jin Shin Jyutzu

Jin Shin Jyutsu is a Japanese form of bodywork that shares some of the same principles as acupuncture. It is a way of harmonizing energy flow in the body through gentle pressure on particular points. It has the additional goal of getting to know one's true self. Like other forms of bodywork, it may have a positive effect on health simply by raising a person's body awareness.

The practice of Jin Shin Jyutsu is ancient, but by the early 1900's, it had fallen into obscurity in Japan. It was rediscovered and revived at that time by Jiro Murai, a philospher who allegedly used it to cure himself of a terminal illness. Jin Shin Jyutsu was introduced in the United States in the 1950's by Mary Burmeister, who learned the technique from Jiro Murai.

The theory behind Jin Shin Jyutsu is that energy, which is believed to flow up the back and down the front of the body, can become blocked in 26 "safety energy locks." Placing the fingertips on the blocked safety energy locks can harmonize and restore the energy flow.

In a typical Jin Shin Jyutsu session, which lasts about an hour, the receiver lies face up and clothed on a cushioned surface. The practitioner first "listens" to the energy pulses in the wrists, then uses a series of hand placement combinations (using the safety energy locks) appropriate for unblocking particular pathways and restoring the person's energy to the energy rhythm of the universe. The points are held with fingertips for a minute or more and then released. As in Reiki, the practitioner is believed to be able to increase the recipient's supply of universal energy without depleting his own supply. Many people report a feeling of deep relaxation after a Jin Shin Jyutsu session.

Jin Shin Jyutsu can also be performed on oneself. Finger placement sequences can be learned from books, such as *The Touch of Healing,* by Alice Burmeister, and self-help classes are offered in some areas. The book *Fun With Happy Hands,* by Mary Burmeister, is written specifically for children and is available through the Web site of Jin Shin Jyutsu, Inc., http://jsjinc.net.

Practitioners of Jin Shin Jyutsu may be certified, indicating they've attended a certain number of hours of classes, but the practice is not licensed. To find a certified Jin Shin Jyutsu practitioner, use the listing on the Web site of Jin Shin Jyutsu, Inc., http://jsjinc.net.

Thought field therapy

Thought field therapy is a mind–body therapy in which the therapist asks a person to think about a troubling situation or event, then to tap with two fingers on a series of acupressure points on the body. The combination of thinking and tapping is believed to eliminate distress by restoring the flow of qi to the relevant meridians. Sometimes a series of eye movements are also performed. If the tapping and eye movements don't resolve the problem, the therapist may search for "energy toxins," such as irritating foods or clothing fabrics that may be interfering with a person's energy field. Once these are removed, the thinking and tapping process is repeated.

Thought field therapy is also known as Callahan Techniques, after psychologist Roger Callahan, who developed the technique in 1981. While he discovered this method essentially by accident, Callahan's explanation for its effectiveness is that when a person thinks of a particular emotional problem (such as a phobia), a "thought field," similar to an electrical field, is generated. The emotional problem results from a blockage in the thought field. The prescribed tapping clears the emotional blockage. Proponents claim that this therapy can work very quickly, sometimes in just one session.

While thought field therapy remains controversial even among practitioners of alternative and complementary medicine, it has been used with some success to treat such mental and physical problems as post-traumatic stress disorder, phobias, anxiety, depression, addictive urges, arthritis pain, and insomnia.

In 1986, Dr. Callahan developed another form of thought field therapy called Voice Technology, which allows practitioners to make a diagnosis and prescribe treatment over the phone. According to Callahan, a person's voice carries a code that reflects the cause of the problem being experienced. His technology uses holographic imaging to extract this information from the voice.

To find a practitioner specifically trained in Dr. Callahan's trade-marked Callahan Techniques, look on his Web site, www.tftrx.com, or call his California office at (760) 564-1008. Since this therapy is used to treat serious psychological problems, look for a licensed behavioral health or medical professional with the training and experience to handle such problems.

Feeling energetic?

There is still much to learn about energy therapies, including just what it is about them that makes them effective when they are effective. Some are known to elicit the relaxation response, which may account for some of their benefits. Those that involve physical touch may be effective for the simple reason that being touched by another person in a nurturing way is known to be healing. It's possible that some people derive psychological benefits from receiving the undivided attention of a biofield therapist. It's also possible that the placebo effect is at work in biofield therapies. Or maybe human beings really do have energy fields that can be manipulated for health benefits.

Most of the therapies that are considered biofield therapies are low-risk interventions. To reap whatever benefits may be had from them, look for a practitioner with training and experience, then judge for yourself whether you feel better and should return for more treatments.

13. Magnets, Light, Color, and Sound

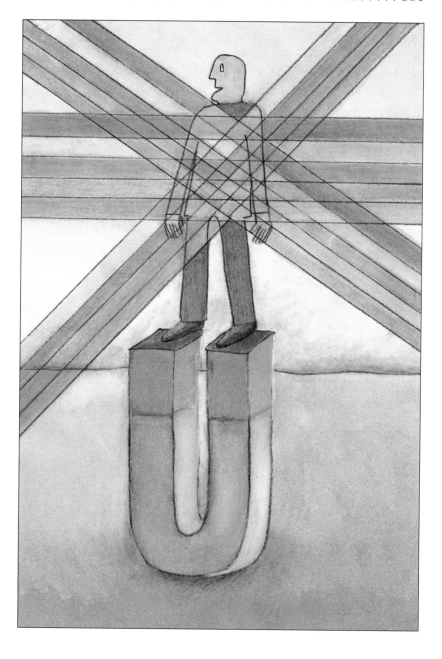

13.
MAGNETS, LIGHT, COLOR, AND SOUND

Magnets, light, color, and sound have been used for hundreds of years—and in some cases, thousands of years—for healing purposes in cultures around the world. Today, all have established conventional medical uses, with certain devices or techniques scientifically proven to help treat various medical conditions. They also have a variety of complementary and alternative uses, some of which seem promising, while others would seem to defy both science and common sense.

What magnetic therapy, light therapy (including colored light therapy), and sound therapy have in common is that, within the field of complementary and alternative medicine, they are all considered "veritable energy" techniques. This means that they employ electromagnetic forces or mechanical vibrations that can be measured: Magnetic fields of specific strengths and light rays and sound waves of specific wavelengths and frequencies may be selected for treatment. In many ways, however, the potential of these therapies is only just beginning to be investigated.

Magnet therapy

Magnets have intrigued humans ever since their discovery. They were employed in the cultures of ancient Greece, Egypt, China, and India to relieve pain and help heal wounds. According to the National Center for Complementary and Alternative Medicine (NCCAM), "Magnets are objects that produce a type of energy called magnetic fields." They are usually made of iron, steel, alloys (mixed metallic substances), or rare-earth elements (scarce metallic elements or minerals). The strength of the magnetic fields they produce is measured in a unit called *gauss*. The strength of the field generated by a typical refrigerator magnet usually ranges from 35 to 200 gauss, while magnets sold for pain relief usually deliver a range from 300 gauss to 5,000 gauss.

All magnets have two poles, where the magnet's power of attraction is strongest. These poles are usually referred to as the north, or negative, pole and the south, or positive, pole. Opposite poles attract each other, but poles of the same type repel each other.

Most magnets marketed for health purposes are *static*, or permanent magnets, which have magnetic fields that don't change. Another type of magnet also used for health purposes is the *electromagnet,* which generates magnetic fields only when electricity flows through it. This type of magnet is usually used at a health-care provider's office or as part of a clinical trial, rather than at home.

Conventional uses

Magnets are used in conventional medicine in several ways. Perhaps their most familiar use is in the technique of *magnetic resonance imaging,* or MRI. This diagnostic procedure uses radio waves and magnets that create a powerful magnetic field (up to 200,000 gauss) to take advantage of the magnetic properties of the body's atoms and produce very detailed images of the body's tissues and organs.

Magnetic technology has also been used in pacemakers, radiation therapy, and other techniques and devices. In 1979, the U.S. Food and Drug Administration (FDA) approved the use of electromagnets to help slowly healing bone fractures heal faster.

More recently, magnets have been used to map areas of the brain with a technique called *magnetoencephalography*.

Complementary and alternative uses

You may know someone who wears magnetic insoles in his shoes, wraps his wrist or back in a magnetic wrap, or sleeps on a magnetic pad. Indeed, there are many magnet-containing products on the market that claim to provide health benefits. Despite the fact that the FDA has not approved the marketing of any magnets promoted for medical uses, a study cited in *The Journal of the American Medical Association* in 2003 estimated that Americans spend $500 million a year on magnets to treat pain.

Is there any evidence that these products actually work? Not much. The few scientific studies of magnets that have been done have been limited and have produced conflicting results, so more are needed before firm conclusions can be drawn.

The chief reason people use magnets outside a conventional health-care context is to relieve pain. Although the mechanism by which magnets may reduce pain has not yet been found, there are several theories about how they may work. For instance, they may affect the nervous system, which uses electrical charges to deliver pain and other signals to the brain. Or, because iron is attracted to magnets and blood contains iron, magnets may increase the flow of blood (and the oxygen and nutrients that come with it) to a certain area of the body. Or they may affect neurotransmitters, such as serotonin, which in turn affect the brain's perception of pain. These theories have yet to be thoroughly tested, but it is known that, while magnets may be able to relieve some pain, they do not treat the underlying source of the pain, so pain may return once magnetic therapy is stopped.

Some other claims for magnets are that they can relieve stress, destroy infections by increasing the body's production of white

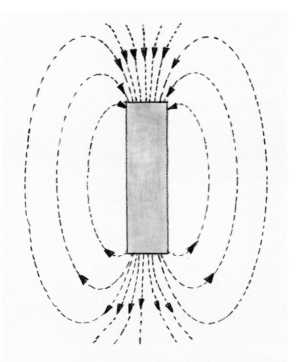

Static Magnets

Static, or permanent, magnets, have an unchanging magnetic field. A magnet's power of attraction is strongest at its opposite ends, usually called the north and south poles. By convention, the north pole of a magnet is the pole that is attracted to the geographic north pole. The north and south poles of a magnet attract each other, but north repels north and south repels south.

blood cells, or relieve central nervous system disorders, such as seizures and panic attacks. There have been few or no clinical trials so far, though, to test these claims.

Static magnetic therapy. Static magnets being used to relieve pain are usually placed either directly on the skin and held in place with tape or an elastic band, or inside clothing or other materials that hold them close to the body. Some products that contain static magnets and are marketed for health purposes include shoe insoles, heel inserts, bracelets and other jewelry, mattress pads, pillows, bandages, belts, and headwear. Static magnets may be applied to a painful area of the body several times per day for several days or weeks. They are left in place for as little as three minutes at a time or for much longer, depending on the severity of the pain.

Findings from published clinical trials have shown some promise for magnetic therapy in the field of pain relief but do not yet support its use. Results for the use of static magnets have been contradictory, with some trials showing that they relieve pain associated with certain conditions and others showing no benefit. Many of the studies of magnetic therapy have been small and of short duration and have had flaws in their design.

One diabetes-related study compared the effect of static magnetic shoe insoles to unmagnetized "placebo" insoles in people with *diabetic peripheral neuropathy,* a complication of diabetes that can cause burning, numbness, and tingling in the feet. Significant reductions in these symptoms occurred in the people who had magnetic insoles, but only during the second half of the four-month study. Further studies are needed to evaluate the long-term or short-term benefit of magnetic insoles.

Electromagnetic therapy. The effectiveness of electromagnetic therapy for treating a variety of painful conditions is currently being studied. Some experimental uses for electromagnets include treatment of arthritis pain, bone and muscle problems, and headaches. Treatment with electromagnets sometimes involves "pulsing," in which the magnetic field is turned on and off very rapidly. Electromagnetic therapy is usually overseen by a health-care professional.

In one specific type of electromagnetic therapy called *transcranial magnetic stimulation,* or TMS, an insulated coil is placed against a person's head, and an electric current then generates a magnetic field in the brain. This technique is used as a diagnostic tool but is also being studied as a method of pain relief. A type of TMS called *repetitive TMS* (or rTMS) may produce longer-lasting pain relief and is being studied as a treatment for a variety of conditions. A related therapy called *repetitive magnetic stimulation* (rMS) involves a coil being placed against a painful area of the body (other than the head) and is being studied as a treatment for musculoskeletal pain.

Clinical trials of electromagnetic therapy have shown more consistent reductions in pain when compared with trials of static magnetic therapy, but their most common conclusion has been that "more research is needed."

Safety concerns

While there is little hard evidence supporting the use of magnets for pain relief, there are also few serious side effects associated with trying them. Some people have reported slight dizziness or light-headedness associated with magnetic therapy, and a few people experience redness, bruising, or irritation of the skin where a static magnet has been worn (this may result from the adhesive used to hold the magnet on the skin). Also, the effects of static magnet therapy on pregnant women have not been researched, so they are discouraged from using this therapy, as are people who use pacemakers, defibrillators, or insulin pumps, because magnets could interfere with the magnetic components of these devices. Finally, people who wear a patch that delivers medicine through the skin, as well as people with an acute sprain, wound, infection, or inflammation, should not use static magnets in case these magnets dilate blood vessels, which could affect the delivery of the medicine or recovery from the acute condition.

There are currently no official training programs or certification credentials in magnetic therapy, so if you are interested in trying this kind of therapy, it is best to see a doctor who specializes in pain management. Such a specialist should be able to guide you through this and other, more proven conventional and alternative treatment options.

Some magnetic devices on the market today are expensive and are not proven to work, despite the manufacturer's claims. Because there are some major multilevel marketing companies selling magnets, caution is needed when accepting the advice of salespeople on the benefits and use of magnets. Multilevel marketing (also called network marketing) is a form of direct sales in which independent distributors sell merchandise, often at a customer's home or by telephone. However, these independent distributors are usually just customers who liked the product and were offered the opportunity to make some money by selling it; they often lack any appropriate professional training or credentials.

The NCCAM suggests that if you do decide to purchase a magnet, you inform your health-care provider about it and look for a magnet with a 30-day return policy and low or no return fees. In most studies that have found benefits for magnetic therapy, the benefits have shown up quickly, so if you do not notice any results within a week or two of using a magnetic device, return it.

Lights and lasers

The field of light therapy encompasses a range of techniques that use visible light or nonvisible rays (such as ultraviolet or infrared waves) to treat different medical conditions. Also included among these techniques is low-energy, or "cold" laser therapy ("laser" is an acronym for "light amplification by stimulated emission of radiation"). All of the forms of light therapy described here originated in the 20th century, although people have been exploring the relationship between light and health for hundreds of years.

Conventional uses

Different types of light therapy are used for many different purposes in conventional medicine. For example, special light boxes that simulate the wavelengths of light produced by the sun (but block harmful ultra-violet waves) and are about 15 times brighter than normal home or office lighting are a proven treatment for a type of depression called *seasonal affective disorder,* or SAD. SAD, which usually affects people during the shorter days of the winter season and produces symptoms such as lethargy, fatigue, overeating, and sleep problems, may result from a disruption of the body's *circadian,* or daily, rhythms due to reduced exposure to sunlight. SAD may also be triggered by over- or underproduction of certain hormones and neurotransmitters that are regulated by sleep and sunlight. Daily light therapy, which consists of sitting near a light box or a special bright lamp for a prescribed amount of time (usually 30 minutes to 2 hours in the morning) has been shown to reduce symptoms for up to 80% of people with SAD. With proper training, people can use light therapy at home and may read or do other tasks in the vicinity of the light box during treatment. Light box therapy is currently being researched as a treatment for other types of depression. It may also be helpful for treating sleep disorders, and it may have therapeutic uses for shift workers who sleep during daylight hours.

Many skin conditions are treated with light therapy. Ultraviolet, or UV, light therapy is used to treat *psoriasis;* a person's eyes and the unaffected areas of his skin are protected while the rest of his skin is exposed to UV light for a prescribed amount of time. People undergoing this treatment may also be prescribed drugs that make their skin more sensitive to the light. This kind of therapy is also used to treat *vitiligo,* an autoimmune condition in which patches of skin lose their pigmentation and which may be more common in people with Type 1 diabetes. UV light therapy is also used to treat a type of skin cancer called *cutaneous T-cell lymphoma.*

Another type of light therapy used to treat certain cancers or precancers is called *photodynamic therapy.* In this type of therapy, a light-activated drug, called a *photosensitiz-*

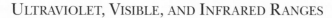

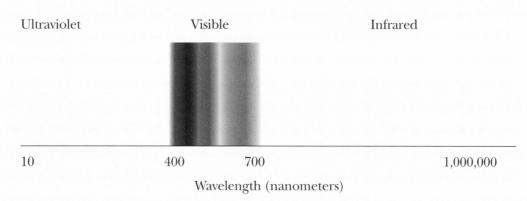

NOTE: Not drawn to scale.

The Electromagnetic Spectrum

The electromagnetic spectrum is composed of ultraviolet waves, visible light waves, infrared waves, gamma rays, x-rays, microwaves, and radio waves. What differentiates one category of wave from another is the wavelength, or the distance from one wave crest to the next. Waves can range in size from several miles, in the case of radio waves, to one-hundredth of a nanometer (which is already one-billionth of a meter), in the case of gamma rays.

Waves that are between 10 nanometers and 400 nanometers fall into the ultraviolet range. Ultraviolet-C light, which has the smallest wavelength in the ultraviolet spectrum, is emitted by the sun, but it is filtered out by the ozone layer before it ever gets to the Earth. Ultraviolet-A and ultraviolet-B light, which are also emitted by the sun, have longer wavelengths and can penetrate the ozone layer. These are the rays that cause a sunburn.

Visible light is the only form of electromagnetic radiation that can be detected by the human eye. This portion of the spectrum has wavelengths that measure from 400 nanometers to 700 nanometers, and ranges in color from violet to red. The perception of color is created by the reflection of particular wavelengths of light off objects and into the eye. A blue sweater, for example, absorbs all of the wavelengths in the visible spectrum except that which corresponds to the color blue; this wavelength is reflected off the object to the eye and interpreted as the sweater's color. Because the sun emits wavelengths for all the colors in the visible spectrum, it appears to us as white.

Wavelengths just beyond the visible spectrum fall into the infrared range, which extends from approximately 700 nanometers to 1,000,000 nanometers (or 1 millimeter). Humans generally do not detect near-infrared energy, which has the shortest wavelengths in the infrared zone. Rather, we observe its effects only indirectly, such as when we use a remote control to operate the television set. Far-infrared energy, on the other hand, is detected directly by the human body every day in the form of heat. When someone holds his hand over a hot stove or a space heater, his sensation of heat is actually caused by his body's absorption of far-infrared energy.

ing agent, is applied to the skin or injected into the bloodstream. Once the drug has been absorbed, the affected area is exposed to a laser or another type of light, and the light in turn activates the drug to destroy cancer cells.

Another procedure called *photopheresis,* or *extracorporeal photochemotherapy,* uses UV light to inhibit the cancer T-cell lymphoma. In this procedure, which takes about 3–5 hours, a person who has taken a light-activatable drug has about a pint of blood removed by a special machine. This machine then separates the blood into different types of cells and treats the white blood cells with UV light. The treated blood is then infused back into the person, where it is believed to trigger an immune response that helps the person battle the cancer. This procedure is now being researched for use in treating other autoimmune conditions.

Finally, a procedure that uses an ultraviolet-energy–emitting laser called the *excimer laser* has recently been shown to help people with diabetes who have severely clogged leg arteries avoid amputation. In this procedure, flexible fiber optic catheters are used to thread the laser into the body, where it uses short bursts of ultraviolet energy to "vaporize" blockages in the leg's arteries. This technique improves blood flow and clears the way for further procedures, such as balloon angioplasty, which can help open clogged arteries.

Complementary and alternative uses

Although light therapy has many proven uses in conventional medicine, less conclusive research has been done on many proposed alternative uses.

Light box and UV therapies. Despite the claims of some supporters, there is no scientific evidence that light boxes or other bright lights can relieve high blood pressure, premenstrual syndrome, migraine headaches, or several other conditions for which they are promoted. Similarly, complementary UV light therapy, sometimes marketed to consumers as sun lamps, has not been proven to neutralize toxins, help the immune system, or fight off infections or cancer, despite claims. And there is no evidence that UV blood irradiation (the alternative medicine counterpart of photopheresis), in which a small tube of blood is removed, treated with UV rays, and returned to the body, kills germs, neutralizes toxins, or stimulates the immune system.

Low-level lasers. More research has been done on procedures involving the use of low-level, or cold, laser therapy, which has been promoted to treat pain and inflammation and speed healing in a variety of medical conditions. Unlike conventional laser therapy, low-level lasers trigger very small temperature elevations, if any, in the areas of the body they are used to treat. These lasers are used directly on or over painful, inflamed, or wounded parts of the body and are thought to stimulate the healing process by triggering enzyme action and bioelectric activity.

The FDA considers low-level laser therapy to be experimental and allows its use in clinical trials; however, many different types of lasers, schedules of treatment, and techniques exist, and many common claims about what low-level lasers can do are unproven. For instance, controlled studies have shown little or no benefit for the use of low-level lasers to stimulate wound healing, as well as no benefit for relieving symptoms of rheumatoid arthritis or musculoskeletal pain. Reviews of multiple studies have also shown that low-level laser therapy provides no benefit in the treatment of tuberculosis, tinnitus, arthritis in general, or carpal tunnel syndrome, for which it is often promoted.

Low-level laser therapy has shown some promise, however, in treating a few specific conditions. For instance, a study showed that people with *Raynaud phenomenon* (a vascular condition in which exposure to cold interrupts blood flow to peripheral parts of the body, like the fingers and toes) who were treated with low-level laser therapy experienced fewer attacks during treatment than those who had received a placebo, or sham therapy. In another study, low-level lasers also helped reduce pain in people who had just had surgery. Low-level lasers are also sometimes used in acupuncture. The laser beams can be used to stimulate the body's acupoints in people who fear the pain of traditional needles. (If you are interested in this kind of therapy, be sure to seek out a licensed acupuncturist who has been trained in laser acupuncture.)

Monochromatic infrared energy therapy. A technique called monochromatic infrared energy therapy, which uses invisible, infrared energy to treat symptoms of diabetic peripheral neuropathy, has been shown to help increase blood flow to the feet and thereby reduce numbness and pain. Generally, this type of therapy is administered by a doctor or physical therapist using an FDA-approved device, although such a device can also be purchased and used at home. The device consists of flexible pads containing diodes that emit infrared waves. During therapy the pads are placed in contact with the feet, strapped or taped in place, and turned on for 20–45 minutes. Sessions are usually scheduled daily at first, then reduced to once or twice a week. An increasing number of doctors and physical therapists now offer this therapy, and it is usually covered by health insurance.

Safety concerns

Light therapy consisting of treatment with only visible light, such as the use of light boxes or special lamps, is generally considered safe, though reported side effects include eye strain, headache, insomnia, and, in a few people being treated for a depressive disorder, symptoms of mania (a hyperactive state). Experts point out that tanning beds or sunlamps are not considered light therapy tools and expose users to

dangerous levels of UV radiation. In fact, any form of therapy that uses UV light raises a person's risk somewhat of developing sunburn, cataracts, and skin-related problems, including premature aging of the skin and skin cancer.

Color therapy

A field related to light therapy is color therapy, also known as *chromatotherapy,* which involves the use of color in several ways to promote health and healing. Visible colors are actually different wavelengths of light in the *electromagnetic spectrum,* and because full-spectrum light (such as sunlight or lamps and light boxes that simulate it) has been shown to have therapeutic uses, many practitioners of color therapy believe that the individual colors that make up light must have specific effects on the body. While traditions of using color for healing go back to the days of ancient Egypt and India, little scientific proof has been found to support such claims.

Conventional uses

One form of colored light therapy has been used in conventional medicine for years to treat newborn babies who have a buildup of the waste product *bilirubin* in their blood, causing jaundice. Exposing the baby's skin to a special blue light, usually for several days, helps him break the bilirubin down into a substance that is more easily cleared from the body. There is currently no evidence, however, that blue or any other type of colored light can effectively treat any other medical conditions or disorders. A couple of small, preliminary studies involving the use of red light in specific ways to treat migraine headaches and knee pain from arthritis have shown promising results, but further research is needed.

Complementary and alternative uses

Color therapy is considered an adjunct to conventional medical treatment, not a replacement for it. Several different techniques may be used, including the shining of colored lights, meditation and visualization involving color, and even the drinking of "colored" water. Practitioners claim that color therapy can affect the production of neurochemicals in the brain and can help treat sleep disorders, diabetes, tuberculosis, impotence, stress, pain, and many other conditions.

In Ayurveda, one of India's traditional systems of medicine, specific colors correspond with each of the seven *chakras*, or physical and spiritual energy "hubs" of the body, and each color has specific healing powers. If you see an Ayurvedic practitioner, he may recommend the use of certain colors in your therapy based on these principles.

In colored light therapy, a light may be shined through a filter of a certain color directly onto the body or part of the body. Colored lights that flash in patterns may also be used. A technique called *esogetic colorpuncture therapy* is an experimental form of acupuncture in which colored light is focused onto acupuncture points. A technique called *hydrochromotherapy* involves sipping water from a colored bottle that has been filled with water and left to sit in the sunlight for several hours, allowing the color to "charge" the water. Other color therapy techniques may include wearing clothes of a certain color, eating foods of a certain color, and visualizing a color or colors while meditating.

While none of these techniques have been proven to have any effect on the body, some of the techniques are relaxing, and, as long as they are used in addition to, not instead of, conventional medicine, should not cause harm. There are currently no programs or organizations that license or accredit color therapists, so if this kind of therapy interests you, it is best to seek out a doctor, psychologist, or counselor who uses color therapy as an adjunct to conventional treatment.

Sound and music

Sound therapy, also known as sound energy therapy or vibrational therapy, is based on the theory that sound waves can help heal and support the body. While the sounds used need not be melodic or harmonic (or, in fact, audible at all), included in this field is music therapy, which uses the listening to and creation of music to promote healing and has been proven effective by several studies.

Conventional uses

One conventional medical use of sound is the technique of *ultrasound*, which uses high-frequency sound waves outside the range of human hearing for diagnostic procedures. During an ultrasound examination, a small handheld device that is pressed against the skin emits sound waves, and the reflection of these sound waves by tissues, bones, and fluids in the body produces detailed images. Some ultrasound examinations, called *invasive ultrasounds*, are done within the body.

Sound waves are also used, of course, in hearing tests, usually administered by a specialist called an *audiologist*.

Complementary and alternative uses

Various theories exist to explain how sound waves and music may help the body heal.
Cymatic and related therapies. Some sound therapy practitioners believe that specific sound frequencies resonate with specific organs in the body. One field, called *cymatic therapy*, claims that illness results when the rhythms of the body's organs are not working harmoniously. Cymatic therapy is an offshoot of *cymatics*, a field of study pioneered by the Swiss doctor Hans Jenny in the mid-20th century in which the effect of sound waves on matter is examined. Cymatic therapy uses computerized instruments to transmit sound waves through the skin, a technique that theoretically restores dis-

eased organs to their natural rhythms; sometimes these devices also contain a magnetic field. Other practices rely on objects such as wind chimes and tuning forks to create sounds and vibrations in connection with Ayurvedic principles. There is, however, no scientific evidence that any of these techniques provide any benefit.

Ultrasound. Ultrasound has also been used as a complementary technique to relieve pain and inflammation resulting from injuries such as sprains, bursitis, and tendonitis, and to speed healing. The rationale behind this therapy is that the high-frequency sound waves used cause tissues to vibrate deep within the injured area, increasing heat and blood flow to the region. However, reviews of many studies have shown little actual benefit for these techniques. Ultrasound has shown some promise, however, in speeding bone fracture repair and will continue to be investigated in this field.

Music therapy. One type of sound therapy that does have scientifically proven benefits is music therapy, a field that in itself encompasses many different techniques. Studies have shown that just listening to music of one's own choosing can help reduce blood pressure, heart rate, and perceived levels of stress, perhaps by affecting brain waves, brain circulation, stress hormone levels, or levels of the body's natural "feel-good" chemicals, such as endorphins and opiates. Music therapy, which may encompass techniques such as making music, writing songs, and discussing music as well as listening to it, has been shown to help reduce pain, anxiety, and nausea in people undergoing chemotherapy. Music therapy can have calming or stimulating effects, and can be used as a complementary therapy for a variety of physical and psychological conditions. (See Chapter 5 for more on music therapy.)

Safety concerns

Sound therapy is generally considered safe as a complementary therapy, as long as it is used in conjunction with, not instead of, conventional medical care. Loud music has been shown to have some detrimental effects on health, and it is possible that musical intervention by a person not trained in music therapy can increase stress or discomfort, so if you are interested in music therapy, seek out a certified music therapist. More than 70 colleges and universities now offer degrees in music therapy, and all certified therapists must undertake a certain number of hours of clinical training as well as an internship. A music therapist will design a program of treatment around an individual's needs.

When to turn to veritable energy therapies

The fields of magnetic, light, color, and sound therapy have shown some promise in treating pain and other side effects resulting from a variety of conditions—in some cases including diabetes. However, many of these techniques have little scientific evidence to back up the health claims associated with their use, especially compared to several better-studied complementary and alternative therapies.

There are few serious safety concerns associated with trying most of the products and therapies currently available in these fields. In fact, the greatest risk is probably that you'll waste your money on a therapy that has not been proven to help in any way. Most experts advise trying tested conventional and alternative therapies first and treating unproven alternative options, like magnets or color therapy, as a last resort. If you do decide to try a less-proven therapy, make sure to do so as a complement to, not a replacement for, your regular medical care. Your doctor should be able to refer you to a reputable pain management specialist, whether that person is a physician, psychologist, acupuncturist, or another type of therapist.

14. CAM THERAPIES FOR DIABETES COMPLICATIONS

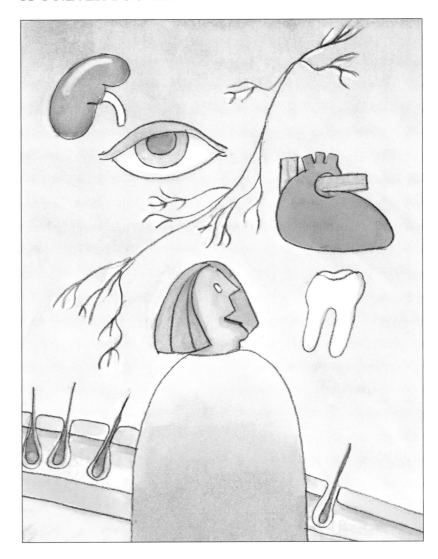

14.
CAM THERAPIES FOR DIABETES COMPLICATIONS

All complications of diabetes, including nerve damage (neuropathy), kidney disease (nephropathy), eye disease (retinopathy and others), and cardiovascular disease, are believed to be related to high blood glucose levels and sometimes high blood pressure levels. Any complementary therapies that help to control blood glucose or blood pressure levels, therefore, will help to prevent or delay the progression of diabetes complications. Keep in mind that if a practice or therapy is effective, you may need to adjust your doses of any medicines, including insulin, that you take for diabetes or blood pressure control to avoid hypoglycemia or blood pressure that is too low.

If you already have any diabetes complications, caution is in order when considering complementary therapies. Therapies or exercises that promote relaxation may help by improving your ability to cope. But radically changing your diet or taking herbal or other dietary supplements without first consulting a health-care provider may actually hurt, particularly if you have kidney disease.

The following suggestions are given as food for thought. Not all therapies will be appropriate for every person. If you're interested in trying complementary therapies to help deal with diabetes complications, discuss what you would like to try with a health-care professional first. Make sure that what you're trying won't make the situation worse or conflict with other drugs or therapies you may be using.

Nerve damage

Diabetic neuropathy can affect pretty much any nerve in the body. Most commonly, however, it affects the nerves in the feet, lower legs, hands, and sometimes arms. This type of neuropathy is called peripheral neuropathy, and it typically causes numbness, pain, or tingling in the affected body part. Neuropathy that affects the nerves that control blood pressure, digestion, sweating, sexual functioning, and other automatic functions is called autonomic neuropathy.

When it comes to neuropathy, first make sure you have a correct diagnosis. While diabetes is a major cause of neuropathy, it is not the only one. Peripheral neuropathy can also be caused by circulatory problems, certain drugs, chemotherapy, alcohol abuse, anemia, AIDS, back problems, surgery, and unknown causes. It's important to have a complete evaluation of any neuropathy symptoms by a doctor to ensure that the treatment is appropriate for the underlying problem.

Exercise is often helpful for improving symptoms of peripheral neuropathy, but care must be taken to choose exercises that are safe. See Chapter 7 for specifics on choosing exercise when you have diabetes complications. If increased blood flow to the feet through exercise or other measures does result in improvement in nerve function, symptoms may actually get worse initially, as the feet regain feeling. That's where techniques like visualization—along with reassurance from your health-care provider—can help.

If you have pain from neuropathy, mind–body techniques that promote relaxation can complement any mainstream pain-reduction therapies you may be using. These include meditation, biofeedback-enhanced relaxation training, hypnosis, guided imagery, various massage techniques, and aromatherapy. Other complementary therapies that may be worth a try include reflexology and acupressure or acupuncture, but check with your health-care provider before allowing any practitioner to apply pressure to your feet. If your skin is fragile, this could do more harm than good. Magnetic therapy, therapeutic touch, Reiki, and healing touch are some other options that have not been proven to help but are unlikely to harm.

Distraction is another way to deal with pain. Focusing your mind on something else, such as a hobby, social activity, or humorous book or movie, can temporarily reduce the pain you feel. Support groups for chronic pain sufferers can also help by offering emotional support and coping strategies.

One botanical-based treatment that has become mainstream is the use of capsaicin-containing cream or ointment on feet affected by painful neuropathy. (Capsaicin is the chemical that makes chili peppers hot.) Capsaicin appears to relieve pain by stimulating the release of substance P, a chemical transmitter of pain, from nerve terminals. Initially, the release of substance P causes pain, but eventually the nerve terminals become depleted of substance P, leading to loss of the pain sensation. When trying capsaicin, keep the following in mind:

■ Try it in one spot first before using it all over your feet to see how it feels and to see if you are allergic to it.
■ If you have a choice of more than one product, try the lower-strength product first. If that doesn't give adequate relief in a week or so, try the higher-strength product.
■ Follow package directions, and wash your hands after use. Don't make the mistake of accidentally rubbing capsaicin in your eyes; it really hurts!

Alpha-lipoic acid supplements have also shown promise for decreasing pain, numbness, and burning in the feet associated with peripheral neuropathy. In studies, people who took 600 milligrams of alpha-lipoic acid per day for a matter of weeks or months experienced these improvements. However, the long-term effects of taking high doses of alpha-lipoic acid are unknown.

Monochromatic infrared energy therapy, which has been shown to help increase blood flow to the feet through the use of invisible, infrared energy, may reduce numbness and pain associated with peripheral neuropathy. It is unlikely to do harm if it doesn't, and it is covered by some health insurance plans. See Chapter 13 for more details on this therapy.

Some forms of foot pain respond to an age-old treatment called contrast bath hydrotherapy, in which the feet are first placed in a cool bath, then in a warm bath, then again in a cool bath. As long as the water used is neither too hot nor too cold, there's no harm in trying this. At the very least, it might be relaxing. Be sure to put some lotion on your feet afterward.

Digestive problems

Diabetes can affect the digestive system in a number of ways. Gastroparesis, for example, is slowed stomach emptying caused by nerve damage. It can cause an early feeling of fullness at meals, nausea, vomiting of undigested food, and difficulty controlling blood glucose levels since food may not reach the small intestine and be absorbed as quickly as expected. If you have symptoms of gastroparesis, get professional help. Improving your blood glucose control may improve stomach functioning. The following measures are also generally recommended for people with gastroparesis:

■ Eat small meals.
■ Avoid high-fiber foods such as whole-grain products and most fruits and vegetables.
■ Avoid high-fat meals.
■ Take a walk after meals to improve stomach emptying.

If you have gastroparesis, be aware that any dietary supplements you take may be

CAM Therapies for Diabetes Complications

Herbs to Avoid in Chronic Kidney Disease

Herbs that may be safe for most healthy people may not be safe for people with chronic kidney disease. The following herbs may be harmful for a number of reasons. Some may directly irritate the kidneys. Some may raise blood pressure. Some have a high likelihood of interacting with prescription drugs. And some contain high amounts of potassium, which is often restricted in the diets of people with kidney disease. Because this list is not exhaustive, always consult your health-care provider before taking any herbal supplements if you have chronic kidney disease.

COMMON NAME	BOTANICAL NAME
Alfalfa	*Medicago sativa*
Aloe	*Aloe barbadensis, Aloe vera*
Bayberry	*Myrica pensylvanica*
Blue cohosh	*Caulophyllum thalictroides*
Broom	*Cytisus scoparius*
Buchu	*Barosma betulina, Barosma serratifolia, Barosma crenulata*
Buckthorn	*Rhamnus frangula*
Capsicum	*Capsicum frutescens, Capsicum annuum*
Cascara	*Rhamnus purshiana*
Coltsfoot	*Tussilago farfara*
Dandelion	*Taraxacum officinale*
Ginger	*Zingiber officinale*
Ginseng	*Panax ginseng, Panax quinquefolius*

COMMON NAME	BOTANICAL NAME
Goldenrod	*Solidago virgaurea*
Horsetail	*Equisetum arvense*
Juniper berries	*Juniperus communis*
Licorice	*Glycyrrhiza glabra, Glycyrrhiza uralensis*
Maté	*Ilex paraguariensis*
Nettle	*Urtica dioica*
Noni juice	*Morinda citrifolia*
Parsley	*Petroselinum crispum*
Rhubarb	*Rheum palmatum, Rheum officinale*
Senna	*Cassia senna, Cassia augustifolia*
Uva ursi	*Arctostaphylos uva-ursi*
Vervain	*Verbena officinalis*

digested slowly and not have the expected effects.

Autonomic neuropathy associated with diabetes can also cause abnormal motility and secretion of fluid in the colon, leading to diarrhea. In some cases, fiber supplementation with bran, bulk laxatives, or high-fiber foods can thicken the consistency of the bowel movement and decrease watery diarrhea. (In other cases, these same measures may worsen diarrhea.) However, not all diarrhea is caused by nerve damage. Sugar alcohols, a type of low-calorie sweetener often used in sugar-free foods, can cause diarrhea in some people. The diabetes drug metformin (brand name Glucophage) is also known to cause diarrhea. If you have frequent or debilitating diarrhea, see your doctor for a diagnosis of the underlying cause and a recommendation for treatment.

Constipation may or may not be caused by diabetes, but plenty of people with diabetes have it. Standard recommendations for treating constipation still include gradually increasing the amount of fiber in your diet (while also increasing the amount of water or other liquids) and engaging in regular physical activity. Having a regular schedule for meals and for waking and sleeping may also help to keep you "regular." It's good to remember, however, that constipation is a common side effect of many drugs. If you are troubled by chronic constipation or develop it suddenly, see your doctor. Do not use dietary supplements that promise "cathartic" effects. They can irritate the colon and may lead to reliance on them for bowel evacuation. Similarly, colon therapy, or colonic irrigation, is not recommended because of its risks and because frequent use of enemas can lead to reliance on them.

Kidney disease

Your kidneys maintain your body's water volume, regulate your blood pressure, remove waste products from the 200 quarts of blood they filter every day, and release essential hormones. Some of the waste products filtered by the kidneys include nitrogen, phosphorus, potassium, sodium, and foreign substances, such as caffeine and drugs.

Many nutrients, including glucose, are initially filtered by the kidneys but then reabsorbed later. When blood glucose levels are normal, most of the glucose that is filtered by the kidneys is reabsorbed, but when blood glucose levels are high, say, over 180 mg/dl, the kidneys are not able to reabsorb it all, and some of it ends up in the urine.

When the kidneys are damaged, their filtering ability is compromised, and wastes can build up in the bloodstream. Because the kidneys help to degrade insulin, people with late-stage kidney disease who use insulin may find that they need less insulin or are more likely to have low blood glucose levels.

Early kidney damage may be prevented from progressing to more severe kidney damage by controlling high blood pressure, high blood glucose levels, and high cholesterol levels and by stopping smoking. Cutting back on sodium, restricting protein intake, and limiting alcohol consumption may help, too.

The effectiveness of dietary protein restriction in protecting the kidneys remains somewhat controversial. Dietary protein restriction has been shown to slow the progression of kidney disease in some animal models. Small clinical studies in people with diabetic kidney disease have shown that people who were able to restrict their dietary protein to 0.8 grams per kilogram of body weight per day (which is the recommended dietary allowance of protein for adults) were able to modestly slow the rate of fall in the glomerular filtration rate (GFR), a measure of how well the kidneys are able to filter waste from the blood. Other studies suggest that red meat, in particular, is more damaging to kidneys, while plant sources of protein have less of an effect.

The use of herbal remedies can be unsafe for people with kidney disease because the kidneys cannot get rid of waste products normally. The National Kidney Foundation cautions against taking any herbs without first consulting a physician or pharmacist. (Common cooking herbs used in moderate amounts to flavor food, however, don't pose a problem.)

Similarly, taking large doses of certain vitamins (such as vitamins A and D and some B vitamins) can be dangerous when the kidneys are not functioning properly. Depending on the degree of kidney damage and type of treatment, your physician may prescribe certain supplements. It is not advised to take others unless you consult your doctor or renal dietitian first.

While caution is needed regarding diet and dietary supplements, both exercise and practicing relaxation techniques can be good for improving the quality of life for people with kidney disease.

Eye diseases

The most common eye complication associated with diabetes is retinopathy, but having diabetes can raise the risk of developing other eye diseases, as well, including cataracts and glaucoma. In addition, people with diabetes are not immune to developing eye problems not associated with diabetes, such as age-related macular degeneration.

Maintaining healthy levels of blood glucose, blood cholesterol, and blood pressure lowers the risk of developing diabetes-related eye diseases. Yearly visits to an eye doctor (an ophthalmologist or optometrist) for a dilated eye exam is recommended to detect any problems early.

While some alternative health providers recommend programs of "eye exercises" for eye health, these are not effective treatment for any eye disease. In addition, you should not do these exercises if you have an eye infection, retinopathy that requires laser treatment, or have been diagnosed with glaucoma.

At this time there are no established complementary therapies for diabetic retinopathy. While certain herbs and other dietary supplements have been suggested at times, none have yet been proven effective. Certain traditional medical systems do have approaches for dealing with eye problems, such as acupuncture. If you wish to try such a program as a complementary therapy, talk to your eye doctor first.

Good nutrition may help to maintain good eye health in more ways than one. For starters, it helps to control blood glucose, blood cholesterol, and blood pressure. Eating foods high in lutein, one of the yellow and orange pigments found in many fruits and vegetables, is believed to help protect against cataracts and macular degeneration. Lutein-rich fruits and vegetables include mangoes, sweet potatoes, watermelon, carrots, squash, tomatoes, and dark-green, leafy vegetables.

Studies also suggest that people with diets high in beta-carotene, zinc, and vitamins C and E are less likely to develop age-related macular degeneration. Good sources of zinc include whole grains, meat, poultry, fish, and dairy products. Good sources of vitamin E include whole grains, vegetable oil, nuts, and eggs. Carrots, kale, and spinach provide beta-carotene. And citrus fruits, broccoli, and bell peppers provide vitamin C.

Heart and other vascular problems

Cardiovascular problems may be the diabetes complications most treatable by complementary therapies. Changes in diet, physical activity programs, and stress-reduction techniques have all proven to be helpful. For guidance on making these changes, talk to your health-care provider, or read up on the Pritikin Program and the Ornish Lifestyle Program, both described in Chapter 10. Be sure to get your doctor's guidance before starting an exercise program if you've been diagnosed with heart disease.

Peripheral arterial disease. In peripheral arterial disease, arteries in the legs (and sometimes arms) narrow and harden as a result of fatty plaque deposits. The result is reduced blood flow to the legs and feet. This disorder can be painful and dangerous, since it can lead to slowed wound healing in the affected areas. Symptoms of peripheral arterial disease include intermittent claudication (cramping leg pain that occurs with walking and stops with rest); numbness, coldness, or tingling in the legs and feet; and slow healing of cuts and sores.

A trade-marked mind–body technique called WarmFeet has been shown to increase blood flow to the feet and reduce pain. The WarmFeet Kit includes an audiotape that prompts the user to release tension through muscle relaxation and breath work. It also includes a visualization segment, during which a person might imagine warmth or the healing process. And it includes a skin thermometer, which works as a biofeedback device. Skin temperature is measured before relaxation and again afterward. A higher temperature afterward indicates that relaxation took place. Paying attention to how a relaxed states feels and remembering that feeling improves a person's ability to achieve that state again.

Daily or even twice daily practice of this technique is recommended for best results. The WarmFeet Kit can be purchased through www.diabetesnet.com ([800] 988-4772) or www.rx4betterhealth.com ([800] 798-6972) for about $20.

Other approaches that can help relieve the pain of peripheral arterial disease include monochromatic infrared energy therapy, which increases blood flow to the feet, and following a prescribed daily exercise program. Most commonly, a person is advised to walk until he feels discomfort in his legs, rest until the discomfort subsides, then walk again for a total of 30 minutes. Daily foot inspections and prompt treatment of any wounds is important to prevent the development of foot ulcers.

High blood pressure. High blood pressure has been shown to respond positively to lifestyle measures, such as following the DASH eating plan, cutting back on sodium in the diet, and cutting back on alcohol intake. Learning and practicing stress management techniques, such as the relaxation response or mindful meditation, can also help. Getting regular exercise is good medicine, too. Doing yoga, in particular, has been shown to reduce blood pressure. However, get your doctor's guidance on how intensely to exercise if you've been diagnosed with high blood pressure.

Skin

Diabetes is associated with a number of skin conditions, with dry skin probably being the most common complaint. Dry skin can be associated with high blood glucose levels. It can also be associated with an absence of

sweating caused by diabetic nerve damage. However, dry skin in a person with diabetes may be the result of dry air and frequent bathing and have nothing to do with diabetes.

Itching is another common complaint. It can be caused by dry skin, fungal infections, such as athlete's foot, and poor blood circulation. The latter tends to cause itchiness in the lower parts of the legs.

There are several things you can do to prevent diabetes-related skin problems, including the following:

■ Take steps to control your blood glucose levels. This can both head off dry skin and improve your ability to fight infections. Over the long term, it lowers your chances of developing complications, such as circulatory and nerve problems.

■ Use a moisturizing lotion regularly. The best time to apply lotion is just after a shower. However, do not put lotion between your toes.

■ Wear gloves when washing dishes or performing other household chores that involve water or cleaning products.

■ Wash your hands before monitoring your blood glucose level. This will help prevent infections at your lancing sites.

■ Be sure to bathe regularly in warm, not hot, water.

■ Wear shower sandals in public showers or locker rooms to avoid picking up athlete's foot and other infections.

■ Keep your feet dry by wearing "wicking" socks for exercise and by changing your socks regularly.

Many skin conditions are worsened by stress, and some conditions such as eczema may even be caused by stress. If you find yourself breaking out in blemishes or getting itchy skin when you're feeling stressed, try practicing one of the stress-reduction techniques described in this book.

Dental health

Diabetes has an unfortunate relationship with periodontal (gum) disease: High

A Walk Through Basic Foot Care

When it comes to foot care, prevention and early detection are the names of the game. These tips will help you to sidestep infections, cuts, and other breaks in the skin and to notice any problems that do develop early, so you can get prompt treatment.

WHAT TO DO	WHY
Keep your blood sugar in your target range as much of the time as possible.	To prevent infection, speed healing, and prevent further damage to blood vessels and nerves.
Do not smoke.	Nicotine impairs blood circulation.
Every day, wash your feet with mild soap and warm water; dry carefully.	To prevent fungal infections (such as athlete's foot) and other infections.
Inspect your feet carefully every day.	To detect any problems early.
Cut toenails straight across (or following the natural curve of the toe) and not too short. A $\frac{1}{16}$-inch to $\frac{1}{8}$-inch rim of white nail beyond the pink nail bed should be clearly visible all the way across the top of the toenail.	To avoid ingrown toenails and to avoid cutting your toes.
Never walk anywhere, even indoors, in bare feet or with socks only, especially if feet are numb. Do not wear open-toed sandals or slippers with soles that can be easily punctured.	To protect feet from being injured by small or sharp objects and to prevent toes from being stubbed.
Do not soak your feet unless your health-care provider has prescribed this for a particular reason.	Soaking removes natural oils, causing feet to dry and crack. In addition, skin is soft and easily injured right after soaking.
If skin on feet is dry, apply lotion to the tops and bottoms.	To prevent skin from cracking.
Do not apply lotion between the toes. (You may apply powder between the toes if desired.)	To prevent fungal infections by keeping the area dry.
Never use commercial corn or callus removers or strong chemical antiseptics. Never perform "home surgery" with sharp cutting tools, and don't use hot water bottles or heating pads on feet.	To prevent burns, cuts, and skin erosion.
Shop for shoes late in the day, when your feet are most swollen, and make sure they fit well.	To avoid injuries when "breaking in" shoes and prevent chronic rubbing from ill-fitting shoes.
Check the insides of shoes daily with your hand before putting them on.	Any object or rough edge in your shoe can cause blisters or breaks in the skin.
Wear socks that keep your feet dry. Avoid knee-high stockings or socks with tight elastic. Change socks often if your feet perspire heavily.	Wet feet are a breeding ground for bacteria. Tight socks constrict circulation.
Don't cross your legs when you sit.	To maintain good circulation.
Take off your shoes at every doctor's visit.	Your doctor or nurse should check your feet.
Contact your doctor, nurse, or podiatrist immediately when you discover a problem.	Most foot problems are much easier to treat when they are attended to promptly.

blood glucose raises the risk of developing periodontal disease, and periodontal disease raises blood glucose levels. Maintaining good oral health and good diabetes care, therefore, requires brushing, flossing, and regular professional dental cleanings (at least every six months), as well as efforts to control blood glucose levels.

High blood glucose lowers the body's ability to fight infection, including periodontal infections. Chronic high blood glucose can also cause dry mouth, which not only feels uncomfortable but also raises the risk of tooth decay and oral infections. Dry mouth can also be a side effect of many drugs, including antidepressants, antihistamines, and medicines for high blood pressure.

Brushing at least twice a day with a gentle brush and flossing at least once a day is recommended. Brushing your tongue with a toothbrush or using a tongue scraper can help prevent bad breath. Sipping water or chewing gum sweetened with xylitol can be helpful for people with dry mouth. Using a mouth rinse is sometimes recommended for killing bacteria, but those that contain alcohol can further dry the mouth. Stress can worsen dental health and lower disease resistance, so using stress-reduction techniques, in addition to all their other benefits, can protect your oral health, as well. Following a nutritious diet is also recommended for good oral health.

If trips to the dentist make you anxious— or dental phobia prevents you from visiting the dentist at all—hypnotherapy may help you to overcome your fear. In fact, dental fear is so common that many dentists have learned hypnotherapy techniques or can refer their patients to a qualified hypnotherapist. Some other ways to relax in the dentist's chair include breathing exercises, progressive muscle relaxation, and visualization. Good oral health is essential for good general health, diabetes care, and quality of life, so don't let fear keep you from having it.

Weight loss or gain

While weight gain or loss is not usually considered a diabetes complication, either can be a consequence of having diabetes. Many people with Type 1 diabetes and some with Type 2 lose a considerable amount of weight before being diagnosed. Usually after starting insulin or oral medicines, they readily regain that weight. But some people continue to be slimmer than they'd like and have trouble putting on weight, while others gain pounds they don't want.

When diabetes goes untreated, the body tries to rid itself of excess glucose in the blood through the urine. When this happens, a person is not absorbing all of the calories he eats. When he begins taking insulin or oral medicines that enable the body to use all of the glucose that enters the bloodstream, he begins to absorb all of the calories he eats. If a person consumes more calories than his body needs, he will put on excess weight.

Whether a person needs to gain or lose weight, attention to diet and exercise are key. In either case, a visit to a registered dietitian is a good idea for individualized guidance.

For those who wish to gain weight, a diet higher in healthful fats may help, since fat is high in calories. However, eating more should be accompanied by exercising more so that the extra calories are turned into muscle, not fat. Resistance exercise tends to build muscle, which is heavier than fat. Regular exercise of any kind may help to perk up a flagging appetite. If eating and exercising more do not cause at least a modest weight gain, see your doctor to be sure you don't have a medical condition such as a thyroid problem affecting your weight.

Preventing weight gain associated with starting diabetes treatment may be as simple as eating slightly smaller servings than you are used to and getting more regular activity, such as a daily walk. Of course, any lifestyle change takes time and practice to make permanent, so even these small changes to your routine will take attention and effort.

Learning to prevent and treat hypoglycemia can also help to prevent unwanted weight gain. In most cases, the recommended treatment for raising a blood glucose level below 70 mg/dl is to consume 15 grams of carbohydrate. (If blood glucose is very low, more carbohydrate may be necessary.) However, many people eat or drink more than 15 grams of carbohydrate in response to low blood glucose. Not only can this lead to high blood glucose later in the day, but over time it can lead to weight gain. If you are experiencing frequent episodes of hypoglycemia, see your doctor or diabetes educator for help in preventing it. A self-help program called Blood Glucose Awareness Training (BGAT) may be of use to you.

If you need to lose weight for improved health, consider the tips in Chapter 9, such as keeping a food diary. You might also consider joining a group such as Overeaters Anonymous or TOPS (Take Off Pounds Sensibly). Outside support can be helpful when you're working on a challenging project like losing weight.

Beware of dietary supplements promoted for weight loss. Most are eventually shown to be useless, and some prove to be dangerous. It's tempting to want a quick fix, but there really are none for weight loss.

It's never too late

Some complications of diabetes, such as heart disease, may be reversible with aggressive lifestyle measures and medical intervention. Others, such as neuropathy and retinopathy, generally are not. However, taking steps now to improve your blood glucose control can prevent the progression of most complications and any further deterioration in comfort or function.

Even if complementary therapies cannot directly treat a diabetes complication, they can help indirectly by helping you to cope. Living with any medical condition is stressful, particularly if it causes pain, discomfort, or difficulty performing daily tasks and other activities. Learning relaxation techniques, making use of other mind–body therapies, and reaching out to others who can help or who are in a similar situation can help you find peace of mind, hope, and energy to face the future.

15. Developing a CAM Program

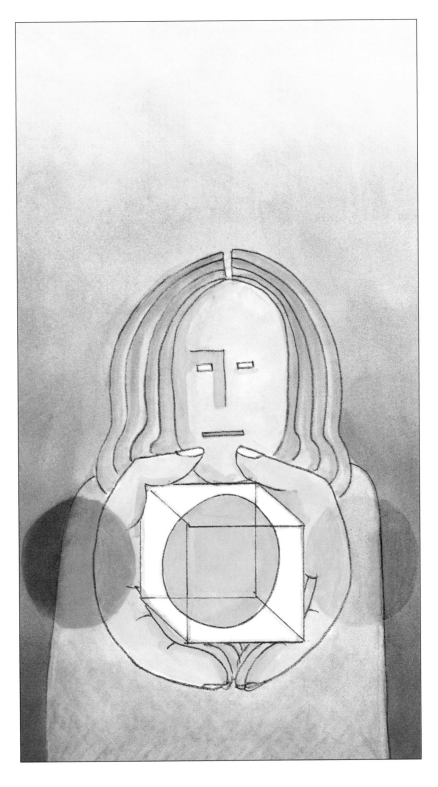

15.
DEVELOPING
A CAM PROGRAM

Ever since diabetes has been recognized as a disease, people have been trying to treat it or, better yet, cure it. Before the causes of diabetes were understood, physicians prescribed such treatments as horseback riding, eating large amounts of sugar, taking opium, and following a near-starvation diet.

With the discovery of insulin in 1921, development of oral drugs to treat Type 2 diabetes in subsequent years, and research leading to a greater understanding of nutrition, modern medicine has extended the life expectancy of people with diabetes. But controlling diabetes still requires carrying out a complex regimen of self-care, and many people have trouble doing this. Quality of life with diabetes remains a serious issue.

The desire for a better quality of life may be one of the main reasons people develop an interest in alternative and complementary therapies. To use such therapies effectively, however, it's important to have realistic expectations. No CAM therapies can cure diabetes, and most take some time and effort to use. But many CAM therapies can help to heal the body, mind, and spirit, leading to better blood glucose control.

Using the PARENT model

One approach to integrating complementary therapies into your diabetes control plan is to use the PARENT model. The acronym PARENT serves as a reminder that in taking care of yourself, you are in some ways acting as your own parent. The individual letters of the acronym stand for Positive thinking, Assertiveness, Relaxation, Exercise, Nutrition, and Touch.

Positive thinking. Maintaining a positive attitude can help you get through life, no matter what problems you face. However, having a positive attitude doesn't mean you can fix any problem. It means having the courage and self-confidence to change what you can change and also accepting that there are things you can't change—and believing that you can live well anyway.

Attitudes are believed to be influenced by both genetics and experience, so the parents you had and the way in which you were raised have a lot to do with the way you see the world as an adult. If positive thinking doesn't come naturally to you, there are various strategies that can help, such as using affirmations to help change your image of who you are. Learning to deal with stress, possibly through techniques such as prayer or meditation, is also invaluable to maintaining a positive attitude. Seeing a psychotherapist who uses cognitive-behavioral techniques or undergoing hypnotherapy can also help to change long-held attitudes that may be holding you back.

If life truly looks hopeless, you may be depressed, and you would do well to seek care from your physician or a mental health professional. Depression is an illness, and while it sometimes resolves with the "tincture of time," the tendency of many things to resolve if you simply wait, it cannot be willed away or "snapped out of," no matter how hard you try. On the positive side, however, it is treatable, and seeking help is an important first step.

Depression can also be a very lonely and isolating condition, but there are many support groups, both online and in-person, dedicated to helping people with depression. Support groups are not a substitute for professional help, but they can help you to feel less alone with your feelings.

Assertiveness. To many people, assertiveness means being able to speak up for yourself. But before you can do that, you need to learn to take your needs seriously so that other people will, too. It's hard to ask for help or ask someone to behave differently unless you truly believe you have the right to have the needs you have. The more comfortable you feel with yourself, the easier it is to express yourself directly, openly, and honestly, without violating the rights or stepping on the feelings of others.

While some people were encouraged as children to express their needs and look out for their own best interests, many were not. Those who were not tend to find it difficult to do so as adults. But it is possible to learn these skills as an adult. One way is to identify your weak spots (such as saying "no"), pick a problem area to work on, make a plan for what you will say or how you will act differently, and practice doing it. As you work on this, it's important to be aware of any negative self-talk and replace it with positive statements that reaffirm your worth as a human being, your right to express your needs and desires, and the importance of what you're doing.

Relaxation. Relaxation is not just about taking an occasional vacation on the beach. It's about finding a way to deal with everyday stresses so they don't damage your health.

Everyone responds to stress in some way, whether it's by pouring themselves a drink, exploding in anger, biting their nails, or taking a "time out" to cool down. The ways in which people deal with stress are usually learned early in life. They are partly patterned after how their parents dealt with stress and partly related to how they as children learned to cope with difficult family or school situations. Unfortunately, many of the ways in which people learn to deal with problems or negative emotions (such as fear or anger) are self-destructive or destructive to those around them. In addition, many common ways of responding to stress don't actually stop the body's stress

response, so real physical harm is done as levels of stress hormones remain high.

It is possible to learn new ways of coping with stress. Methods of relaxation training can be mind-based, such as meditation, or body-based, such as progressive relaxation. When practiced regularly—usually while a person is not feeling a large amount of stress—they can cause a person to react much more calmly when confronted with a problem.

Vacations on the beach, or simply taking some time for yourself occasionally to do something you enjoy, are important, too. Listening to music you like can both cheer you up and reduce feelings of anxiety. Taking the time to enjoy the aroma of a few drops of an essential oil in a bowl of warm water can have the same effect. Whatever you do to lower your stress reaction will have mental and physical payoffs.

Exercise. The benefits of physical activity for diabetes control are many, so it's worth the effort to choose an activity and do it regularly. You can often combine exercise with relaxation, particularly if you practice yoga or tai chi, which have a meditative aspect. But many forms of physical activity can have a mentally relaxing effect, particularly if being active gets your mind off work or other stressful thoughts.

What if you hate to exercise? Sometimes being a good parent means insisting on things that kids really don't want but that parents know won't hurt them and could be important later on. For example, few kids like getting shots, taking tests at school, or doing chores or homework when they'd rather be playing. But letting them avoid all that is unpleasant or difficult in life can lead to their getting sick, failing academically, and never learning how to take care of themselves or communicate well with others.

Making yourself exercise when you don't enjoy it takes discipline, but not self-abuse. Calling yourself "lazy" or berating yourself for missed workouts won't help. Just as a good parent shows compassion for a child who is anxious about auditioning for the school play—then insists that he go through with it anyway—so must you show compassion for your feelings, then find a way to deal with them so they don't stop you from getting the physical activity you need.

Nutrition. Feeding your body well may be the ultimate parenting task. What parent doesn't worry about whether his child is getting adequate nutrients for proper growth and development? As an adult, you need those nutrients to maintain what you've got and stay healthy into old age. Eating right may also help to stave off chronic conditions such as heart disease, cancer, and a variety of eye diseases.

Not eating correctly may mean that you are not taking the time to care for yourself properly. A hectic lifestyle is not a healthy lifestyle. Taking supplements cannot make up for a healthy lifestyle, but it can serve as a cue that you may need to readjust your priorities and slow down. When you take more time to plan and prepare meals, you may also find you enjoy the food more, and that's good for you, too.

Touch. Human touch often gets overlooked in a health-care plan, but it can be important to physical and mental health. Once again, this is an area in which the way you were raised can strongly influence how you feel and behave as an adult. People who were touched affectionately as children may be more comfortable with affectionate touching as adults. People who were not touched much or who were abused in some way are likely to be less comfortable with physical contact.

Culture also affects how readily or easily adults touch each other. In a culture that "allows" touch only between intimate partners or parents and their children, adults who don't have those types of relationships may have little touch in their lives.

Healing therapies that involve a nurturing, socially acceptable form of touch include massage in its various forms, bodywork, and some forms of biofield therapies. In addition to physical touch, getting in touch, or becoming more emotionally intimate with others—through support groups, for example—can be healing.

Stopping to smell the roses

In many ways, using alternative and complementary therapies is about really tuning in to yourself and your body to determine what you need and how best to meet those needs in constructive ways. It's about getting to know yourself and learning to take care of yourself. It's important to include your health-care providers in your decisions about the use of complementary therapies. While they may not always agree with you about your priorities or choices of therapies, they should be willing to discuss your choices with you, review the facts that support the therapy (you may need to do some homework on your own to provide them with information), express their concerns in a respectful way, and support you in your efforts to take responsibility for your health and well-being.

GLOSSARY OF TERMS

ACUPRESSURE The stimulation of specific points on the body using the fingers, elbows, or various devices. The goal of acupressure is the same as that of acupuncture: unblocking or balancing of the flow of vital energy, leading to a balancing of yin and yang.

ACUPUNCTURE The stimulation of specific points on the body by a variety of techniques, the most common being insertion of very fine needles. The goal of acupuncture is the unblocking or balancing of the flow of vital energy, leading to a balancing of yin and yang.

AFFIRMATION A positive statement.

ALEXANDER TECHNIQUE A technique for reeducating the neuromuscular system, allowing the release of habitual tension.

ALLOPATHIC A word sometimes used as a synonym for "conventional" or "Western" when speaking of medicine.

ALTERNATIVE MEDICINE A medical system, practice, or product used in place of conventional Western medicine.

AROMATHERAPY The use of essential plant oils for healing purposes.

ART THERAPY A therapeutic approach that uses art to address emotional and behavioral problems.

AURA The energy field that is said to emanate from living beings.

AUTOGENIC THERAPY A method of relaxation that combines visualization with self-suggestion.

AUTOIMMUNE DISORDER A disorder in which the immune system reacts against the body's own tissues and produces abnormal antibodies to attack those tissues. Type 1 diabetes is an example of an autoimmune disorder.

AYURVEDA The traditional healing system of India.

BARBARA BRENNAN HEALING SCIENCE A form of hands-on energy healing developed by one-time physicist Barbara Brennan.

BIOFEEDBACK A technique that uses various monitoring devices to help a person learn to voluntarily alter normally involuntary body functions or reactions such as brain activity, blood pressure, muscle tension, or heart rate.

BIOFIELD A field of energy believed by some to be in and around the physical body. In biofield therapies, the practitioner attempts to smooth, strengthen, or otherwise affect a person's biofield, usually with hand motions and sometimes touch.

BOWEN TECHNIQUE A gentle bodywork system that involves a unique "muscle rolling" technique. It was developed in Australia in the 1950's by Thomas Bowen.

CHAKRAS Centers of physical or spiritual energy in the body.

CHELATION THERAPY The use of intravenous infusions of a man-made amino acid called EDTA. In conventional medicine, chelation therapy is used to remove toxic metals from the blood. Unproven uses include using it to prevent heart disease or treat atherosclerosis.

There is also a technique in healing touch called chelation, whose purpose is to rid the body of energy blockages. It does not involve injecting substances into the body.

CHIROPRACTIC A medical system that uses manipulations of the spine and other joints to align the body and reduce any interference in nerve flow and function.

COGNITIVE-BEHAVIORAL THERAPY A form of psychotherapy that focuses not on past traumas but rather on present "cognitive distortions," or errors in perception, that would lead a person to conclude that life is hopeless or everyday life unmanageable.

COLON THERAPY The practice of using enemas or laxatives to clean or "detoxify" the colon. Also known as colonic irrigation.

COLOR THERAPY The use of color to alter mood, encourage relaxation, or otherwise support the healing process.

COMPLEMENTARY MEDICINE A medical practice or product that is used along with (not in place of) conventional treatment.

COMPRESS A pad soaked in hot or cold water or in an herbal infusion and applied to the body for relief from pain, inflammation, and swelling.

CONTRAINDICATION Reason not to take a particular drug, engage in a particular activity, or make use of a particular form of treatment. A contraindication could include taking another drug that would interact with the drug in question or having a medical condition that could be worsened by taking a particular drug or using a particular treatment.

CORTISOL A stress hormone produced by the adrenal glands that causes blood glucose levels to rise.

CRANIOSACRAL THERAPY A complementary, hands-on therapy intended to enhance the flow of cerebrospinal fluid through gentle palpation of the bones of the skull.

CUPPING A traditional Chinese practice of heating the air in a cup or similar vessel and placing it on the body to improve circulation or decrease pain in that area.

CYMATICS The study of the effects of sound waves on matter. The term "cymatic therapy" has been adopted by some holistic healers who believe that sound waves transmitted through the human body can normalize imbalances and synchronize the cells' frequencies, bringing them back to their natural, healthy state.

DAN TIEN In tai chi, the body center, from which all movement originates. It is located below the navel, centered between the front and back of the body. It can also be thought of as the body's center of gravity.

DECOCTION An herbal preparation similar to an infusion.

DIETARY SUPPLEMENT As defined in a law passed by Congress in 1994, a dietary supplement is a product intended to supplement the diet that contains vitamins, minerals, herbs or other botanicals, amino acids, or a combination of these substances. To be considered a dietary supplement, it must be intended to be taken as a tablet, capsule, powder, softgel, gelcap, or liquid. It cannot be marketed as a meal replacement.

DOSHAS In Ayurveda, the three primary life forces, called vata, pitta, and kapha, found in each cell of every human being.

EMETIC A substance such as an herb or medicine that stimulates vomiting.

EMOLLIENT Something that softens or soothes, such as a skin-moisturizing lotion.

ENDORPHINS Chemicals made by the body that have a chemical composition similar to that of morphine. They are released during exercise and laughter.

ENERGY THERAPY A therapy that is intended to affect a person's biofield (energy believed to be in and around the body) or that makes unconventional use of electromagnetic fields to influence health and healing.

ESSENTIAL OIL Concentrated extract taken from the roots, leaves, or blossoms of a plant.

EXTRACT A solution obtained by steeping or soaking a substance such as an herb, usually in water.

EYE MOVEMENT DESENSITIZATION AND REPROCESSING A psychological treatment technique that involves moving the eyes in a specific sequence or pattern while focusing the thoughts on personal concerns and fears.

FASCIA Connective tissue that holds the structures of the body together. Some forms of bodywork, such as Rolfing, specifically target tightness in the fasciae.

FELDENKRAIS METHOD A method of releasing habitual tension and learning to move more freely. This method can be done in group classes with verbal instructions or one-on-one, with the practitioner guiding a person's body through various motions.

FUNCTIONAL FOOD A food or component of food that may provide health benefits beyond the basic nutrition it provides.

GLYCEMIC INDEX A ranking of carbohydrate-containing foods on a scale of 0 to 100 based on how quickly the food raises blood glucose levels after eating. The higher the number, the more rapidly digested and absorbed the food.

GLYCEMIC LOAD The glycemic index of a food multiplied by the number of grams of carbohydrate in a serving, divided by 100. Calculating the glycemic load of a food portion helps to predict the effect it will have on blood glucose level.

GUIDED IMAGERY A technique that uses the imagination to achieve personal goals, reduce pain, and bring about emotional and physical healing.

HEALING TOUCH A type of energy therapy developed by nurse Janet Mentgen.

HELLERWORK A form of bodywork that integrates techniques from Rolfing along with movement reeducation and dialogue to increase awareness of the connection between body and mind.

HERBAL MEDICINE The use of plants for healing purposes.

HOLISTIC MEDICINE An approach to medicine that treats the whole person, including the body, mind, and spirit.

HOMEOPATHY An alternative medical system in which individuals are given highly diluted substances called "remedies" that purportedly would produce the same or similar symptoms of illness in a healthy person if given in larger doses. These remedies are believed to stimulate the body's defenses to prevent or treat illness.

HOMEOSTASIS The body's dynamic state of equilibrium. In spite of continuous changes in the external environment, the body is able to maintain relatively stable internal conditions.

HYDROTHERAPY The scientific use of water to treat disease.

HYPNOTHERAPY A form of therapy that makes use of hypnosis, a state of focused concentration in which a person is more open to suggestion.

INFUSION The most common way of preparing herbs for consumption; usually referred to as a tea.

INTERCESSORY PRAYER A prayer said by an individual or group on behalf of another person.

JIN SHIN JYUTSU A way of harmonizing energy flow in the body through gentle pressure on particular points.

KETONES Acidic by-products of fat metabolism. Trace amounts of ketones in blood and urine are normal, but large amounts may indicate that a person's diabetes is out of control. Large amounts of ketones in combination with very high blood glucose levels and dehydration can lead to diabetic ketoacidosis, a life-threatening condition.

KI The Japanese word for life force or vital energy.

KINESIOLOGY The study of the principles of mechanics and anatomy in relation to human movement. "Applied kinesiology" is an unproven system of determining health imbalances through the identification of weakness in specific muscles.

KIRLIAN PHOTOGRAPHY A photographic technique that purportedly captures an object's aura, or energy field.

LABYRINTH An intricate path with no dead ends. Walking through a labyrinth can have a meditative quality.

LYMPHATIC SYSTEM The system of organs that return fluid leaked from the blood (called lymph) to the blood vessels and that help cleanse the blood. These organs also house cells involved in immunity.

MACROBIOTIC A way of life as well as of eating. The mostly vegetarian diet involves balancing yin foods with yang foods. Despite claims, it has not been shown to cure cancer, and it can be nutritionally unbalanced.

MANTRA A word or phrase used as an object of concentration and repeated aloud or silently during transcendental meditation.

MEDITATION A way of focusing the attention on a sound, word, image, or process such as breathing for the purpose of quieting the mind and body.

MEGADOSE A large dose. When speaking of vitamins, a megadose is usually one that is much larger than the recommended dietary allowance.

MELATONIN A hormone secreted by the pineal gland that appears to regulate the sleeping-waking cycle. It is also sold as a dietary supplement and taken to help with sleep problems caused by shift work or jet lag, although studies have shown it to be largely ineffective for these uses.

MERIDIANS Channels in the body through which vital energy, or qi, is believed to circulate.

METABOLISM A broad term referring to all the chemical reactions within the body that are necessary to maintain life. It includes the breakdown of food into simpler substances as well as the building of larger molecules or structures from smaller ones.

MONOCHROMATIC INFRARED THERAPY A treatment in which a device that emits infrared light is placed on areas of the body, such as the feet, with the goal of increasing nitric oxide concentration, and therefore blood circulation, to that area. The best-known device for delivering this form of treatment is the Anodyne Therapy system.

MOXIBUSTION A traditional Chinese medicine technique in which dried mugwort, an herb, is burned over a specific acupuncture point to expel cold, warm the meridians, and increase the flow of energy.

MUSIC THERAPY The therapeutic use of music to explore psychological problems, enhance relaxation, alter mood, or affect heart rate, blood pressure, breathing, or other bodily functions.

MYOTHERAPY Also known as Bonnie Prudden myotherapy, this form of massage uses deep finger pressure on specific points to control muscle spasms and other muscle-related conditions.

NATUROPATHY An alternative medical system that places emphasis on supporting the body's natural healing ability and on treating the causes of ill health rather than just the symptoms.

NEPHROPATHY The type of kidney disease most commonly associated with diabetes.

NEUROPATHY Nerve damage. Diabetic neuropathy is believed to be caused primarily by high blood glucose levels.

NUTRACEUTICAL A food or part of a food thought to provide medical or health benefits. While this term is used to market various products, it has no regulatory definition in the United States.

ORTHOMOLECULAR MEDICINE A medical system that focuses on the use of proper nutrition to maintain and restore health. It uses combinations of vitamins, minerals, and amino acids normally found in the body to treat specific conditions. It is sometimes referred to as megavitamin therapy.

OSTEOPATHIC MEDICINE A mainstream (not alternative) medical system that places emphasis on the role of the musculoskeletal system in bodily functioning. A system of manipulation is used to restore proper structure and therefore function.

PALPATE To examine by touch.

PANACEA A remedy for all ills and difficulties; a cure-all.

PATENT The grant of a property right to an inventor. A patent gives the inventor the right to exclude others from making, using, offering for sale, selling, or importing his invention. The fact that a dietary supplement or device is patented does not mean that it has been proven safe or effective or that it is endorsed by the U.S. Patent and Trademark Office.

PHYTOCHEMICALS Chemicals found in plants. Some phytochemicals may have health benefits for humans, which is one of the reasons nutrition experts recommend eating a variety of fruits and vegetables and not relying solely on supplements for vitamin intake.

PILATES METHOD A system of body conditioning known particularly for strengthening the core (abdominal) muscles.

PLACEBO An inactive substance or sham procedure. Placebos are often used in research studies to test the efficacy of the real drug or procedure.

PLACEBO EFFECT Improvement in a person's condition that cannot be considered due to the treatment. It is well known that believing in a remedy can lead to recovery or an improvement in symptoms, even if the remedy is inert.

POLARITY THERAPY A healing approach based on the idea that there are areas on the body that hold positive and negative charges, which drive electromagnetic currents in and around the body. The therapy incorporates a variety of techniques, from reflexology to nutrition to massage, to balance the energy field.

PROGRESSIVE RELAXATION A relaxation technique in which a person tenses then relaxes his muscles in a particular sequence. It is hoped that by paying attention to the sensation of a relaxed versus a tensed muscle, the person will eventually be able to relax tense muscles at will, without going through the whole sequence.

POULTICE A soft, warm, moist mass—of herbs, for example—spread between layers of cloth and applied to the skin to relieve pain and inflammation.

PRANA The term used in Indian medicine for life force or vital energy.

PRANAYAMA The name for breathing exercises in yoga.

PROBIOTICS Foods or supplements that contain helpful living microorganisms that support and maintain a healthy digestive tract.

PURGATIVE A medicine that causes the evacuation of the bowels; a laxative.

QI The Chinese word for life force or vital energy, pronounced "chee."

QIGONG A Chinese form of exercise that includes breathing exercises, visualizations, meditation, and physical exercises.

REFLEXOLOGY A bodywork system in which pressure is applied to points on the feet, hands, and ears to unblock energy flow and enhance health in other parts of the body.

REIKI A way to activate the universal life force for the purposes of healing. In Reiki, energy is believed to flow from the universal to the practitioner to the person needing healing. Most Reiki treatments do not involve physical contact between healer and the person being healed.

ROLFING METHOD FOR STRUCTURAL INTEGRATION A system for stretching tight fasciae to increase freedom of movement, reduce chronic pain and tension, and improve body alignment.

ROSEN METHOD A form of bodywork that combines gentle massage with verbal observations about patterns of muscle tension in a person's body. The purpose is to increase awareness of the mind–body connection and tap into the unconscious.

SHAMANISM A religion characterized by belief in an unseen spirit world. Priests, or shamans, are able to call upon the spirit world for guidance in healing or curing people who are ill.

SHIATSU A type of Japanese massage in which pressure is applied with the fingers to acupuncture points to promote healing as well as relaxation.

SPORTS MASSAGE A variety of massage developed to meet the needs of athletes.

STANDARDIZED On a dietary supplement label, "standardized" means the product contains a set amount of an active compound.

SWEDISH MASSAGE The type of massage most commonly used in the United States. Massage has been found to relieve stress and muscular tension, reduce pain from injuries, and speed healing from certain acute and chronic conditions.

TAI CHI An exercise system that evolved from an ancient Chinese form of martial art. Its movements are slow and flowing.

TENS (transcutaneous electrical nerve stimulation) An approach to pain relief in which an electric current is applied to certain nerves to stop them from conducting pain messages to the brain. TENS may also stimulate the body to produce natural painkillers.

THERAPEUTIC TOUCH A touch-free form of bodywork in which the healer "manipulates" a person's energy field by passing his hands over the person's body while feeling compassion for him.

THOUGHT FIELD THERAPY (Callahan Technique) A mind–body therapy in which the therapist asks a person to think about a troubling situation or event, then tap with two fingers on a series of acupressure points on the body. The combination of thinking and tapping is believed to eliminate distress.

TINCTURE A usually alcohol-based herbal preparation, with the alcohol acting as a natural preservative.

TOXIN Poisonous substance.

TRAGER APPROACH A method of bodywork in which the therapist rocks, rotates, pulls, or shakes various parts of a person's body to undo patterns of chronic muscle tension.

TRANCE In hypnosis, a state of focused concentration.

TRIGGER POINTS Areas of tightness or tenderness in the muscles. Trigger points are known to refer pain to other areas of the body.

ULTRASOUND Ultra-high-frequency sound above the range that can be heard by humans. It is used to produce images of the insides of the body and to break up kidney stones.

VASOCONSTRICTION Narrowing of the blood vessels.

VASODILATION Dilation, or enlargement, of the blood vessels.

VIBRATIONAL THERAPY Also known as sound energy therapy, this approach is based on the belief that sound waves of various frequencies can help heal the body.

VISUALIZATION A mind–body technique in which a person visualizes a particular scene or allows his mind to flow freely and notices what images come in.

YOGA A system of exercise to bring together the physical, mental, and spiritual energies for the enhancement of health and well-being. Yoga combines physical movements with meditation, breathing exercises, and sometimes chanting.

ZONE THERAPY A practice that led to the development of reflexology. In zone therapy, the body is divided into ten zones. Each zone is believed to correspond to points in the hands and feet. Applying pressure to these points is believed to bring relief to organs in the corresponding zone.

COMPLEMENTARY AND ALTERNATIVE THERAPIES AT A GLANCE

Many of these therapies and practices make use of the mind–body connection to relieve both mental and physical symptoms of stress. The safety of those that are not strictly self-help measures depends on finding practitioners that are properly trained and appropriately certified or licensed in their area of expertise.

THERAPY	USED FOR	PRECAUTIONS
Acupressure	Pain and stress reduction.	Pressure should not be applied to wounds, scars, or areas of inflammation. Extra caution is needed when used by people with blood vessel disease or by pregnant women.
Acupuncture	Nausea, pain, addiction, asthma, stroke rehabilitation.	Generally considered safe.
Affirmations	Thinking more positively about yourself.	Care is needed to create positive affirmations; negative affirmations will not help change beliefs or behaviors.
Alexander Technique	Release of habitually held muscle tension.	Requires many lessons to unlearn old habits; increased awareness of old, "bad" habits can cause increased physical and emotional discomfort if new habits are not yet learned.
Applied kinesiology	Diagnosing medical conditions.	Unproven technique; should not be used in place of conventional medical care for serious health concerns.
Aromatherapy	Relaxation, stimulation, improved mood, pain reduction.	Essential oils should not be ingested. Women who are pregnant and people with asthma or epilepsy should use extra caution. Sensitivity to oils can develop.

THERAPY	USED FOR	PRECAUTIONS
Art therapy	Expressing and processing feelings through creation of art, developing personal insight.	Can provoke strong emotional reactions.
Auriculotherapy	Pain reduction, substance abuse.	May cause ear soreness.
Autogenic therapy	Mental and physical relaxation.	People with abnormal blood pressure or heart disease should consult a doctor before using this technique.
Biofeedback	Controlling blood pressure, asthma, incontinence, and other medical conditions.	Generally considered safe.
Bowen Technique	Pain and stress relief.	Generally considered safe.
Breathing techniques	Relaxation, more effective exercise practice, minimizing asthma or panic attacks.	Generally considered safe.
Chelation	Removal of toxic chemicals from the blood; atherosclerosis.	Use as a treatment for atherosclerosis unproven.
Chiropractic	Some types of chronic low back pain.	Use of chiropractic manipulations is not appropriate treatment for all forms of neck or back pain; having an accurate diagnosis is a must.
Cognitive-behavioral therapy	Emotional distress caused by negative thinking patterns.	None, as long as the therapist is properly trained and licensed.
Colon therapy	Detoxification.	No proven need for colon cleansing. Frequent use of enemas can cause dependency on them for bowel movements.

THERAPY	USED FOR	PRECAUTIONS
Color therapy	Any number of conditions.	Generally considered safe.
Craniosacral therapy	Relaxation.	Safe, but should not be used in place of conventional medicine for serious illness.
Cymatic therapy	Healing diseased organs through sound waves.	Safe, but should not be used in place of conventional medicine for serious illness.
Dance therapy	Expressing and processing feelings through movement. Improved self-esteem and body image.	None, as long as physical limitations are respected.
Drumming	Improved mood, improved physical fitness, enhanced communication skills.	None.
Eye Movement Desensitization and Reprocessing	Treatment of post-traumatic stress disorder.	This treatment method should only be practiced by properly trained, licensed psychotherapists.
Feldenkrais Method	Pain relief, freedom of movement.	None.
Guided imagery	Achieving personal goals, improving sports performance, reducing stress.	None.
Healing touch	Pain relief, relaxation.	Generally considered safe.
Hellerwork	Greater awareness of the mind–body connection.	Should not be used by people with serious bone or blood diseases or cancer.
Homeopathy	Used for any number of ailments.	Relying on homeopathy rather than seeking conventional treatment for a serious illness is not recommended.
Hug therapy	Promoting happiness and feelings of human connection.	Sensitivity to your and to other people's comfort level with physical touching is required.

THERAPY	USED FOR	PRECAUTIONS
Hydrotherapy	Muscle relaxation, pain relief.	Hot water and hot compresses should not be applied to the feet and lower legs of people with peripheral neuropathy.
Hypnotherapy	Changing old habits and thought patterns, reducing pain and nausea, overcoming phobias.	Generally considered safe.
Jin Shin Jyutsu	Stress reduction.	Generally considered safe.
Joint mobilization	Increasing range of motion.	Safe, as long as therapy is provided by a trained practitioner.
Journaling	Increased self-knowledge, stress management.	None.
Labyrinth walking	Developing personal insight.	None.
Laughter	Reducing stress, improving mood.	None.
Light therapy	Reducing pain and inflammation, speeding healing.	Generally considered safe but may cause eyestrain, headache, and insomnia.
Low-level laser	Pain reduction, speeding wound healing.	Considered an experimental therapy.
Magnet therapy	Pain relief	Pregnant women; people who use pacemakers, defibrillators, or insulin pumps; people who wear patches that deliver medicine; and people with acute sprains, wounds, or infections are discouraged from using magnet therapy.
Massage	Stress relief, relief of muscle tension, pain relief.	Massage therapist must be informed of all health conditions before treatment so that precautions can be taken.
Mindfulness meditation	Reducing stress.	None, as long as a person has no serious mental disorders.

Therapy	Used for	Precautions
Monochromatic infrared energy therapy	Painful neuropathy.	Safe if used correctly.
Music therapy	Stress reduction, pain reduction, improved mood, improved physical fitness, enhanced communication skills.	None.
Orthomolecular medicine	Any number of medical problems.	Should be practiced only by qualified practitioners.
Pilates	Strengthening the abdominal muscles.	Some postures may not be recommended for people with some forms of retinopathy.
Polarity therapy	Pain and stress relief.	Dietary recommendations may affect blood glucose control.
Positive thinking	Feeling more in control in life.	None.
Prayer	Stress-related conditions.	None, as long as a person has no serious mental disorders.
Progressive relaxation	Mental and physical relaxation.	If tensing and relaxing the muscles causes pain or muscle spasms, some other relaxation technique should be used.
Qigong	Physical conditioning and mental relaxation.	Not recommended for people with serious mental disorders.
Reflexology	Encouraging energy flow in the body.	People who have circulation problems or foot problems should consult a health-care provider before using reflexology.
Reiki	Reducing anxiety and depression, speeding healing, counteracting the side effects of various cancer treatments.	Generally considered safe.
Relaxation response	Reducing stress.	None, as long as a person has no serious mental disorders.

THERAPY	USED FOR	PRECAUTIONS
Rolfing	Stretching tight fasciae (connective tissue) to improve body alignment.	Should not be used by people with serious bone or blood diseases or cancer.
Rosen Method	Becoming aware of emotions through patterns of muscle tension.	Not a substitute for psychotherapy.
Shiatsu	Neck, shoulder, and lower back problems; arthritis; depression; and anxiety,	Shiatsu practitioner must be informed of all health conditions before treatment so that precautions can be taken.
Tai chi	Physical conditioning and improved balance.	Generally considered safe, but people with serious health issues should consult a doctor first.
Therapeutic touch	Relaxation, wound healing, pain reduction.	Generally considered safe.
Thought field therapy	Post-traumatic stress disorder, phobias, anxiety, depression.	This treatment method should only be practiced by properly trained, licensed behavioral health or medical professionals.
Trager Approach	Releasing patterns of tension in movement and posture.	Generally considered safe.
Trigger point therapy	Relief of soft-tissue pain and dysfunction.	Therapist must be informed of all health conditions before treatment so that precautions can be taken.
Ultrasound	Reducing pain and inflammation resulting from injuries. Speeding bone fracture repair.	Generally considered safe.
Visualization	Reducing stress.	None.
Yoga	Physical fitness, mental relaxation.	Some postures may place too much pressure on the feet; others may not be recommended for people with some forms of retinopathy.

SETTING UP AN EXERCISE PROGRAM

There are at least three components to physical fitness: strength, endurance, and flexibility. Resistance training can help to build muscular strength and endurance. Stretching can help to build and maintain flexibility. Both have numerous benefits, not least of which is simply feeling better and making it easier to perform activities of daily living.

To be on the safe side, see your doctor before beginning an exercise program to check for any heart problems or other conditions that might affect your choice of activity. Keep in mind that any activity that burns calories can affect your blood glucose level, and the only way to know how a particular type of exercise affects your blood glucose level is to monitor before and after the activity. Always keep glucose in some form with you when you exercise, and wear an identification bracelet or necklace saying that you have diabetes.

RESISTANCE EXERCISES FOR STRONGER MUSCLES

Resistance exercises can be done at home with small dumbbells, rubber exercise bands, your own body weight, or ordinary household objects such as small cans of soup. While resistance exercises are safe for most people, those with retinopathy should speak with their ophthalmologist before starting. In addition, people who have moderate or proliferative retinopathy should avoid doing any exercises that place the head below the heart.

Start with a weight that you can lift easily 12–15 times in a row without stopping. You may find you need lighter weights for some exercises and heavier weights for others. Wherever you are now is fine. As you gain strength, you can increase the weight.

As you lift (or push or pull), engage your abdominal muscles to support your back. If you need to arch your back to perform an exercise or you develop back pain after your workout, you are probably trying to lift too much and should lighten your load.

FRONT RAISE
1. Use small, unopened soup cans, filled water bottles, or small dumbbells for this exercise.
2. Start with your arms at your sides. With your palms facing down, lift arms to the front until they are parallel to the floor. Return to starting position.
3. Repeat 12–15 times.

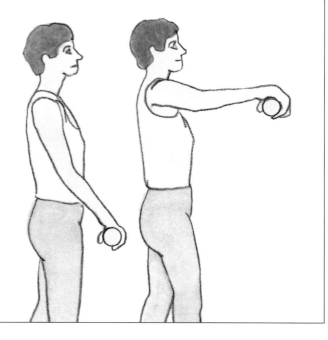

SIDE LATERAL RAISE

1. Use small, unopened soup cans, filled water bottles, or small dumbbells for this exercise.

2. Start with your arms at your sides. With palms facing down, lift arms to sides until they are parallel to the floor. Return to starting position.

3. Repeat 12–15 times.

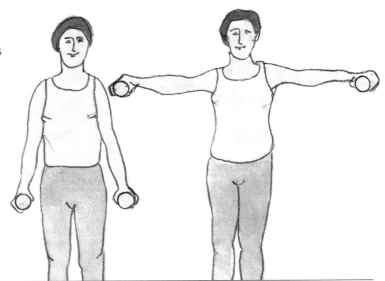

PUNCHES

1. Use small, unopened soup cans, filled water bottles, or small dumbbells for this exercise.

2. Start with your elbows bent, hands at chest level. Extend one arm forward, pull it back, and extend the other arm, keeping your palms facing down.

3. Repeat 12–15 times.

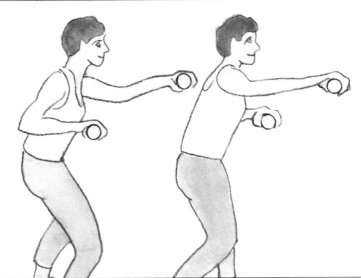

KICKBACKS

1. Use small, unopened soup cans, filled water bottles, or small dumbbells for this exercise.

2. Bend forward slightly from the hips and bend your knees slightly. Hold your weights at hip height, and elbows pointing back. Straighten your elbows, extending your forearms and hands back. With arms extended, raise your weights as high as you can (another couple of inches). Return to starting position.

3. Repeat 12–15 times.

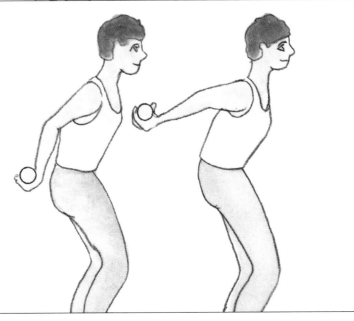

WALL PUSH-UP

1. Stand 24–36 inches from a wall and extend your arms towards the wall, keeping your hands lower than your shoulders.

2. Lean against the wall with your arms straight.

3. Bend your elbows and touch your nose to the wall, *keeping your back straight.* Push back to starting position.

4. Repeat 12–15 times. This exercise uses your body weight as the source of resistance.

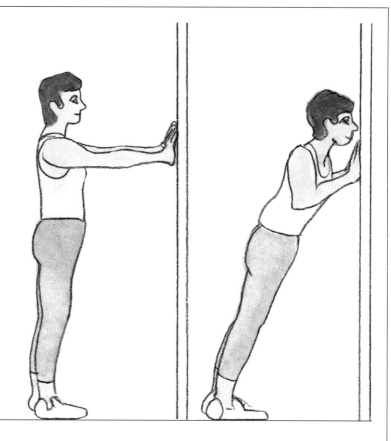

TOE TOUCH

1. Stand with your feet shoulder-width apart and your arms out to each side, parallel to the floor.

2. Bend your knees, then bend forward from the hips and touch your left foot with your right hand.

3. Return to starting position and repeat with your left hand and right foot.

4. Repeat 12–15 times. This exercise uses your body weight as the source of resistance.

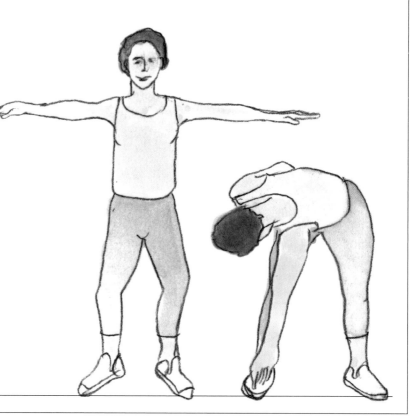

For these exercises, pick a weight you can lift or press 12–15 times without stopping to rest. If you have a history of frozen shoulder or other shoulder problems, start with very light weights or no weight at all.

OVERHEAD PRESS
1. For beginners, a good starting weight is 1 to 5 pounds.
2. Hold your weights to either side of your head, elbows at shoulder height. Extend your arms overhead, straightening your elbows. Return to starting position.
3. Repeat 12–15 times.

4. If this exercises hurts, stop doing it and don't resume until you have talked to your doctor about it.

UPRIGHT ROW
1. Start by holding your dumbbells in front of your thighs. Pull the weights up to your armpits; your elbows should be slightly above shoulder height. Return to starting position.
2. Repeat 12–15 times.

BICEPS
1. Stand with your arms at your sides, knees bent slightly. Keeping your upper arm still, bring your hands toward your shoulders, bending only at the elbow. Lower your hands slowly to starting position.
2. Repeat 12–15 times.

OVERHEAD EXTENSION
1. Hold one weight behind your head, elbow pointing to the side. Extend your arm upward by straightening your elbow; your arm will be at a slight angle, not perpendicular to the floor. Return to starting position.
3. Repeat 12–15 times.
4. Repeat exercise with your other arm.

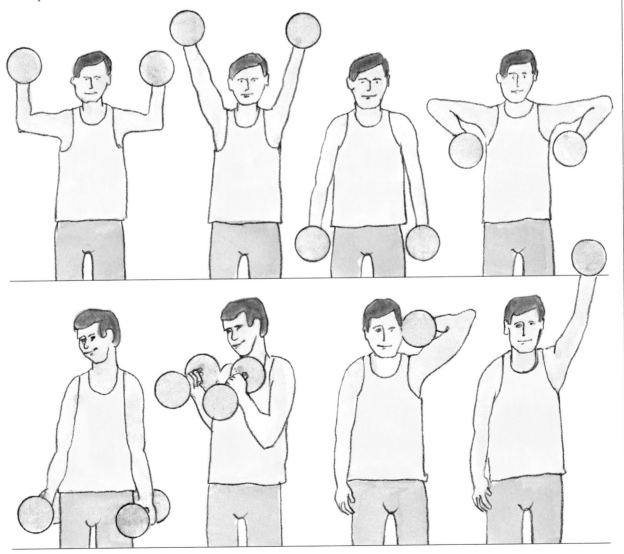

Use a rubber exercise band for these exercises.

DOOR PULL

1. Select a resistance you can pull 15 times in a row, and be careful to release the resistance in a slow, controlled manner. Allowing the band to "snap" your arm back to its starting position can injure your joints.
2. To maintain your balance, stand with one foot ahead of the other (as if you were taking a step).

3. Place one end of the rubber band around the doorknob of an open door (or have a partner hold it), and hold the other end in your hand.
4. Keeping your arm bent at a 90-degree angle, pull away from the door (or your partner), then return to your starting position, releasing the tension slowly.
5. Repeat 12–15 times, then switch hands.

DOOR PUSH

1. Place one end of the band around the doorknob of an open door, and hold the other end in your right hand. Standing with your right side to the door, hold your right hand at shoulder height in front of you, elbow bent, palm facing toward you. Push the band forward until you feel resistance. Return to your starting position, releasing the tension slowly.
2. Repeat 12–15 times, then place your left side to the door and do the exercise with your left hand.

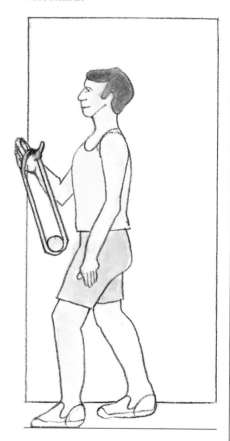

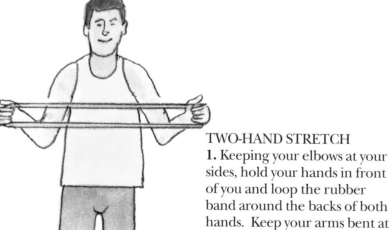

TWO-HAND STRETCH

1. Keeping your elbows at your sides, hold your hands in front of you and loop the rubber band around the backs of both hands. Keep your arms bent at a 90-degree angle.

2. Slowly move your hands away from each other so that you feel resistance from the band.
3. Return to your starting position, releasing the tension slowly.
4. Repeat 12–15 times.

SEATED RESISTANCE EXERCISES

These exercises are particularly good for people who use a wheelchair, because they help to build the pelvic, abdominal, and upper-body strength needed to sit with good alignment and transfer oneself in and out of the chair.

UPPER BACK, ARM, AND NECK STRENGTHENER

This exercise will help you improve your posture, feel more in control of your balance, and present a more assertive image. Because it places the head below the level of the heart, however, it may not be appropriate for people with retinopathy.

1. Sit squarely on your chair. Visualize and try to position your ears directly over your shoulders, shoulders over hips, and thighs firmly on the chair seat. Your shins should be perpendicular to the floor. As you do this exercise, focus on your balance and the sensations you feel in your arms, legs, torso, and feet.

2. Raise both arms straight overhead so they are pointing to the ceiling. With your mouth closed, breath in deeply through your nose. Exhale through your nose and bend forward, hinging at your hips, until your torso is resting on your thighs; allow your arms to drop toward the floor. Relax your neck, and lower your head.

3. Inhale, raising your arms alongside your ears and elevating your head slightly until your face and arms are parallel with the floor. Raise your torso up one or two inches off your thighs. Visualize and hold your spine as straight as possible. Stretch your head, arms, and shoulders as far beyond your knees as you comfortably can.

4. Hold this off-balance position for three full in-and-out breaths. Return to the beginning, upright, seated position.
5. Repeat this exercise three or more times every other day. You should see an improvement in your balance in two to three months.

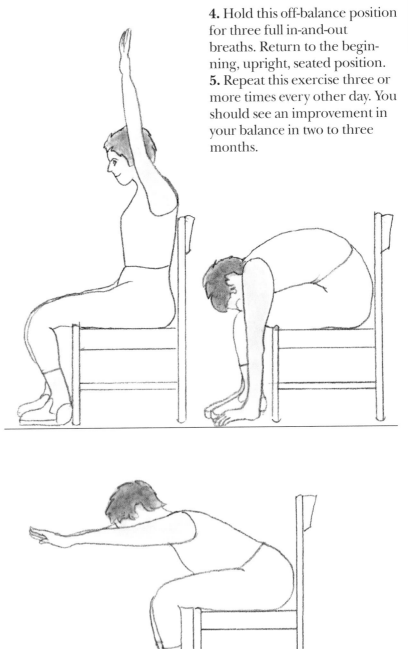

LOWER TORSO STRENGTHENER

This exercise is for people who have control of the muscles in their abdomen, pelvis, and buttocks.

1. Sit as tall and straight as possible. Using your abdominal muscles, pull your navel toward your spine until you feel the middle of your back straighten toward the chair back. You may need to tilt your pelvis forward to get your back to straighten. Tighten your abdomen and buttocks. Hold this position for up to six seconds. Release and relax.

2. Repeat five more times for a total of six. It may take several practice sessions to engage all of the muscles in the area or to keep them contracted for six seconds.

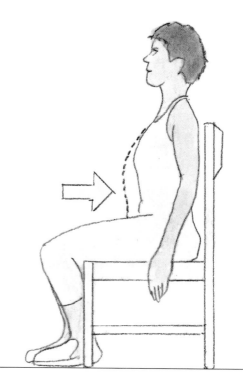

ABDOMEN AND THIGH STRENGTHENER #1

This exercise requires the ability to lift your thighs.

1. Sitting erect, lift your right thigh toward your chest using only your thigh and abdominal muscles. Do not assist with your hands. Hold your thigh off the seat for up to six seconds, then relax.

2. Repeat five more times with your right leg, then switch to the left leg. It may require several sessions before you can repeat or hold this position while counting to six.

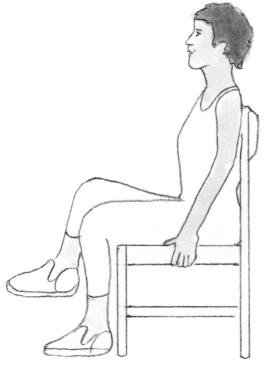

Setting Up an Exercise Program

ABDOMEN AND THIGH STRENGTHENER #2

Choose this method if your abdomen protrudes over your thighs.

1. Sit erect. Press down firmly with the sole of your right foot onto the floor or a footrest. Continue pressing and hold for a count of six.

2. Alternatively, extend your right leg so the knee is straight. Press forward firmly with the sole of your right foot against a wall or other stationary object. Hold for a count of six. Release and relax.

3. Repeat either exercise a total of six times with the right leg, then repeat with the left leg. It may require several sessions to develop the ability to do the exercise six times or to hold it for six counts.

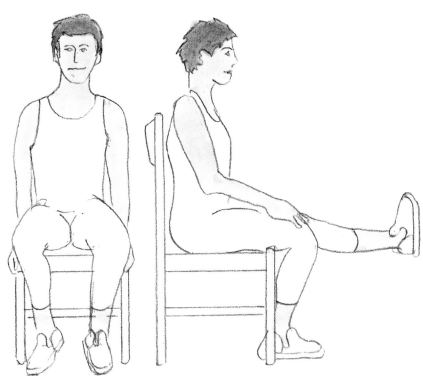

UPPER ARM STRENGTHENER

This exercise makes transferring to and from a wheelchair easier; it can also make lifting objects easier. Practice this on a firm seat, not on a soft cushion.

1. Place your right hand on the edge of the seat beside your right thigh, palm down, fingers pointed toward floor, and left hand beside your left thigh, palm down, fingers pointed toward floor.

2. Push down with the heels of your hands to lift yourself slightly off the seat. Hold for up to six seconds. Release and relax.

3. Repeat five more times for a total of six times. It may take several sessions to gain sufficient strength to repeat or to get to a six-second count.

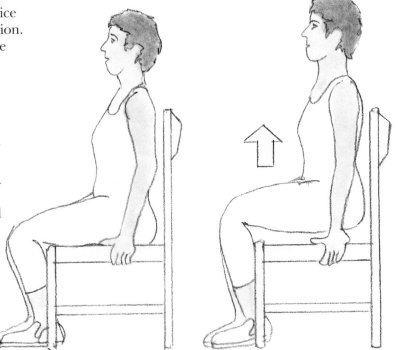

SHOULDER FLEXIBILITY

1. While seated, place your right hand on your left knee and your left hand on your right knee. (Alternatively, place your hands on the forward ends of opposite chair arms.)

2. Open both arms out to your sides just above the chair arms.

3. Bringing your arms up to shoulder level, cross extended arms in front of you.

4. Open your arms out to sides again, this time above shoulder level.

5. Cross your extended arms again in front of you at shoulder level.

6. Open your arms again out to sides just above the chair arms.

7. Return to beginning position, with hands on opposite knees or chair arms.

8. Repeat this series of movements for a total of six times.

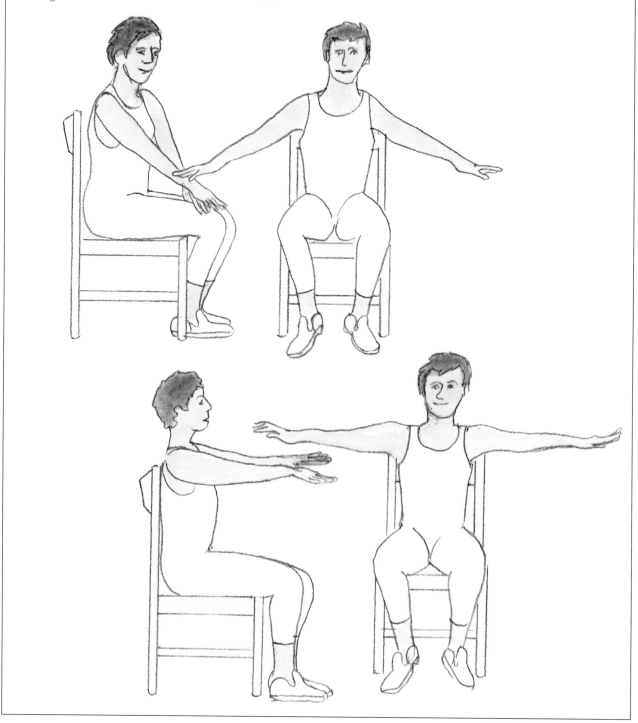

ARM CIRCLES

1. Sitting upright, extend your arms out to your sides at shoulder level.

2. Keeping them straight, move both of your arms in large circles backward five times, then in large circles forward five times.

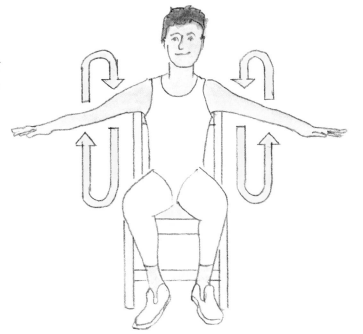

WRIST FLEXER AND STRENGTHENER

1. Rest your forearms, palms down, on your thighs or chair arms; your hands should be extended beyond the ends of your knees or the arms of the chair. Curl your hands into a loose fist. Raise your hands, bending only at the wrists; keep forearms in resting position. Relax wrists, returning fists to level position. Repeat five more times.

2. Turn arms over so palms are facing up. Curl your hands into loose fists. Raise your hands, bending only at the wrists. Return hands to level position. Repeat five more times.

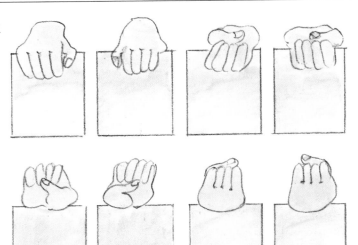

FINGER STRENGTHENER

1. Make a circle with your little finger and thumb. Press the end of the finger and the end of the thumb tightly together to strengthen the finger muscles.

2. Then make a circle with your ring finger and thumb, pressing them together tightly.

3. Repeat with middle finger and forefinger, then do the same on other hand.

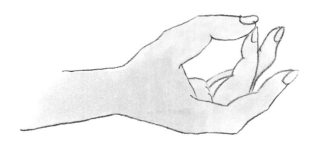

EXERCISES FOR IMPROVED BALANCE

Many people with diabetes have balance problems, sometimes due to aging and sometimes due to complications of diabetes such as peripheral neuropathy, which can cause a loss of sensation in the feet. Without balance, it's hard to get around and to pursue an active lifestyle. The good news is that balance can often be improved. The exercises that follow can help.

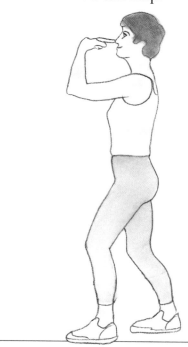

NOSE TOUCHER

1. Stand with your right leg approximately 24 inches in front of your left, bend your knees slightly, and try to touch your nose with one finger. The more in line your feet are with each other, the more challenging this will be. Repeat 10 times.
2. Switch your left leg to the front. Repeat 10 times.
3. Once you can do it well with either leg in front of the other, try this with your eyes closed.

HEEL RAISES

1. Hold on to a sturdy chair for balance, rise up onto your toes, then lower your heels back to the ground. Repeat 10–15 times.
2. Progress to touching the chair with one finger for balance, not holding on at all, and doing the exercise with your eyes closed.

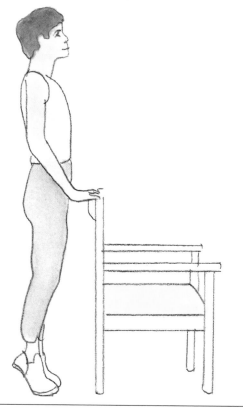

MARCHING

1. Hold on to a sturdy chair for balance and lift your right knee up toward your chest, then lower it to the floor. The left knee can be bent slightly while you do this. Repeat 10–15 times with the right leg, then do it with the left leg.
2. Progress to touching the chair with one finger for balance, not holding on at all, and doing the exercise with your eyes closed.
3. For more of a challenge, alternate the marching between the left and right leg instead of doing sets with one leg at a time.

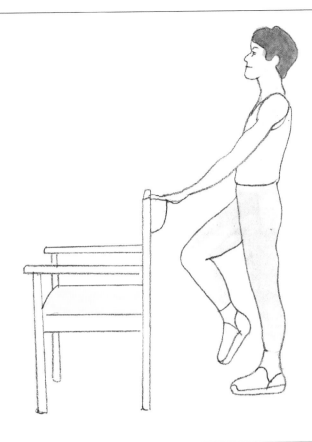

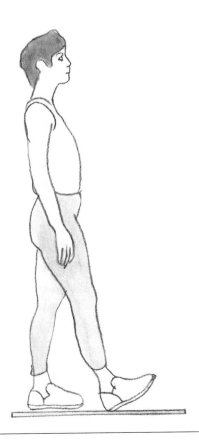

WALK A STRAIGHT LINE

1. Look for a straight line on the floor (such as a line of floor tiles) and try to walk along it. The key here is to land with one foot directly in front of the other and also to land on your heel first. Hold on to the wall if necessary.
2. For variety, try walking with your arms extended out then relaxed at your sides.
3. For more of a challenge, try walking forward to one end then backward to the other.
4. For even more of a challenge, try walking with your eyes closed, but only walk with your eyes closed if someone is there to assist you.

Setting Up an Exercise Program

SIDE LEG RAISE

1. Hold on to a sturdy chair for balance and lift your right leg out to the side. Your left knee can be bent slightly while you do this. Repeat 10–15 times with the right leg, then do the left leg.

2. Progress to touching the chair with one finger for balance, not holding on at all, and doing the exercise with your eyes closed.

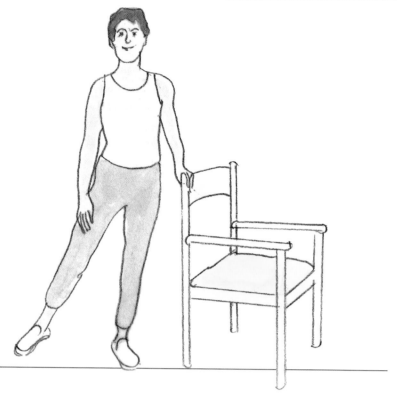

STEP-UPS

1. Stand in front of a staircase and step up with your right foot, then up with your left, then down with your right, then down with your left. Repeat 10 times.

2. If you need a little support, hold on gently to the railing, or just touch the wall with a fingertip. You may be surprised at how much balance that gives you.

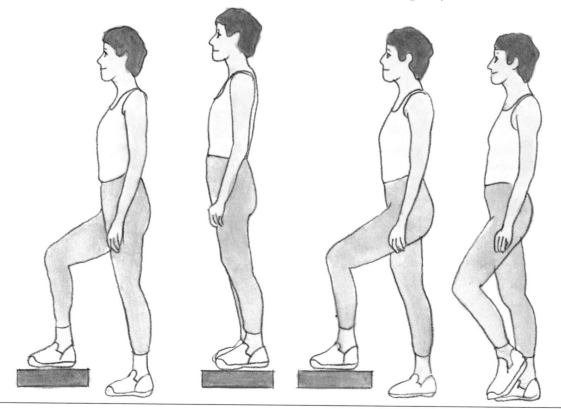

SIT–STANDS

1. Sit on the edge of a sturdy chair and stand up without swinging your arms forward. Sit back down slowly. Repeat 10 times.

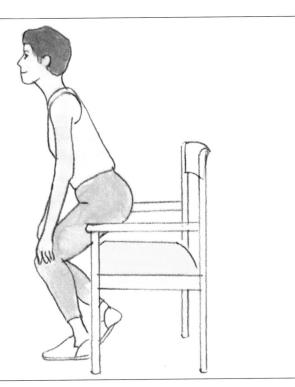

BIRD-DOG

1. Start on your hands and knees. Your knees should be right below your hips, and your hands right below your shoulders.

2. Contract your abdominal muscles and lift one arm, holding it out in front of you for 2–5 seconds. Place it back on the floor and lift the other arm, holding it out in front of you for 2–5 seconds. Next lift one leg, holding it out straight for 2–5 seconds. Place it back on the floor and lift the other leg for 2–5 seconds.

3. For a more advanced exercise, contract your abdominal muscles and simultaneously lift one arm and the opposite leg. Hold for 2–5 seconds, then switch. Repeat 5–10 times on each side.

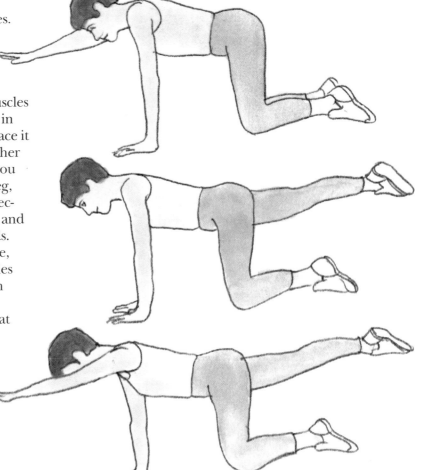

Setting Up an Exercise Program

FOUR-SQUARE STEP TEST

This is an advanced exercise. Only do this if someone is there to assist you.

1. Lay two towels or ropes on the floor to form a cross, as illustrated.
2. Stand in square 1 facing square 2.
3. Step forward into square 2, sideways into square 3, backward into square 4, sideways into square 1, sideways into square 4, forward into square 3, sideways into square 2, and backward into square 1.
4. Move slowly at first until you get the hang of it. As your skill improves, move faster.

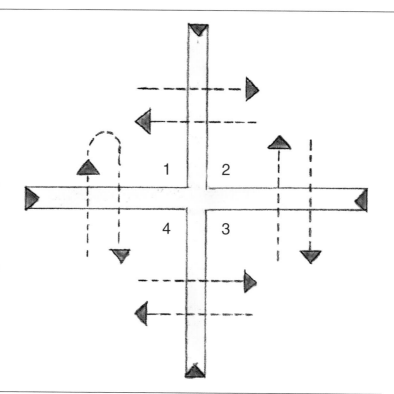

WOBBLE BOARD EXERCISES

A wobble board is a wooden or plastic board with a rise on the bottom, which makes the board unstable. Standing on the board and attempting to balance will improve your balance.

1. Hold onto the back of a chair or lightly touch a wall with your hand for balance. Step onto the board with both feet and balance.
2. While standing on the board, slowly rock from side to side without letting the front or the back of the board touch the floor. Keep your torso upright and your neck, shoulders, and arms relaxed. Rock from side to side for 30–60 seconds.
3. Now rock from front to back for 30–60 seconds.
4. Once you get the hang of it, try doing these exercises without holding onto anything with your hand.
5. For the most advanced step, try doing these exercises with your eyes closed. However, only do this with your eyes closed if someone is there to assist you.

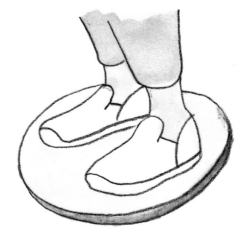

STRETCHES

The stretches shown here are *static* stretches. The proper technique is to stretch the muscle or muscle group until you feel mild tension, hold that position until the muscle feels looser, then stretch a little further.

Stretching is safe for most people, but people who have moderate or proliferative retinopathy should check with their health-care provider before starting any exercise or stretching program. If given the go-ahead, they should avoid doing any stretches that place the heart lower than the waist or that involve holding the breath and straining, which can raise blood pressure.

SIDE BEND
1. Stand with legs shoulder width apart, toes pointing forward, and knees slightly bent.
2. Place one hand on your hip and reach the other hand straight up, toward the ceiling.
3. Slowly bend to the side, toward the hand that's on your hip.
4. Repeat on the other side.

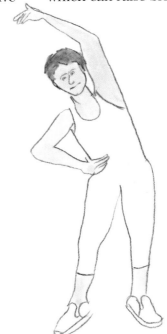

TORSO ROTATION
1. Stand 12–24 inches in front of a wall with your back to the wall.
2. With feet shoulder width apart and toes pointing forward, slowly turn your torso toward the wall until you can place both hands on the wall at shoulder height. Rotate back to facing forward.
3. Turn in one direction and then the other.

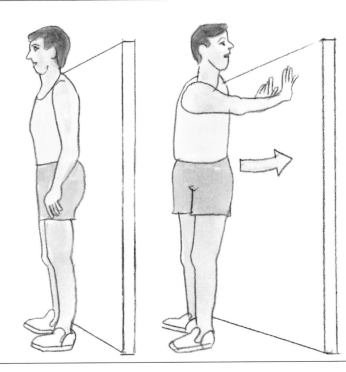

FORWARD BEND

1. Start in a standing position with legs shoulder width apart and toes pointing forward.

2. Keeping the knees slightly bent, bend forward from the hips until you feel a slight stretch in the backs of your legs. Let your head and arms hang freely, and don't bounce.

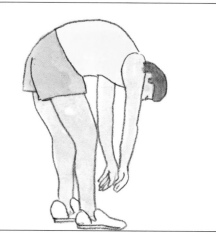

TOTAL BODY STRETCH

1. Lie on your back and extend your arms overhead.

2. Reach your arms and legs in opposite directions as far as is comfortable. Hold for several seconds then relax. This stretch can also be done in a standing position.

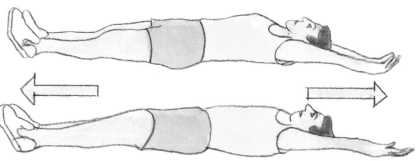

KNEES TO CHEST

1. Lie on your back and pull your knees into your chest with your hands for a stretch in the hip and buttock region.

2. To vary the stretch, pull one knee in at a time.

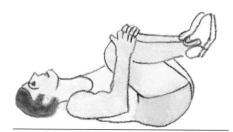

ARM AND SHOULDER STRETCH

1. Interlace your fingers then push your hands out in front of you, palms facing out and arms straight, with hands at about eye level.

2. Hold for a few seconds, then release.

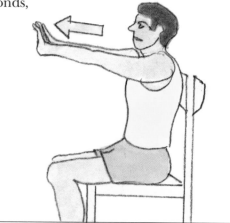

Setting Up an Exercise Program

SEATED SIDE STRETCH

1. Extend both arms overhead, then grasp the outside of your left hand with your right hand.
2. Lean to the right, feeling the stretch along your left side.
3. Return to center, then grasp the outside of your right hand with your left hand and lean left.

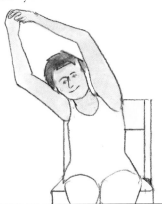

CHEST STRETCH

1. Interlace your hands behind your head, keeping your elbows pointed out to the sides.
2. Imagine pulling your shoulder blades together across your back so that your elbows point even further back.

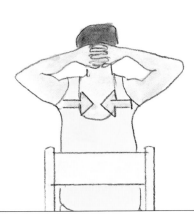

SEATED BACK STRETCH

1. With feet resting firmly on the floor, bend forward from your hips and rest your torso on your thighs as your arms and head hang freely.

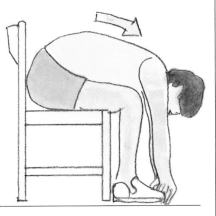

NECK STRETCHES

1. Keeping your back straight, slowly lean your head to the left, as if you were reaching your left ear toward your left shoulder.
2. Repeat on your right side, reaching your right ear toward your right shoulder.
3. Bend your head forward, feeling the stretch in the back of your neck and upper back.

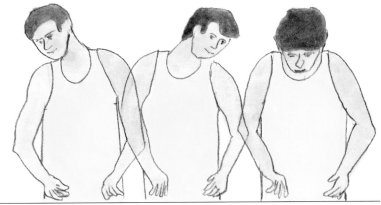

CALF STRETCH

1. Stand facing a wall or other solid support and place your forearms on the wall, head resting on hands if desired.
2. Place one foot several inches from the wall and bend the knee of that leg. Place the other foot 12–24 inches behind you and keep that leg straight. Both heels should remain on the floor at all times, and toes should be pointing forward.
3. Gently move your hips forward, toward the wall, keeping your back leg straight and your lower back flat.
4. Switch legs and repeat.

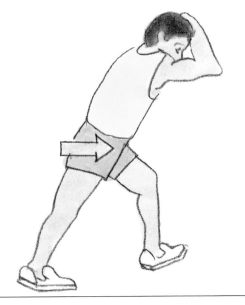

QUADRICEPS STRETCH

1. Position yourself between two chairs, one in front of you to hold onto for balance and one in back of you to place your foot on.
2. Extend one leg behind you and place your foot on the chair (or table or couch). Keep the knee of the leg you're standing on slightly bent.
3. Flex your buttocks so that the elevated thigh comes forward a bit and you feel a stretch on the front of your elevated thigh.
4. Switch legs and repeat.

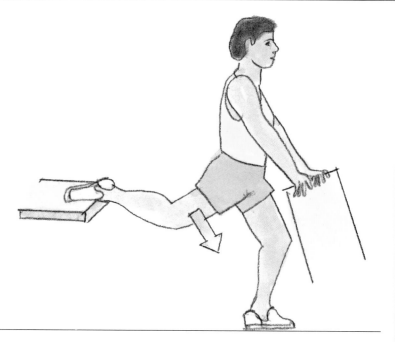

SEATED HAMSTRING STRETCH

1. Sit on the floor with one leg extended to the side and one leg bent so that the foot touches the inner thigh of the straight leg.
2. Rotate your torso toward the extended leg and bend at the hips toward that leg until you feel a stretch along the back of your leg.
3. For more of a stretch, loop a towel around the ball of your foot and gently pull your toes toward your knee.
4. Repeat with the other leg extended.

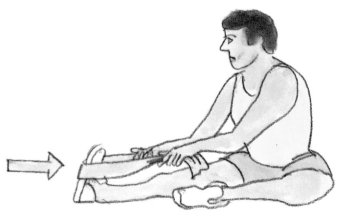

KNEE CROSSOVER

1. Lie on your back and bend one knee at a 90-degree angle. Extend the arm on that side of your body out to the side (resting on the floor).
2. Grasp the bent knee with the opposite hand and pull it across your body.
3. Keeping your shoulders and head on the floor, turn your head away from the bent knee, toward the extended arm.
4. Pull the bent knee toward the floor until you feel a stretch in your hip and lower back.
5. Repeat on the other side.

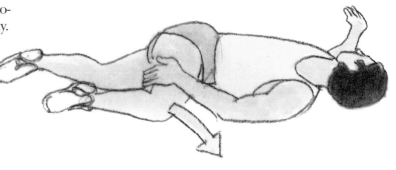

SUPER FOODS

Do you want to get the most nutrients possible from the foods you eat? If so, you need to know about super foods. Super foods are ordinary foods with extraordinary benefits. They have been shown to prevent disease, enhance health, and possibly extend the life span. In most cases, super foods are unprocessed, so they retain their naturally occurring nutrients.

BEANS AND LEGUMES

ADZUKI BEANS (*also called* AZUKI, ADUKI)

Serving size: ½ cup, cooked

Per serving:
Calories:. 147
Carbohydrate: . . . . 28 g
Protein:. . . . . 9 g
Fat:. . . . . 1 g
Saturated fat: . . . . 0 g
Cholesterol:. . . . . 0 mg
Sodium:. 1 mg
Fiber:. . . . . 7 g
Calcium: . . . . 43 mg
Folate: . . . . 128 mcg

Good source of:

folate, fiber, protein, potassium, phosphorus, iron, zinc, copper, manganese

Description:
Adzuki beans are small, dark red, roundish-oval beans, with a whitish "seam" on one side where the bean attaches to its pod. Adzukis originally hailed from Asia, and they are very important in Chinese and Japanese cuisine and culture, as evidenced by their appearances in festival dishes. Adzuki beans are somewhat sweet, and in Japan they are often used to make red bean paste, or sweet, dense, bean-based confections called *wagashi*. Adzuki beans are also cooked with rice.

Health benefits:
For centuries, beans and other legumes have been a cornerstone of the human diet. Scientists are showing a new interest in these nutritional powerhouses, which are now understood to have a host of health-promoting benefits.

Beans are low in fat, rich in protein, and high in both soluble and insoluble fiber. They are also packed with micronutrients and phytochemicals. As an additional boon, a serving of beans provides complex carbohydrate that has both a low glycemic index and a low glycemic load. Beans also contain so-called "resistant starch," which is not readily converted to glucose. Research suggests that these factors promote improved blood glucose control and insulin responses among bean eaters. In addition, beans help promote heart health and appear to fight cancer risk. The revised 2005 USDA Dietary Guidelines for Americans recommend that Americans consume at least 3 cups of beans each week. In recognition of beans' importance to health promotion, the FDA recently issued the following dietary guidance message: "A diet including beans may help reduce the risk of heart disease and certain cancers."

Selection tips:
Adzuki beans are easiest to find in health-food stores, Asian markets, and some gourmet shops or by mail order. They are available both dried and canned.

Although dried beans are shelf-stable, they taste best the fresher they are. (Old beans might also take longer to cook.) When purchasing dried adzuki beans, look for uniformly shaped, deeply colored, smooth beans with unshriveled skins.

Canned beans should be purchased only in cans that have no dents or evidence of bulging or rust. Check the expiration date on both dried and canned beans.

Storage tips:
Store dried beans in an airtight container in a cool, dry place, preferably out of direct light, for up to one year.

Canned beans should also be stored in a cool, dry place and used before their expiration date.

Once cooked, beans can be kept in a covered container in the refrigerator for up to five days. Leftover canned beans should be transferred to a covered container before being stored in the refrigerator.

Cooked, drained beans can be frozen in a well-sealed container in the freezer for up to six months.

Preparation tips:
Sort through dried beans before cooking and remove any foreign matter (such as pebbles) or any beans that are shriveled, broken, oddly shaped, or split. Rinse the sorted beans well.

Next, soak the beans. Place them in a large bowl and cover with at least 3 inches of cold water. Leave them to soak in the refrigerator for at least six hours or overnight. Drain and rinse before cooking.

Alternatively, if you haven't planned ahead for a long cold soak, you can use the quicker hot-soak method. Place sorted, rinsed beans in a large saucepan or pot. Add enough cold water to cover the beans by at least 3 inches. Place the pot over medium heat and bring the beans to a boil. Skim off and discard the foam that usually forms, along with any beans that rise to the surface of the water. Boil the beans for two minutes, then remove the pot from the heat and cover it. Allow the beans to soak in the cooking water for one hour, then drain and rinse before cooking.

After soaking and rinsing the beans, place them in a saucepan and cover with a generous amount of cold water (there should be at least 3 inches of water over the top of the beans).

It's fine to season the water with fresh herbs, garlic, or a small amount of oil, but do not add salt or acidic ingredients such as citrus juice, tomatoes, or vinegar at this point because doing so will harden the outer wall of the beans, and they will not cook properly.

Bring the beans to a boil over medium heat. Once the beans come to a boil, lower the heat, cover partially, and simmer. Periodically skim off any foam that forms on the surface of the cooking water and discard.

About three-quarters of the way into the cooking time, begin to test the beans. (You can add any acidic or salty ingredients at this point.) Simply bite into a bean—if it is uniformly cooked inside and has a soft, tender texture, the beans are ready. Avoid overcooking beans, or they will become mushy.

Adzuki beans take approximately 1 to 1½ hours to cook.

Beans can also be cooked in a pressure cooker. They will cook much faster, but might be less flavorful and the texture mushier. The foam from the cooking beans can clog the valve on the pressure cooker, so it's critical to first bring the beans to a boil without the cover and skim off any foam. Add one to two teaspoons of oil to the water before attaching the cover to prevent more foam from forming while the beans are under pressure.

Try adzuki beans with rice or other grains. Or play up their sweet side and stir mashed, cooked adzuki beans into vanilla frozen yogurt or low-fat ice cream for a homemade version of red bean ice cream. Adzukis are also a nice textural contrast to fruit and an interesting addition to baked goods.

Precautions:
Adzuki beans are rich in potassium, providing 612 milligrams per half-cup serving. Those on potassium-restricted diets should consult a registered dietitian or doctor before consuming adzuki beans.

Beans can cause harmless but potentially unpleasant gastrointestinal distress, usually in the form of gas, if they aren't soaked and drained. This is because beans are rich in oligosaccharides, a class of sugar molecules that humans can't digest easily.

The fresher the beans and the longer they are soaked, the more oligosaccharides will be removed. Don't forget to drain the beans and use fresh cooking water, or you'll end up keeping all of the oligosaccharides that were in the soaking water. Skimming off and discarding any foam that forms on the surface of the water as the beans cook will further reduce the oligosaccharides.

BLACK BEANS (*also called* TURTLE BEANS and *FRIJOLES NEGROS*)

Serving size: ½ cup, cooked

Per serving:
Calories:. 114
Carbohydrate: . . . . 20 g
Protein:. . . . . 8 g
Fat:. . . . . 1 g
Saturated fat: . . . . 0 g
Cholesterol:. . . . . 0 mg
Sodium:. 4 mg
Fiber:. . . . . 4 g
Calcium: . . . . 24 mg
Folate: . . . . 128 mcg

Good source of:
protein, fiber, iron, magnesium, phosphorus, potassium, manganese, copper, zinc, anthocyanins

Description:
Black beans are small to medium, plump oval-shaped beans that have a small white spot where the bean attaches to its pod. The skins are a deep, purplish black, while the interior is a creamy white color.

Black beans are native to Central and South America and are important in the cuisines throughout those regions, as well as in Mexico and the Caribbean. They are one of the integral ingredients in *feijoada*, the national dish of Brazil.

Health benefits:
Researchers are now learning that like other plant foods, beans are an excellent, though previously overlooked source of antioxidants. It appears that the darker the bean's seed coat, the greater antioxidant activity it possesses. Black beans take the cake in that arena, thanks to their high concentration of anthocyanins.

Among beans' myriad health benefits, they are linked to lower cancer rates; the antioxidants they contain are likely a factor.

Low-fat, high-protein beans are rich in both soluble and insoluble fiber, which benefits lipid profile, blood pressure, and overall heart health. The resistant starch in beans helps to promote improved glycemic control and insulin response.

The revised 2005 USDA Dietary Guidelines for Americans recommend that Americans consume at least 3 cups of beans each week, and the FDA recently issued the following dietary guidance message: "A diet including beans may help reduce the risk of heart disease and certain cancers."

Selection tips:

Black beans are commonly found in supermarket or health-food stores. They are available both dried and canned.

Although dried beans are shelf-stable, they taste best the fresher they are. (Old beans might also take longer to cook.) When purchasing dried black beans, look for uniformly shaped, smooth beans, with unshriveled skins.

Canned beans should be purchased only in cans that have no dents and no evidence of bulging or rust. Check the expiration date on both dried and canned beans.

Storage tips:

Store dried beans in an airtight container in a cool, dry place, preferably out of direct light, for up to one year.

Canned beans should also be stored in a cool, dry place and used before their expiration date.

Once cooked, beans can be kept in a covered container in the refrigerator for up to five days. Leftover canned beans should be transferred to a covered container before being stored in the refrigerator.

Cooked beans can be frozen in a well-sealed container in the freezer for up to six months.

Preparation tips:

Sort through dried beans before cooking and remove any foreign matter (such as pebbles) or any beans that are shriveled, broken, oddly shaped, or split. Rinse the sorted beans.

Next, soak the beans. Place them in a large bowl and cover with at least 3 inches of cold water. Leave them to soak in the refrigerator for at least six hours, or overnight. Drain and rinse before cooking.

Alternatively, if you haven't planned ahead for a long cold soak, you can use the quicker hot-soak method. Place sorted, rinsed beans in a large saucepan or pot. Add enough cold water to cover the beans by at least 3 inches. Place the pot over medium heat and bring the beans to a boil. Skim off and discard the foam that usually forms along with any beans that rise to the surface of the water. Boil the beans for 2 minutes, then remove the pot from the heat and cover it. Allow the beans to soak in the cooking water for one hour, then drain and rinse before cooking.

After soaking and rinsing the beans, place them in a saucepan and cover with a generous amount of cold water (there should be at least 3 inches of water over the top of the beans).

It is fine to season the water with fresh herbs, garlic, or a small amount of oil, but do not add salt or acidic ingredients such as citrus juice, tomatoes, or vinegar, at this point because this will harden the outer wall of the beans, and they will not cook properly.

Bring the beans to a boil over medium heat. Once the beans come to a boil, lower the heat, cover partially, and simmer. Periodically skim off any foam that forms on the surface of the cooking water and discard it.

About three-quarters of the way into the cooking time, begin to test the beans. (Any acidic or salty ingredients can be added at this point.) Simply bite into a bean—if it is uniformly cooked inside and has a soft, tender texture, the beans are ready. Avoid overcooking beans, or they will become mushy.

Black beans take approximately 1½ hours to cook.

Beans can also be cooked in a pressure cooker. They will cook much faster but might be less flavorful and the texture mushier. The foam from the cooking beans can clog the valve on the pressure cooker, so it is critical to first bring the beans to a boil without the cover and skim off any foam. Add one to two teaspoons of oil to the water before attaching the cover to prevent more foam from forming while the beans are under pressure.

Black beans are great in burritos or quesadillas, but they're so pretty it seems a shame to hide them. Mix them into salsas or serve over rice. Cooked, rinsed black beans are wonderful tossed with corn kernels, diced peppers, avocado, and lime vinaigrette, and served chilled.

Black beans are a nice addition to zucchini fritters and make amazing veggie burgers.

Play up black beans' inherent purple pigments by pureeing them into a dip or soup. Or emphasize their sweet quality by cooking them into rice pudding or by adding black bean puree to brownie recipes.

Precautions:
Beans can cause harmless though potentially unpleasant gastrointestinal distress, usually in the form of gas, if they aren't soaked and drained. This is because beans are rich in oligosaccharides, a class of sugar molecules that humans can't digest easily.

The fresher the beans, and the longer they are soaked, the more oligosaccharides will be removed. Don't forget to drain the beans and use fresh cooking water, or you'll end up keeping all of the oligosaccharides that were in the soaking water. Skimming off and discarding any foam that forms on the surface of the water as the beans cook will further reduce the oligosaccharides.

Adding baking soda to the soaking or cooking water is not recommended. This practice can destroy thiamine (vitamin B_1), decrease the overall nutrient availability of the beans, and make them taste soapy.

CHICKPEAS (*also called* GARBANZO BEANS and CECI)

Serving size: ½ cup, cooked

Per serving:
Calories:.....................134
Carbohydrate: ....21 g
Protein:.......................7 g
Fat:..........................2 g
Saturated fat: ....0 g
Cholesterol:..................0 mg
Sodium:.....................6 mg
Fiber:........................6 g
Calcium: ....40 mg
Folate: ....141 mcg

Good source of:
protein, fiber, folate, iron, copper, zinc, manganese, calcium

Description:
Since antiquity, chickpeas—which are believed to have originated in the Middle East-have been important in the cuisines there and throughout North Africa, India, and the Mediterranean. Chickpeas have a unique appearance that is unlike most other legumes. The ridged seeds have a roundish heart shape, with a divot on one side and a raised spine on the other. Buff-colored chickpeas are most commonly consumed in the United States, but there are darker brown, red, and green varieties as well. The chickpea's botanical name is a nod to its unusual appearance—*Cicer aretinum* refers to the zodiacal sign Aries, which means "ram" in Latin.

Health benefits:
Studies have found that chickpeas or breads made with chickpea flour raised blood glucose and insulin levels less than white bread among people who don't have diabetes.

Numerous other studies have found that bean consumption also promotes improved blood glucose control among those with diabetes. That beans seem to universally help keep blood glucose and insulin levels in check has important implications for both diabetes prevention and control.

For the above reasons and because they are so fiber-rich, beans are also helpful for weight management. Bean eaters tend to feel more satisfied after a meal that contains legumes and to go longer between meals.

A 2004 Spanish study found that chickpeas have a component that appears to significantly inhibit the growth of a certain type of cancerous cell and recommended further study into the legumes' potential cancer-fighting properties.

The revised 2005 USDA Dietary Guidelines for Americans recommend that Americans consume at least 3 cups of beans each week. In recognition of beans' importance to health promotion, the FDA recently issued the following dietary guidance message: "A diet including beans may help reduce the risk of heart disease and certain cancers."

Selection tips:
Chickpeas are commonly found in supermarkets or health-food stores. They are available both dried and canned.

Although dried beans are shelf-stable, they taste best the fresher they are. (Old beans might also take longer to cook.) When purchasing dried chickpeas, look for uniformly shaped beans.

Canned chickpeas should be purchased only in cans that have no dents and no evidence of bulging or rust. Check the expiration date on both dried and canned beans.

Storage tips:
Store dried chickpeas in an airtight container in a cool, dry place, preferably out of direct light, for up to one year.

Canned chickpeas should also be stored in a cool, dry place and used before their expiration date.

Once cooked, chickpeas can be kept in a covered container in the refrigerator for up to five days. Leftover canned chickpeas should be transferred to a covered container before being stored in the refrigerator.

Cooked, drained chickpeas can be frozen in a well-sealed container in the freezer for up to six months.

Preparation tips:
Sort through dried chickpeas before cooking and remove any foreign matter (such as pebbles) or any chickpeas that are shriveled, broken, oddly shaped, or split. Rinse the sorted beans.

Next, soak the chickpeas. Place them in a large bowl and cover with at least 3 inches of cold water. Chickpeas benefit from a longer soak than other beans. Soak them in the refrigerator for at least eight hours, and preferably overnight. Drain and rinse before cooking.

Alternatively, if you haven't planned ahead for a long cold soak, you can use the quicker hot-soak method. Place sorted, rinsed beans in a large saucepan or pot. Add enough cold water to cover the chickpeas by at least 3 inches. Place the pot over medium heat and bring the beans to a boil. Skim off and discard the foam that usually forms, along with any chickpeas that rise to the surface of the water. Boil the beans for 2 to 3 minutes, then remove the pot from the heat and cover it. Allow the chickpeas to soak in the cooking water for one hour, then drain and rinse before cooking.

After soaking and rinsing the beans, place them in a saucepan and cover with a generous amount of cold water (there should be at least 3 inches of water over the top of the beans).

It is fine to season the water with fresh herbs, garlic, or a small amount of oil, but do not add salt or acidic ingredients such as citrus juice, tomatoes, or vinegar at this point because this will harden the outer wall of the beans, and they won't cook properly.

Bring the beans to a boil over medium heat. Once the beans come to a boil, lower the heat, cover partially, and simmer. Periodically skim off any foam that forms on the surface of the cooking water and discard it.

About three-quarters of the way into the cooking time, begin to test the beans. (Any acidic or salty ingredients can be added at this point.) Simply bite into a bean—if it is uniformly cooked inside and has a soft, tender texture, the beans are ready. Avoid overcooking beans, or they will become mushy.

Chickpeas take approximately 2 to 2½ hours to cook.

Beans can also be cooked in a pressure cooker. They will cook much faster but might be less flavorful and the texture mushier. The foam from the cooking beans can clog the valve on the pressure cooker, so it is critical to first bring the beans to a boil without the cover and skim off any foam. Add one to two teaspoons of oil to the water before attaching the cover to prevent more foam from forming while the beans are under pressure.

Hummus, a Middle Eastern dip made from pureed chickpeas, can now be found in virtually every supermarket. Homemade hummus is infinitely more delicious, and it is remarkably easy to make. Just puree or food process cooked or canned chickpeas with garlic, lemon juice, olive oil, and whatever spices you prefer (cumin and coriander are traditional additions). Or, for a more rustic texture, simply mash the ingredients together with a fork. Stir in sesame tahini if you'd like. Use hummus as a dip for vegetables or as a spread for sandwiches and wraps. Hummus is also great with the fried chickpea patties known as falafel.

Try chickpeas in a Moroccan vegetable stew served over whole wheat couscous, or look to India for inspiration and add them to curried spinach and potatoes.

Toss chickpeas into pasta with sautéed greens or broccoli rabe, or add them to soups. Dress them with garlic, herbs, extra-virgin olive oil, and a generous squeeze of lemon and serve cold. Roasted chickpeas are a great party snack—toss the cooked legumes with olive oil and spices. Spread the chickpeas evenly on a cookie sheet and roast in a 450°F oven, stirring periodically until they are lightly browned and beginning to get crisp. Remove from the oven, place in a bowl, and serve with lemon wedges.

Precautions:

Beans can cause harmless though potentially unpleasant gastrointestinal distress, usually in the form of gas, if they aren't soaked and drained. This is because beans are rich in oligosaccharides, a class of sugar molecules that humans can't digest easily.

The fresher the beans and the longer they are soaked, the more oligosaccharides will be removed. Don't forget to drain the beans and use fresh cooking water, or you'll end up keeping all of the oligosaccharides that were in the soaking water. Skimming off and discarding any foam that forms on the surface of the water as the beans cook will further reduce the oligosaccharides.

Serving size: ½ cup, cooked

Per serving:
Calories:. 105
Carbohydrate: . . . . 19 g
Protein:. 7 g
Fat:. . . . . 1 g
Saturated fat: . . . . 0 g
Cholesterol: . . . . 0 mg
Sodium:. . . . . 2 mg
Fiber:. . . . . 5 g
Calcium: . . . . 61 mg
Folate: . . . . 91 mcg

Good source of:

calcium, iron, folate, fiber, protein, potassium, zinc, thiamine

Description:

Great northern beans are large, white, oblong beans related to kidney and pinto beans. They are the bean of choice in traditional Boston baked beans and are a key component in the classic French dish cassoulet. Great northerns are a good recipe stand-in for navy beans or cannellini beans if those varieties are unavailable.

Health benefits:

Beans are low in fat, rich in protein, and high in both soluble and insoluble fiber. They are also packed with micronutrients and phytochemicals. As an additional boon, a serving of beans provides complex carbohydrate that has both a low glycemic index and low glycemic load. Beans also contain so-called "resistant starch," which is not readily converted to glucose. Research suggests that these factors promote improved blood glucose control and insulin responses among bean eaters. What's more, beans help promote heart health and appear to fight cancer risk. The revised 2005 USDA Dietary Guidelines for Americans recommend that Americans consume at least 3 cups of beans each week. In recognition of beans' importance to health promotion, the FDA recently issued the following dietary guidance message: "A diet including beans may help reduce the risk of heart disease and certain cancers."

Selection tips:

Great northern beans are commonly found in supermarket or health-food stores. They are available both dried and canned.

Although dried beans are shelf-stable, they taste best the fresher they are. (Old beans might also take longer to cook.) When purchasing dried great northern beans, look for uniformly shaped, smooth beans with unshriveled skins.

Canned beans should be purchased only in cans that have no dents or evidence of bulging or rust. Check the expiration date on both dried and canned beans.

Storage tips:

Store dried beans in an airtight container in a cool, dry place, preferably out of direct light, for up to one year.

Canned beans should also be stored in a cool, dry place and used before their expiration date.

Once cooked, beans can be kept in a covered container in the refrigerator for up to five days. Leftover canned beans should be transferred to a covered container before being stored in the refrigerator.

Cooked beans can be frozen in a well-sealed container in the freezer for up to six months.

Preparation tips:

Sort through dried beans before cooking and remove any foreign matter (such as pebbles) or any beans that are shriveled, broken, oddly shaped, or split. Rinse the sorted beans.

Next, soak the beans. Place them in a large bowl and cover with at least 3 inches of cold water. Leave them to soak in the refrigerator for at least six hours or overnight. Drain and rinse before cooking.

Alternatively, if you haven't planned ahead for a long cold soak, you can use the quicker hot-soak method. Place sorted, rinsed beans in a large saucepan or pot. Add enough cold water to cover the beans by at least 3 inches. Place the pot over medium heat and bring the beans to a boil. Skim off and discard the foam that usually forms and any beans that rise to the surface of the water. Boil the beans for two minutes, then remove the pot from the heat and cover it. Allow the beans to soak in the cooking water for one hour, then drain and rinse before cooking.

After soaking and rinsing the beans, place them in a saucepan and cover with a generous amount of cold water (there should be at least 3 inches of water over the top of the beans).

It's fine to season the water with fresh herbs, garlic, or a small amount of oil, but do not add salt or acidic ingredients such as citrus juice, tomatoes, or vinegar, at this point, as this will harden the outer wall of the beans and they will not cook properly.

Bring the beans to a boil over medium heat. Once the beans come to a boil, lower the heat, cover partially, and simmer. Periodically skim off any foam that forms on the surface of the cooking water and discard.

About three-quarters of the way into the cooking time, begin to test the beans. (You can add any acidic or salty ingredients at this point.) Simply bite into a bean—if it's uniformly cooked inside and has a soft, tender texture, the beans are ready. Avoid overcooking beans or they will become mushy.

Great northern beans take approximately 1½ to 2½ hours to cook.

Beans can also be cooked in a pressure cooker. They will cook much faster but might be less flavorful and the texture mushier. The foam from the cooking beans can clog the valve on the pressure cooker, so it is critical to first bring the beans to a boil without the cover and skim off any foam. Add one to two teaspoons of oil to the water before attaching the cover to prevent more foam from forming while the beans are under pressure.

Great northern beans are beautifully versatile and are complemented by a wide range of savory herbs and spices. Try them in classic or vegetarian versions of cassoulet or make a stew of roasted vegetables and great northerns. Look to the Mediterranean for inspiration and serve them alongside ratatouille, or mash or puree them with lemon juice, garlic, and a drizzle of extra-virgin olive oil for a wonderful dip or sandwich spread. Puree great northern beans with broth for a simple and elegant soup, or try a more rustic approach and toss them into minestrone. Great northerns are also wonderful simply tossed with lemon-herb vinaigrette.

Precautions:

Beans can cause harmless but potentially unpleasant gastrointestinal distress, usually in the form of gas, if they aren't soaked and drained. This is because beans are rich in oligosaccharides, a class of sugar molecules that humans can't digest easily.

The fresher the beans, and the longer they are soaked, the more oligosaccharides will be removed. Don't forget to drain the beans and use fresh cooking water, or you'll end up keeping all of the oligosaccharides that were in the soaking water. Skimming off and discarding any foam that forms on the surface of the water as the beans cook will further reduce the oligosaccharides.

KIDNEY BEANS

Serving size: ½ cup, cooked, light red variety

Per serving:

Calories:................... 110
Carbohydrate: .... 20 g
Protein:.................... 8 g
Fat:....................... 0 g
Saturated fat: .... 0 g
Cholesterol: .... 0 mg
Sodium:................... 4 mg
Fiber:..................... 4 g
Calcium: .... 58 mg
Folate: .... 66 mcg

Good source of:

protein, fiber, folate, calcium, iron, potassium, copper

Description:

Kidney beans take their name from their distinctive shape and red color. There are both light and dark red kidney beans. The varieties have similar nutrient profiles, though light red kidney beans are slightly higher in calcium and iron. Kidney beans are often featured in chili, in red beans and rice, or in cold bean salads. Kidney beans can be used in place of small red beans.

Health benefits:

Beans are low in fat, rich in protein, and high in both soluble and insoluble fiber. They are also packed with micronutrients and phytochemicals. As an additional boon, a serving of beans provides complex carbohydrate that has both a low glycemic index and low glycemic load. Beans also contain so-called "resistant starch," which is not readily converted to glucose. Research suggests that these factors promote improved blood glucose control and insulin responses among bean eaters. Plus, beans help promote heart health and appear to fight cancer risk.

The revised 2005 USDA Dietary Guidelines for Americans recommend that Americans consume at least 3 cups of beans each week. In recognition of beans' importance to health promotion, the FDA recently issued the following dietary guidance message: "A diet including beans may help reduce the risk of heart disease and certain cancers."

Selection tips:

Kidney beans are commonly found in supermarket or health-food stores. They are available both dried and canned.

Although dried beans are shelf-stable, they taste best the fresher they are. (Old beans might also take longer to cook.) When purchasing dried kidney beans, look for uniformly shaped, smooth beans with unshriveled skins.

Canned beans should be purchased only in cans that have no dents and no evidence of bulging or rust. Check the expiration date on both dried and canned beans.

Storage tips:
Store dried beans in an airtight container in a cool, dry place, preferably out of direct light, for up to one year.

Canned beans should also be stored in a cool, dry place and used before their expiration date.

Once cooked, beans can be kept in a covered container in the refrigerator for up to five days. Leftover canned beans should be transferred to a covered container before being stored in the refrigerator.

Cooked beans can be frozen in a well-sealed container in the freezer for up to six months.

Preparation tips:
Sort through dried beans before cooking and remove any foreign matter (such as pebbles) or any beans that are shriveled, broken, oddly shaped, or split. Rinse the sorted beans.

Next, soak the beans. Place them in a large bowl and cover with at least 3 inches of cold water. Red kidney beans require longer soaking than other beans to reduce the risk of red kidney bean poisoning (see Precautions, below). They should be left to soak in the refrigerator for at least eight hours, and preferably overnight. Drain and rinse before cooking.

After soaking and rinsing the beans, place them in a saucepan and cover with a generous amount of cold water (there should be at least 3 inches of water over the top of the beans).

It is fine to season the water with fresh herbs, garlic, or a small amount of oil, but do not add salt or acidic ingredients such as citrus juice, tomatoes, or vinegar, at this point because this will harden the outer wall of the beans, and they will not cook properly.

Bring the beans to a brisk boil over medium heat. To ensure the destruction of the potentially toxic phytohaemagglutinin in red kidney beans, they must be boiled for at least 10 minutes and should be stirred periodically. After the beans have been adequately boiled, lower the heat, cover partially, and simmer for 45 to 60 minutes. Periodically skim off any foam that forms on the surface of the cooking water and discard it.

About three-quarters of the way into the cooking time, begin to test the beans. Slice a kidney bean in half—if it is still opaque inside, the beans should continue to cook. Properly cooked kidney beans should be tender throughout, with a soft, creamy texture.

Kidney beans take approximately 1½ to 2 hours to cook.

Kidney beans can also be cooked in a pressure cooker, which will achieve a high enough temperature to destroy the phytohaemagglutinins. They will cook much faster but might be less flavorful and the texture mushier. The foam from the cooking beans can clog the valve on the pressure cooker, so it is critical to first bring the beans to a boil without the cover and skim off any foam. Add one to two teaspoons of oil to the water before attaching the cover to prevent more foam from forming while the beans are under pressure.

Kidney beans complement rice well and are good additions to soup. Add them to burritos, or mash them to use as a sandwich filling. Kidney beans are a perfect choice for chili.

Precautions:
Consuming as few as four or five raw or improperly cooked red kidney beans can cause severe, rapid-onset food poisoning

characterized by nausea, vomiting, and diarrhea. Red kidney beans have a high concentration of phytohaemagglutinin (or lectin), which is toxic unless destroyed by high temperatures. Be sure to follow soaking and cooking directions carefully and boil red kidney beans for at least 10 minutes. Red kidney beans should not be cooked in slow cookers, which do not achieve sufficiently high temperatures to destroy the phytohaemagglutinins and might actually increase their toxicity. Red kidney beans should not be sprouted.

Adding baking soda to the soaking or cooking water is not recommended. This practice can destroy thiamine (vitamin B_1), decrease the overall nutrient availability of the beans, and make them taste soapy.

LENTILS, BROWN

Serving size: ½ cup, cooked

Per serving:
Calories:................... 115
Carbohydrate: .... 20 g
Protein:..................... 9 g
Fat:......................... 0 g
Saturated fat: .... 0 g
Cholesterol: .... 0 mg
Sodium:................... 2 mg
Fiber:...................... 8 g
Calcium: .... 19 mg
Folate: .... 179 mcg

Good source of:

protein, fiber, iron, folate, magnesium, potassium, thiamine, zinc

Description:
Archaeological evidence tells us that lentils—which originated in the Fertile Crescent—were among the earliest crops cultivated by Neolithic peoples. The small, round, lens-shaped seeds were important in many ancient cultures. They figure prominently in the biblical story of Esau, who sold his birthright to his brother Jacob for some lentil soup. Lentils were buried in the tombs of Egyptian pharaohs, and the ancient Greeks and Romans regarded them as both food and medicine. According to the Roman writer Pliny, lentils made an unconventional appearance in shipping; during Caligula's reign hundreds of thousands of bushels of the tiny pulses were used as ballast on the massive barge that transported an Egyptian obelisk to Rome. (The obelisk now stands in St. Peter's Square at the Vatican.) Lentils spread throughout the Mediterranean into Europe, North Africa, and Asia. They remain a staple in India, where they figure prominently in the cuisine as an important source of protein. In the United States, folks in Pullman, Washington, have celebrated the little seeds at the annual National Lentil Festival for almost two decades.

Health benefits:
Like other legumes, lentils are high in protein, fiber, micronutrients, and phytochemicals. The many components in lentils work together to promote a healthy lipid profile,

normal blood pressure, and overall heart health. Lentils have a sustained beneficial effect on postprandial glucose levels, which might benefit those with diabetes. The fiber and protein in lentils contribute to feelings of after-meal fullness, which plays a role in successful weight loss and weight management. Researchers at the Harvard School of Public Health discovered a lower risk of breast cancer among lentil eaters that they believed warranted further investigation. And a study conducted in Australia discovered that habitual lentil consumption was a predictor of long life expectancy, with significant reduction in mortality risk for each incremental increase in daily legume intake.

Selection tips:

Brown lentils are sold whole in supermarkets, ethnic markets, and health-food stores. Look for whole lentils that are uniformly shaped and fairly consistent in color. Packaged lentils should carry an expiration date. For those sold in boxes, there should be no evidence of moisture damage in the packaging. When purchasing bulk lentils, choose a store that has high stock turnover and make sure the bins are covered.

Storage tips:

Store dried lentils in an airtight container in a cool, dry, preferably dark place for up to one year.

Canned lentils should also be stored in a cool, dry place and used before their expiration date.

Preparation tips:

Brown lentils do not require soaking. Sort and rinse the lentils. Place them in a saucepan with cold water, using 2 cups of water for each cup of lentils. Bring the lentils to a boil, then reduce the heat and simmer until tender. Brown lentils take approximately 20–25 minutes to cook.

Brown lentils are often used in soups, where they work well either whole or pureed, depending on the desired texture. They make hearty stews and are a good accompaniment to poultry and other meats. Whole or partially mashed brown lentils are a good addition to veggie burger recipes, too.

Brown lentils hold their shape nicely when cooked, so they work well in salads. Try adding diced vegetables such as tomatoes, carrots, peppers, and onions, and toss with balsamic, lemon, or red wine vinaigrette. Top with a bit of crumbled Feta or goat cheese, if desired, and serve with greens as a light, yet satisfying meal.

Precautions:

Be sure to sort and rinse lentils before cooking, as there are often small stones hiding among them.

Lentils are high in purine, and some with gout might find that lentils exacerbate their symptoms.

LENTILS, FRENCH GREEN (*also called LENTILLES du PUY*)

Serving size: ½ cup, cooked

Per serving:
Calories:. 120
Carbohydrate: . . . . 20 g
Protein:. . . . . 10 g
Fat:. . . . . 0 g
Saturated fat: . . . . 0 g
Cholesterol: . . . . 0 mg
Sodium:. . . . . 5 mg
Fiber:. . . . . 5 g
Calcium: . . . . 20 mg

Good source of:

protein, fiber, iron, folate, magnesium, potassium, thiamine, zinc

Description:

French green lentils are small, delicate lentils with bluish-grey mottling on the skin and a refined, peppery flavor. Epicures adore French green lentils, which hold their shape beautifully and are firmer than other lentil varieties. Although green lentils are now grown in North America and Italy, they are often referred to as French lentils. But those grown in the volcanic soils of Le Puy, in the Haute-Loire region of France, are particularly special. They were the first dry vegetable to earn the French government's AOC (Appellation d'Origine Contrôlée) designation, which guarantees that French green lentils bearing the AOC label were produced in Le Puy in a traditional manner and according to designated standards.

Health benefits:

Like other legumes, lentils are high in protein, fiber, micronutrients, and phytochemicals. The many components in lentils work together to promote a healthy lipid profile, normal blood pressure, and overall heart health. Lentils have a sustained beneficial effect on postprandial glucose levels, which might benefit those with diabetes. The fiber and protein in lentils contribute to feelings of after-meal fullness, which plays a role in successful weight loss and weight management. Researchers at the Harvard School of Public Health discovered a lower risk of breast cancer among lentil eaters that they believed warranted further investigation. And a study conducted in Australia discovered that habitual lentil consumption was a predictor of long life expectancy, with significant reduction in mortality risk for each incremental increase in daily legume intake.

Selection tips:

French green lentils are sold whole in supermarkets, ethnic markets, and health-food stores. Look for whole lentils that are uniformly shaped and fairly consistent in color (the mottling on Le Puy lentils is normal and desirable). Packaged lentils should carry an expiration date. For those sold in boxes, there should be no evidence of moisture damage in the packaging. When purchasing bulk lentils, choose a store that has high stock turnover, and make sure the bins are covered. French green lentils carrying the AOC designation are the best bet for the highest quality, most flavorful lentils.

Storage tips:
Store dried lentils in an airtight container in a cool, dry, preferably dark place for up to one year.

Canned lentils should also be stored in a cool, dry place and used before their expiration date.

Preparation tips:
Green lentils do not require soaking. Sort and rinse the lentils. Place them in a saucepan with cold water, using 2 cups of water for each cup of lentils. Bring the lentils to a boil, then reduce the heat and simmer until tender. French green lentils take approximately 20–25 minutes to cook.

Although they can certainly be used in soups and stews, French green lentils hold their shape so well and have such a pretty appearance that they are especially nice in recipes that show them off. Try them in rice or grain pilafs. Create green lentil salads with chopped raw or roasted vegetables and Dijon mustard vinaigrette. Simply sautéed, with a touch of olive oil, garlic, shallots, herbs, and tiny diced carrots, they make a great accompaniment to meats or grilled fish.

Precautions:
Be sure to sort and rinse lentils before cooking because small stones are often hiding among them.

Lentils are high in purine, and some people with gout might find that lentils exacerbate their symptoms.

LENTILS, RED (*also called* EGYPTIAN LENTILS or ORANGE LENTILS)

Serving size: ½ cup, cooked

Per serving:
Calories:. 170
Carbohydrate: . . . . 28 g
Protein:. . . . . 13 g
Fat:. . . . . 1 g
Saturated fat: . . . . 0 g
Cholesterol: . . . . 0 mg
Sodium:. . . . . 5 mg
Fiber:. . . . . 7 g
Calcium: . . . . 20 mg

Good source of:
protein, fiber, iron, folate, magnesium, potassium, thiamine, zinc

Description:
Red lentils are commonly used in the Middle East and India. They are available whole, with their brownish skins intact, though in the United States they are more often sold hulled (without their skins). Hulled red lentils actually look more orange than red, and they are smaller than unhulled red lentils. Red lentils are used as a base for the Indian *dal* (or *dhal*) dishes and the Middle Eastern lentil and rice stew called *mujaddarah*.

Health benefits:
Like other legumes, lentils are high in protein, fiber, micronutrients, and phytochemicals. The many components in lentils work together to promote a healthy lipid profile, normal blood pressure, and overall heart health. Lentils have a sustained beneficial effect on after-meal blood glucose levels,

which might benefit those with diabetes. The fiber and protein in lentils contribute to feelings of post-meal satiety, which plays a role in successful weight loss and weight management. Researchers at the Harvard School of Public Health discovered a lower risk of breast cancer among lentil eaters that they believed warranted further investigation. And a study conducted in Australia discovered that habitual lentil consumption was a predictor of long life expectancy, with significant reduction in mortality risk for each incremental increase in daily legume intake.

Selection tips:

Red lentils are sold whole in supermarkets, ethnic markets, and health-food stores. Look for whole lentils that are uniformly shaped and fairly consistent in color. Packaged lentils should carry an expiration date. For those sold in boxes, there should be no evidence of moisture damage in the packaging. When purchasing bulk lentils, choose a store that has high stock turnover, and make sure the bins are covered.

Storage tips:

Store dried lentils in an airtight container in a cool, dry place for up to one year.

Canned lentils should also be stored in a cool, dry place and used before their expiration date.

Preparation tips:

Red lentils do not require soaking. Sort and rinse the lentils. Place them in a saucepan with cold water, using 2 cups of water for each cup of lentils. Bring the lentils to a boil, then reduce the heat and simmer until tender. Red lentils take approximately 25–35 minutes to cook.

Red lentils—especially when hulled—disintegrate easily when cooked. This works to advantage in soups and dal, where a pureed texture is desirable. Red lentils have a great affinity for ginger and are delicious over rice (try brown basmati) or with braised greens. Red lentils even work as an unconventional pasta topping—add them whole to whole wheat fusilli with sautéed spinach, olive oil, and garlic. Or cook them until they reach a pureed texture and use them like a sauce. For parties or as a snack, mash red lentils with freshly squeezed lemon juice, extra-virgin olive oil, garlic, and spices and use as a dip for crudités or as a spread for crackers.

Precautions:

Be sure to sort and rinse lentils before cooking because small stones are often hiding among them.

Lentils are high in purine, and some with gout might find that lentils exacerbate their symptoms.

NAVY BEANS (*also called* BOSTON BEANS and PEA BEANS)

Serving size: ½ cup, cooked

Per serving:
Calories:. 130
Carbohydrate: . . . . 24 g
Protein:. . . . . 8 g
Fat:. . . . . 1 g
Saturated fat: . . . . 0 g
Cholesterol: . . . . 0 mg
Sodium:. . . . . 1 mg
Fiber:. . . . . 5 g
Calcium: . . . . 64 mg
Folate: . . . . 128 mcg

Good source of:

protein, fiber, folate, calcium, iron, manganese, potassium, phosphorus

Description:

Navy beans are small, white, oval-shaped beans that earned their name thanks to their service as a staple ration on naval vessels. They are often used in commercial baked beans or in traditional recipes for Boston baked beans. According to statistics kept by the Michigan Bean Commission, navy beans are the second most popular bean consumed in the United States.

Health benefits:

Beans are low in fat, rich in protein, and high in both soluble and insoluble fiber. They are also packed with micronutrients and phytochemicals. As an additional boon, a serving of beans provides complex carbohydrate that has both a low glycemic index and low glycemic load. Beans also contain so-called "resistant starch," which is not readily converted to glucose. Research suggests that these factors promote improved glycemic control and insulin responses among bean eaters. Plus, beans help promote heart health and appear to fight cancer risk. The revised 2005 USDA Dietary Guidelines for Americans recommend that Americans consume at least 3 cups of beans each week. In recognition of beans' importance to health promotion, the FDA recently issued the following dietary guidance message: "A diet including beans may help reduce the risk of heart disease and certain cancers."

Selection tips:

Navy beans are commonly found in supermarket or health-food stores. They are available both dried and canned.

Although dried beans are shelf-stable, they taste best the fresher they are. (Old beans might also take longer to cook.) When purchasing dried navy beans, look for uniformly shaped, smooth beans with unshriveled skins.

Canned beans should be purchased only in cans that have no dents and no evidence of bulging or rust. Check the expiration date on both dried and canned beans.

Storage tips:
Store dried navy in an airtight container in a cool, dry place, preferably out of direct light, for up to one year.

Canned navy beans should also be stored in a cool, dry place and used before their expiration date.

Once cooked, beans can be kept in a covered container in the refrigerator for up to five days. Leftover canned beans should be transferred to a covered container before being stored in the refrigerator.

Cooked beans can be frozen in a well-sealed container in the freezer for up to six months.

Preparation tips:
Sort through dried beans before cooking and remove any foreign matter (such as pebbles) or any beans that are shriveled, broken, oddly shaped, or split. Rinse the sorted beans.

Next, soak the beans. Place them in a large bowl and cover with at least 3 inches of cold water. Leave them to soak in the refrigerator for at least six hours, or overnight. Drain and rinse before cooking.

Alternatively, if you haven't planned ahead for a long cold soak, you can use the quicker hot-soak method. Place sorted, rinsed beans in a large saucepan or pot. Add enough cold water to cover the beans by at least 3 inches. Place the pot over medium heat and bring the beans to a boil. Skim off and discard the foam that usually forms along with any beans that rise to the surface of the water. Boil the beans for 2 minutes, then remove the pot from the heat and cover it. Allow the beans to soak in the cooking water for one hour, then drain and rinse before cooking.

After soaking and rinsing the beans, place them in a saucepan and cover with a generous amount of cold water (there should be at least 3 inches of water over the top of the beans).

It is fine to season the water with fresh herbs, garlic, or a small amount of oil, but do not add salt or acidic ingredients such as citrus juice, tomatoes, or vinegar, at this point because this will harden the outer wall of the beans, and they will not cook properly.

Bring the beans to a boil over medium heat. Once the beans come to a boil, lower the heat, cover partially, and simmer. Periodically skim off any foam that forms on the surface of the cooking water and discard it.

About three-quarters of the way into the cooking time, begin to test the beans. (Any acidic or salty ingredients can be added at this point.) Simply bite into a bean—if it is uniformly cooked inside and has a soft, tender texture, the beans are ready. Avoid overcooking beans, or they will become mushy.

Navy beans take approximately 1 to 1½ hours to cook.

Beans can also be cooked in a pressure cooker. They will cook much faster but might be less flavorful and the texture mushier. The foam from the cooking beans can clog the valve on the pressure cooker, so it is critical to first bring the beans to a boil without the cover and skim off any foam. Add one to two teaspoons of oil to the water before attaching the cover to prevent more foam from forming while the beans are under pressure.

Navy beans are a perfect choice for baked bean recipes, and they make an unexpected but delicious choice for chili. Navy beans can stand in for other white beans, so try them in cassoulet or puree them for white bean dips or soups. Drizzle navy beans with a little extra virgin olive oil, lemon, fresh oregano, and sage, toss with chopped tomatoes, and serve alongside grilled fish. Add them to baby green salads or sautéed spinach, toss them in pasta, or mash them and use as a filling for wraps.

Precautions:
Beans can cause harmless though potentially unpleasant gastrointestinal distress,

usually in the form of gas, if they aren't soaked and drained. This is because beans are rich in oligosaccharides, a class of sugar molecules that humans can't digest easily.

The fresher the beans and the longer they are soaked, the more oligosaccharides will be removed. Don't forget to drain the beans and use fresh cooking water, or you'll end up keeping all of the oligosaccharides that were in the soaking water. Skimming off and discarding any foam that forms on the surface of the water as the beans cook will further reduce the oligosaccharides.

Adding baking soda to the soaking or cooking water is not recommended. This practice can destroy thiamine (vitamin B_1), decrease the overall nutrient availability of the beans, and make them taste soapy.

PINTO BEANS

Serving size: ½ cup, cooked

Per serving:
Calories:................... 118
Carbohydrate: .... 22 g
Protein:..................... 7 g
Fat:......................... 1 g
Saturated fat: .... 0 g
Cholesterol: .... 0 mg
Sodium:.................... 2 mg
Fiber:....................... 6 g
Calcium: .... 41 mg
Folate: .... 147 mcg

Good source of:
protein, fiber, folate, selenium, potassium, iron, thiamine

Description:
Pinto beans are medium-size beans with a slight kidney shape. These pretty beans have a beige background and are mottled with brownish-red spots, hence the name "pinto," which means "painted" in Spanish. As the beans cook, the mottling disappears and the skin becomes a uniform pinkish color. Cooked pintos have a creamy texture that is used to advantage in bean dips and refried beans. They are also used frequently in chili and work well in recipes that call for red beans or kidney beans. Pintos are the most popular variety of bean in the United States, according to the Michigan Bean Commission.

Health benefits:
Beans are low in fat, rich in protein, and high in both soluble and insoluble fiber. They are also packed with micronutrients and phytochemicals. As an additional boon, a serving of beans provides complex carbohydrate that has both a low glycemic index and low glycemic load. Beans also contain so-called "resistant starch," which is not readily converted to glucose. Research suggests that these factors promote improved blood glucose control and insulin responses among bean eaters. In addition, beans help promote heart health and appear to fight cancer risk. The revised 2005 USDA Dietary Guidelines for Americans recommend that Americans consume at least 3 cups of beans each week. In recognition of beans' importance to

health promotion, the FDA recently issued the following dietary guidance message: "A diet including beans may help reduce the risk of heart disease and certain cancers."

Selection tips:

Pinto beans are commonly found in supermarket or health-food stores. They are available both dried and canned.

Although dried beans are shelf-stable, they taste best the fresher they are. (Old beans might also take longer to cook.) When purchasing dried pinto beans, look for uniformly shaped, smooth beans with unshriveled skins.

Canned beans should be purchased only in cans that have no dents and no evidence of bulging or rust. Check the expiration date on both dried and canned beans.

Storage tips:

Store dried pinto beans in an airtight container in a cool, dry place, preferably out of direct light, for up to one year.

Canned pinto beans should also be stored in a cool, dry place and used before their expiration date.

Once cooked, beans can be kept in a covered container in the refrigerator for up to five days. Leftover canned beans should be transferred to a covered container before being stored in the refrigerator.

Cooked beans can be frozen in a well-sealed container in the freezer for up to six months.

Preparation tips:

Sort through dried beans before cooking and remove any foreign matter (such as pebbles) or any beans that are shriveled, broken, oddly shaped, or split. Rinse the sorted beans.

Next, soak the beans. Place them in a large bowl and cover with at least 3 inches of cold water. Leave them to soak in the refrigerator for at least six hours, or overnight. Drain and rinse before cooking.

Alternatively, if you haven't planned ahead for a long cold soak, you can use the quicker hot soak method. Place sorted,

rinsed beans in a large saucepan or pot. Add enough cold water to cover the beans by at least 3 inches. Place the pot over medium heat and bring the beans to a boil. Skim off and discard the foam that usually forms along with any beans that rise to the surface of the water. Boil the beans for 2 minutes, then remove the pot from the heat and cover it. Allow the beans to soak in the cooking water for one hour, then drain and rinse before cooking.

After soaking and rinsing the beans, place them in a saucepan and cover with a generous amount of cold water (there should be at least 3 inches of water over the top of the beans).

It is fine to season the water with fresh herbs, garlic, or a small amount of oil, but do not add salt or acidic ingredients such as citrus juice, tomatoes, or vinegar at this point because this will harden the outer wall of the beans, and they will not cook properly.

Bring the beans to a boil over medium heat. Once the beans come to a boil, lower the heat, cover partially, and simmer. Periodically skim off any foam that forms on the surface of the cooking water and discard it.

About three-quarters of the way into the cooking time, begin to test the beans. (Any acidic or salty ingredients can be added at this point.) Simply bite into a bean—if it is uniformly cooked inside and has a soft, tender texture, the beans are ready. Avoid overcooking beans, or they will become mushy.

Pinto beans take approximately 1 to 1½ hours to cook.

Beans can also be cooked in a pressure cooker. They will cook much faster but might be less flavorful and the texture mushier. The foam from the cooking beans can clog the valve on the pressure cooker, so it is critical to first bring the beans to a boil without the cover and skim off any foam. Add one to two teaspoons of oil to the water before attaching the cover to prevent more foam from forming while the beans are under pressure.

Pintos make great refried beans. Cook the pintos and reserve some of the cooking water (or use canned beans and keep the liquid). Heat olive oil in a skillet and sauté a chopped onion until it is translucent. Add garlic, chili, and oregano and sauté for 10–15 seconds, then add the cooked pinto beans. Sauté the beans, then add some of the cooking liquid and bring to a boil. Reduce the heat and let the beans simmer for about 10 minutes. Mash them roughly with a spatula, and serve as a side dish or burrito filling. Use pinto beans in chili or soup, serve them over rice, or try them in baked bean recipes. Pinto beans add color to three-bean salads and salsas and taste great with corn—try mixing the beans, corn kernels, and chopped tomatoes, toss with red wine vinaigrette, and chill.

Precautions:
Beans can cause harmless though potentially unpleasant gastrointestinal distress, usually in the form of gas, if they aren't soaked and drained. This is because beans are rich in oligosaccharides, a class of sugar molecules that humans can't digest easily.

The fresher the beans, and the longer they are soaked, the more oligosaccharides will be removed. Don't forget to drain the beans and use fresh cooking water, or you'll end up keeping all of the oligosaccharides that were in the soaking water. Skimming off and discarding any foam that forms on the surface of the water as the beans cook will further reduce the oligosaccharides.

Adding baking soda to the soaking or cooking water is not recommended. This practice can destroy thiamine (vitamin B_1), decrease the overall nutrient availability of the beans, and make them taste soapy.

BEVERAGES

COCOA

Serving size: 1 tablespoon cocoa powder

Per serving:
Calories:. 12
Carbohydrate: . . . . 3 g
Protein:. 1 g
Fat:. . . . . 1 g
Saturated fat: . . . . 0 g
Cholesterol: . . . . 0 mg
Sodium:. . . . . 1 mg
Fiber:. . . . . 2 g
Calcium: . . . . 7 g

Good source of:
magnesium, iron, copper, flavanols

Description:
The cacao tree, from which chocolate and cocoa are derived, has been cultivated for over 3,000 years. The tree and the seeds it produces played an enormous role in Aztec, Mayan, and Toltec culture, religion, and society. The Maya were the first to harvest and process cacao beans and turn them into a beverage. The Aztecs later adopted this bitter drink, which they blended with chili peppers, spices, and water.

Spanish conquistador Hernán Cortés encountered cacao in Mexico and took it back to Spain in the 1500's. Conquistadores spread cultivation through the Caribbean, and by the 1800's, cacao was also being produced in Africa and South America.

In the 1600's, Europeans began importing cacao and adding sugar—another expensive, status-boosting import—to it. This beverage was the forerunner of today's milk-laced hot cocoa.

Before they can be eaten, cacao beans are fermented, dried, roasted, cooled, and cracked to obtain the chocolate liquor (really a paste) inside. Cocoa powder is made by pressing out most of the cocoa butter component of the chocolate liquor and grinding the resulting paste.

Contrary to popular belief, Dutch cocoa doesn't refer to the powder's origin. "Dutched" indicates that the cocoa underwent further processing to make it more soluble. Dutched cocoa is also more alkaline, so when baking with cocoa, adhere to the recipe's specifics with regard to the type of cocoa and leavening agent for the best results.

Health benefits:

Studies have shown that cocoa products are protective of heart health. Authors of a 2005 study published in the journal *Hypertension* believe the flavanols in cocoa contribute to the beneficial effects they observed among study subjects with essential hypertension, including reduced blood pressure and LDL cholesterol, and improved insulin sensitivity.

Other studies have shown that the flavonols in cocoa, including epicatechin and catechin, have antioxidant capacity. Cacao beans and the products made from them also contain theobromine, an effective cough suppressant, which might explain why traditional healers in Latin America use cocoa to treat bronchitis.

Although modern cocoa and chocolate preparations tend to be abundant in cavity-causing sugar, cocoa itself appears to have antibacterial components that actually fight tooth decay. For cavity-fighting benefits, take a cue from ancient Mesoamerican culture and try an unsweetened cocoa drink.

It should be noted that in several studies, heavy processing or the addition of milk diminished the beneficial effects of chocolate or cocoa consumption. Choose natural cocoa or dark, minimally sweetened chocolate with a high cocoa content to reap the potential health benefits of the beans.

Selection tips:

Look for natural cocoa, unless a recipe specifically calls for Dutch-processed cocoa. Natural cocoa tends to be made from higher-quality cacao beans, is lighter in color, and has a deeper, more complex flavor than Dutch-processed cocoa.

Storage tips:

Store cocoa powder in an airtight container in a cool, dark place. Cocoa powder will keep for up to two years.

Preparation tips:

Forgo the over-sweetened cocoa mixes (which often contain partially- hydrogenated oils) and make your hot cocoa from scratch. To mix the cocoa powder into liquid with the greatest ease, start with a slurry: place 1 tablespoon of unsweetened cocoa powder into a small saucepan. Add 1 tablespoon of cold water and whisk together to form a paste. Add one teaspoon sugar, maple syrup, or honey, if you prefer sweet cocoa (remember to account for the approximately 5 grams of carbohydrate that each teaspoon of these nutritive sweeteners provides). Place the saucepan over low heat, and slowly add 1 cup of skim or low-fat (1%) milk or soy milk, whisking constantly. (You can also use a combination of water and milk or soy milk, in whatever proportion you prefer.) Heat until very warm, but do not boil. Remove from heat and stir in a drop of vanilla extract if desired.

Try adding cinnamon and a dash of powdered chili or cayenne pepper to the cocoa powder slurry for a modern take on ancient Mayan and Aztec cocoa—as a bonus, you'll add even more disease-fighting phytochemicals in the process!

Precautions:

Humans might love chocolate, but don't share it with pets—the theobromine it contains can be fatal to cats and dogs.

COFFEE

Serving size: 8 ounces, brewed

Per serving:

Calories:. 2
Carbohydrate: . . . . 0 g
Protein:. . . . . 0 g
Fat:. . . . . 0 g
Saturated fat: . . . . 0 g
Cholesterol: . . . . 0 mg
Sodium:. . . . . 5 mg
Fiber:. . . . . 0 g
Calcium: . . . . 5 mg

Good source of:

polyphenols

Description:

Coffee beans grow on shrubs indigenous to Africa. Common lore states that humans began experimenting with coffee consumption when goatherders noticed that their charges got frisky after nibbling on the bushes. By the late 1500's, Arab growers began cultivating coffee. Thanks to the popularity of the stimulating beans, coffee is now grown in tropical regions worldwide and is one of the most heavily traded commodities on the planet.

Health benefits:

For a long time, coffee got a bad rap due to its caffeine content. Studies have found that excessive coffee and caffeine consumption appear to be detrimental to human health and might be implicated in infertility and miscarriage, for example. But moderate coffee consumption might have significant health benefits. In other words, drinking 8 cups of coffee per day is not advisable, but 1 to 2 cups per day can actually protect one's health.

In a 2004 study published in the *Annals of Internal Medicine,* Harvard researchers reported that among both men and women, long-term coffee drinkers enjoyed a statistically significant reduced risk of developing Type 2 diabetes. Other studies found similar results; improved insulin sensitivity and response among coffee drinkers appear to be factors in this reduced risk. For coffee lovers with a family history of Type 2 diabetes, drinking this beverage might be a wise move.

In multiple studies, researchers have observed decreased risk of various gastrointestinal cancers among regular coffee drinkers. Various antioxidants in coffee might play a role in this protective effect.

As for the caffeine in coffee, it seems to play a role in a significantly reduced risk of Parkinson disease among coffee drinkers.

Selection tips:

As with wine, there is enormous variety in the flavors, aromas, and depth of coffee beans. Beans are roasted before consumption, and the length of the roast adds still more variation to the complexity and nuance of various coffees.

Some diehard coffee lovers buy their beans green and roast them at home. If, like most people, you buy preroasted, ground coffee beans, make sure they are in a vacuum-packed container. Ground coffee loses flavor and desirable aroma quickly, so only purchase it from stores with quick turnover. Better yet, buy whole beans and have the store or coffee shop grind them, or invest in a small home coffee grinder. That way, you can grind beans as needed, for maximum freshness and flavor.

In terms of the type of beans to choose, coffee selection is highly personal. Some people prefer smoother, milder beans and roasts, while others like astringent coffees, and some are dedicated to deep, complex flavors. Many people like blends of beans. Taste different coffees to get a feel for your own signature bean or blend.

Consider seeking out Fair Trade Certified coffee. Most coffee workers are subjected to arduous working conditions yet are paid less for their coffee yield than the cost of production. Fair Trade Certification ensures that coffee producers receive reasonable prices for their beans and economic support for their farming, health care, and education. Increasingly, these farmers are able to convert to organic production, another boon both environmentally and health-wise.

Storage tips:

Whole roasted beans will keep at room temperature for one to two weeks. Beans purchased in coffee shops and supermarkets are often packaged in bags with a small valve. This is desirable because it allows carbon dioxide gas to escape from the bag without letting oxygen in. If your coffee shop scoops your beans into a paper bag, transfer them to an airtight ceramic or glass container before storing. The beans' quality will suffer in the light, so if you choose a glass container, store it in a cool, dark cupboard or in the freezer.

Whole coffee beans can be stored in the freezer for one to two months. Refrigerator storage can compromise the quality of coffee beans and is not a good option.

Roasted ground coffee has the shortest shelf life. It should be stored in a cool, dry place. It will taste best in the first few days, so it is best to buy small quantities. You can extend the shelf life to a week or two by storing it in an airtight container in the freezer.

Green coffee beans have the longest shelf life. They will last in an airtight container in a cool, dry place for at least a year. Of course, coffee devotees willing to roast their own beans probably won't have them around that long!

Preparation tips:

There are many ways to prepare coffee, and preferences are as individual as favorite coffee bean choices.

Perhaps the most popular method is to brew with a drip coffee maker, although home espresso makers are gaining a strong following. Press pots are another simple way to brew coffee—ground beans are added to a carafe and boiling water is poured over them. After a few minutes, the plunger in the carafe's lid is depressed and the coffee is ready. (There tends to be more caffeine in coffee made this way).

Try adding a dash of cinnamon, cardamom, or unsweetened cocoa powder (or all three) to coffee for a different flavor. Pour brewed coffee over ice for a more refreshing version of a wake-up standard.

Precautions:

Coffee is high in caffeine and other stimulants and should be consumed in moderation. Coffee consumption might disrupt sleep patterns, particularly if drunk shortly before bedtime. Some people find that coffee exacerbates symptoms of gastro-esophageal reflux disease (GERD).

Caffeine is also a diuretic, meaning that it tends to increase the flow of urine. Be sure to stay well hydrated when drinking coffee—try to drink an extra glass of water for each glass of coffee consumed. If you take diuretic medicines, ask a doctor or pharmacist about coffee consumption.

If you are pregnant or nursing, discuss coffee safety with a doctor, midwife, or registered dietitian. Many authorities feel one 6-ounce cup of coffee per day is fine. Those with a history of miscarriage, however, should consider forgoing coffee when trying to conceive or during pregnancy.

Take care with coffee additions. Cream or full-fat milk, sugars, and artificial sweeteners, especially when used with a heavy hand, can render an otherwise healthy beverage far less so.

GREEN TEA

Serving size: 6 ounces, brewed

Per serving:

Calories:. 2
Carbohydrate: . . . . 1 g
Protein:. 0 g
Fat:. . . . . 0 g
Saturated fat: . . . . 0 g
Cholesterol: . . . . 0 mg
Sodium:. . . . . 5 mg
Fiber:. . . . . 0 g
Calcium: . . . . 0 mg

Good source of:
flavonoid antioxidants

Description:
Green tea has been drunk in China and Japan for thousands of years and remains a major part of diet and culture in those countries. Although black tea is usually associated with Britain's tea-drinking culture, green tea was initially England's favored brew. Until the early 1900's, the majority of the tea imported into America also was green; today, as scientists learn more about the health benefits of green tea, the beverage has enjoyed a renaissance in Europe and the United States.

All tea, whether green or black, comes from the same plant, the Camellia sinensis. Green tea comes from the new buds and young leaves of the plant. Green tea is unoxidized (or unfermented), and the leaves and buds are sometimes withered (or dried in bamboo racks) and then steamed or baked immediately after harvest. The green tea is rolled and then dried to prevent oxidation. It retains its green color and produces a pale golden or greenish brew.

Health benefits:
Green tea is high in antioxidants, including a catechin called epigallocatechin gallate (EGCG) that appears to inhibit the growth and spread of cancer cells without damaging healthy cells. A Japanese study found that in women with early stage breast cancer, the disease spread more slowly in those who drank at least five cups of green tea per day.

EGCG appears to work synergistically with the caffeine in green tea to boost the metabolic rate. This might confer weight management benefits upon habitual green tea drinkers and possibly aid in weight loss.

Green tea might also play a role in the prevention of Alzheimer disease. Studies have found that green tea inhibits the action of certain enzymes that appear to factor into the disease's development.

Green tea boosts the body's insulin activity, which might be beneficial for prevention or management of diabetes, or both.

Selection tips:

The flavor of green tea depends on where it was grown, when it was picked, whether it was machine-harvested or hand-harvested, and how it was processed. Hand-harvested and rolled teas are of the best quality, while machine-harvested and processed teas tend to be inferior. Loose teas will generally produce the best cups of tea. It is increasingly possible to find loose teas in fabric tea sachets, marrying the convenience of the tea bag with the high quality of teas brewed from loose leaves.

Storage tips:

Store loose green tea in an airtight container in a cool, dry place. Properly stored, tea leaves will keep for six months to one year. Rolled leaves, such as gunpowder green tea, will keep the longest because less of the leaf is exposed to the air.

Tea bags should also be kept in a dark, cool, and dry place, such as a cupboard that is located away from a heat source.

Preparation tips:

For the best tasting tea, run your water through a filter pitcher, or use bottled spring water. However, if your municipal tap water is pleasant tasting, by all means use it, but run the cold water for a moment first so you don't end up making your tea from standing water.

Heat 6 ounces of cold water for each cup of tea. Use about a teaspoon of leaves per cup if you are using loose tea or one tea bag per cup.

Loose tea can go into a teapot with a built-in strainer, into a press pot, or into a tea ball. If you opt for a tea ball or paper tea sachets that you fill yourself, be sure to leave enough room for the tea leaves to unfurl as they brew.

Green tea is delicate, so it shouldn't be subjected to boiling water. For those who like to get technical, heat the water to between 160°F and 175°F. Green tea should be brewed for 1 to 3 minutes.

Try pouring green tea over ice, or, for a grown-up version of a favorite summertime treat, pour freshly brewed green tea into Popsicle molds and freeze until solid.

Experiment with green tea as you would a spice. Invest in powdered matcha green tea and use it in spice rubs for poultry or fish or whisk it into vinaigrettes. (You can also try pulverizing tea leaves with a mortar and pestle or grind them in a spice grinder). Or stir green tea powder into softened low-fat vanilla frozen yogurt for a "homemade" version of a Japanese restaurant favorite.

RED WINE

Serving size: 5 ounces

Per serving:
Calories:. 125
Carbohydrate: . . . . 4 g
Protein:. 0 g
Fat:. . . . . 0 g
Saturated fat: . . . . 0 g
Cholesterol: . . . . 0 mg
Sodium:. . . . . 6 mg
Fiber:. . . . . 0 g
Calcium: . . . . 12 mg

Note: Most of the calories in red wine come from alcohol, which has 7 calories per gram. However, alcohol is metabolized differently from other calorie sources, and not all of the calories from alcohol are available for energy use.

Good source of:

phenolic compounds, resveratrol, catechins, other antioxidants

Description:

Next to water, wine may be among the oldest libations known to humankind. Most commonly made from the fermentation of grapes, the first winemaking efforts may have involved wild fruits, and likely occurred in the Neolithic period. But wide-scale wine production probably didn't occur until sometime after the fruits were domesticated, over 5,000 years ago.

Since antiquity, wine has played an important role in the cultures, religions, and medicinal traditions of winemaking regions throughout the world. Wines once contained less alcohol than their modern counterparts, and were often diluted with water. When safe water was scarce and cholera and other water-borne diseases rampant, wine appears to have literally saved lives. The effect may have had to do with antibacterial compounds present in wine. Research has demonstrated that even diluted wines are effective against various disease-causing bacteria.

The potentially intoxicating effects of alcohol didn't go unnoticed, of course. Truly moderate drinkers tend to report only feelings of relaxation or mildly increased sociability, but throughout history, alcohol has inspired many outspoken activists. The temperance movement in the United States, which began in the early 1800's, eventually set the political stage for Prohibition and did much to cast alcohol consumption in a negative light. Even after the repeal of Prohibition, alcohol's image as an illicit substance tied to crime, amoral behavior, and ill health persisted in the minds of many.

Science, however, is providing an ever-broadening body of evidence about the potential health benefits of moderate alcohol use. Generally speaking, people who enjoy a glass of wine with dinner may be doing themselves a healthful favor.

New and Old World wineries are thriving, and many turn out high-quality, extremely affordable vintages. The vast majority of wines produced today are meant to be enjoyed while they are still young (or at the time of purchase), so one need not have a wine cellar or any special wine storage knowledge to drink them at their best. There has also been a renaissance in interest about wine, which makes it easier than ever to find consumer-friendly information and advice about wine selection and enjoyment.

Health benefits:

There has been a tremendous volume of research examining the health effects of alcohol—including red wine—in recent years. Overall, people who drink moderate amounts of alcohol on a regular basis appear to enjoy multiple health benefits. Moreover, making red wine one's drink of choice may be especially beneficial, since compounds unique to the beverage offer additional benefits.

Nevertheless, many people in the medical community take an extremely conservative stance when it comes to alcohol. Perhaps out of fear that the average person will take any endorsement of alcohol as license to drink excessively, practitioners and health agencies go on record with the assertion that people who don't already drink shouldn't start.

That position may err on the side of caution. For people who enjoy wine but have historically abstained out of fear that consuming any amount of alcohol carries negative health consequences, it may be fine to give that glass of red the green light. A wise strategy is to first discuss your individual medical history, including any drugs you take, as well as any family history of alcoholism with a doctor before adding wine or other forms of alcohol to your diet.

Population studies suggests that moderate alcohol consumption may promote improved insulin sensitivity, thereby helping to decrease the risk of developing Type 2 diabetes. According to a small, short-duration study published in 2005 in the journal *Metabolism,* study subjects with diabetes who drank moderate amounts of red wine experienced decreased insulin resistance. This suggests that the potential benefits of improved insulin sensitivity associated with alcohol consumption may extend beyond the general population to people who have diabetes.

Studies have shown that moderate alcohol intake improves blood lipid levels by increasing HDL ("good") cholesterol. Compounds called *saponins* in red wine may also decrease total cholesterol, while the antioxidant *resveratrol* helps prevent LDL ("bad") cholesterol oxidation.

Moderate amounts of alcohol also have a protective effect against blood clots and stroke. These factors appear to promote cardiovascular health and lower the risk of heart-disease–related deaths among people with and without diabetes. In fact, British cardiologist William McCrea made news in 2003 for prescribing red wine to many of his cardiac patients at Swindon & Marlborough Great Western Hospital in an effort to decrease their likelihood of a second heart attack or stroke.

Other studies suggest that the antioxidants in red wine appear to have anti-inflammatory effects and may also contribute to cancer prevention.

Should you get approval to include alcohol in your diet, the key is to stick to a moderate intake. Just what does that mean? As it turns out, "moderate" means different things for different people. For women, moderate intake is one unit of alcohol per day—in the case of wine, that translates to one 4- to 5-ounce glass. Men are permitted up to two units, or two 4- to 5-ounce glasses of wine per day.

It is very important to recognize that a person can't safely "save up" his intake and drink three glasses of wine every other day or a week's worth of alcohol over the weekend. Excessive drinking or binge drinking obliterates any potential health benefits and can have devastating short- and long-term consequences, including liver disease, diabetes complications, cancer, and potentially fatal accidents resulting from impaired judgment.

Selection tips:

Younger wines tend to be higher in antioxidant capacity. Cabernet Sauvignon, Petite Syrah, and Pinot Noir are rich in antioxidants, while Merlot, red zinfandel, and white wines are weaker choices when it comes to antioxidant power.

If you are new to wine, selecting a bottle can be baffling. Choose a reputable wine shop and ask for assistance. Describe flavors and scents you find pleasant and tell the clerk about the meal you plan to enjoy with the wine. Don't be afraid to set a budget—there are plenty of great wines priced under $10.

Try wines made from different grapes and take notes so you can hone in on personal flavor preferences over time. If you find you're intrigued by Pinot Noir, for example, taste bottles from different wineries or of different prices to see how they compare.

Don't fret about rules—when it comes to wine, none are hard and fast. You can, for instance, drink red wine with fish. Learn a bit about the wines you enjoy most and you'll glean great information about how best to prepare the meals to serve alongside them.

Wine Enthusiast (www.winemag.com), *Wine Spectator* (www.winespectator.com), and *Food & Wine* (www.foodandwine.com) magazines are good sources for wine information, reviews, and food pairing suggestions. Kevin Zraly's *Windows on the World Complete Wine Course* and Andrea Immer's *Great Wine Made Simple: Straight Talk from a Master Sommelier* are excellent, accessible resources for wine novices and connoisseurs alike.

Storage tips:

Store wine in a cool, preferably dark place. Choose a spot with a relatively stable temperature (ideally between 50° and 55°F for red wine). Store unopened bottles on their sides to help keep the seal airtight and prevent the cork from drying out. If the unopened wine will be stored for more than six months, the ambient humidity should be around 70% and the storage area free of vibration.

Once it has been opened, it is best to consume a bottle of wine within a couple of days. To save it, recork the wine or use a vacuum sealer or stopper. Refrigerate the bottle, but bring red wine back to room temperature before serving.

Preparation tips:

Wine experts are often particular about using glassware that is specially tailored to particular styles of wine. The rationale is that certain shapes are best for allowing wines to "breathe" and for directing the distinctive aromas of different wines to the taster's nose.

But don't worry if you don't have special glassware—after all, wine served in short tumblers or juice glasses lends the table a casual European look. What's most important is that the glasses be very clean, as soap residue and other contaminants can ruin the taste of wine.

Serve red wines at room temperature. To prevent drips when pouring, twist the bottle slightly from the wrist as you finish each pour. Before tasting, give the wine a little swirl in its glass if you desire—that helps aerate the wine, allowing the flavors to develop.

Typically full-bodied and complex, Cabernet Sauvignon generally pairs well with roasted meats, hard cheeses, and spicy foods.

The fruit and spice notes in Syrah/Shiraz (these are two names for the same grape varietal) are great with pasta, pizza, grilled meats, and chocolate.

Lighter, softer Pinot Noir is a great red to serve with grilled fish or vegetarian entrees.

There are plenty of other varietals to try and countless pairings that work beautifully. One way to explore them is to host a "blind" tasting. Assemble a group of friends and four to six different bottles of wine. Cover the bottles with wine bags so the labels are not visible. Give each guest a notepad and pour everyone a small amount of the first wine. Smell, taste, and discuss the wine and have everyone record a guess about the wine's identity. Have a drink of water or a palate-clearing snack such as a plain cracker or piece of bread, then repeat with the other bottles and fresh glasses. If you like a bit of competition, turn the evening into a game—whichever guest identifies the most wines accurately wins. Send him home with a book about wine, a corkscrew, or a set of wine stoppers.

Incidentally, wine needn't be restricted to a glass—try using it in marinades, sauces, compotes, or granita (a semifrozen dessert).

Precautions:

People who have a personal or family history of alcoholism, have liver disease, or are pregnant should avoid alcohol. Women with a personal or family history of breast cancer should discuss their situation and the potential risks and benefits of alcohol with a doctor and should be especially careful about sticking to one drink per day at most.

Do not drink alcohol, including wine, if your diabetes is poorly controlled. If your doctor approves alcohol intake, monitor your blood glucose closely to avoid low or high blood glucose levels, and do not drink on an empty stomach.

People who take prescription or over-the-counter drugs should check with a doctor or pharmacist to see if it is safe to consume alcohol with the drugs in question.

Never drive immediately after drinking alcohol, no matter how you feel, and never ride with an intoxicated driver, even if that person assures you he is fit to drive.

WATER

Serving size: 8 fluid ounces

Per serving:
Calories:......................0
Carbohydrate: ....0 g
Protein:....................0 g
Fat:........................0 g
Saturated fat: ....0 g
Cholesterol: ....0 mg
Sodium:..................5 mg
Fiber:......................0 g
Calcium:................5 mg

Note: Values are averages for municipal tap water.

Good source of:

water (Note, however, that many mineral waters can be significant sources of important nutrients, such as calcium and magnesium. Check the labels on different brands of mineral water for more information.)

Description:

It provides no calories, few nutrients (usually in trace amounts), and isn't even considered a food by most authorities. Yet, in an important sense, it nourishes us and is absolutely essential. "It" is water, and we can't live without it. In fact, our bodies are comprised of approximately 50% to 75% water, depending on age and body composition.

Our need for water must have been among the first recognized by primitive humans. We can live for weeks without food, but even in temperate climates, adults cannot survive for more than about 10 days without water, and children cannot go longer than 5 days without water.

Agricultural societies—indeed, civilization itself—necessarily bloomed in close proximity to water sources. Human beings' vital need for water drove the development in ancient societies of sophisticated irrigation systems and engineering feats like the aqueduct. Many world religions employ water in their rituals, and curative or therapeutic powers have long been associated with water. The earliest spas grew around mineral springs and natural hot baths; people suffering from a variety of ailments (or simply seeking health) made pilgrimages to "take the waters." Today's booming spa trend is rooted in that tradition.

Health benefits:

Water is an elemental part of our very being—it is an essential, multifunctional component of our cells, blood, and every body tissue. Water is a conduit for inter- and intracellular communication and is essential to all metabolic processes. It lubricates our joints, helps regulate body temperature, and helps ensure proper organ function.

Studies have found that people with higher water intakes tend to have lower rates of certain cancers, including bladder and colon cancer. Adequate fluid intake is also associated with decreased risk of kidney stone development. Conversely, inadequate water intake compromises optimal metabolic functioning and the ability to exercise effectively. Chronic mild dehydration can contribute to fatigue, appetite changes, low blood pressure, difficulty concentrating, and increased sensitivity to temperature changes.

Just how much water humans require is a source of debate. The American Dietetic Association continues to recommend that adults drink 8–10 eight-ounce glasses of water per day. Other experts believe that drinking when you feel thirsty is adequate. However, many conditions, as well as the use of some drugs, can interfere with a person's thirst mechanism, such that he rarely feels thirsty and may not drink enough. A person's size, activity level, and the weather are all important factors that help determine how much water a person needs.

There's no question, however, that water should be our primary beverage. Studies have shown that most people do not compensate for extra calories consumed in beverages by eating less at meals. Caloric beverages like juice, soda, whole or 2% milk, and sweetened teas or coffees can make weight management difficult for people who drink them throughout the day or in large quantities. Sugary beverages may also raise triglyceride levels and can cause blood

glucose levels to spike. Replacing these drinks with water, however, often translates into weight loss and may help improve lipid levels profile and blood glucose control.

Selection tips:

Obtaining water can be as simple as turning on the tap. For drinking and cooking, it is best to use water from the cold tap only—hot water can leach metals from the pipes. Allow the water to run for a moment to clear standing water from the pipes as well.

If there is concern about water safety in your area, or if you prefer bottled water, read labels to ascertain information about mineral content, purity, and water source. Select bottles that are undamaged and properly sealed, and look for the bottling and expiration dates—believe it or not, water does have a shelf life!

If you are traveling in a country with unsafe water, stick to bottles of spring water from a recognizable brand, make sure that the bottle is properly sealed, and steer clear of ice. Use bottled water for drinking, toothbrushing, and face washing.

Storage tips:

Unopened bottles of water can be stored at room temperature in a cool, dry place. Once opened, store water bottles in the refrigerator. If you chill water in pitchers, cover them with a lid or plastic wrap. Water to which you've added fruit or vegetable slices or herbs should be refrigerated and consumed within 1–2 days.

Preparation tips:

Some people feel that all waters taste the same. Others with very sensitive noses and palates can discern differences in the mineral contents of different bottled waters, and have very firm opinions about their favorites. But many people—especially those accustomed to drinking sodas and juices frequently—complain that they find water boring or that they dislike the taste.

The key is starting with good water. Municipal waters vary in quality—some are superb, while others have metallic notes or taste of chlorine. A good-quality filter pitcher is an inexpensive solution; faucet-mounted or under-sink systems are other options.

There are many home delivery services for bottled water as well, though bottled water isn't necessarily a safer or healthier option than tap. Be aware that not all bottled waters are spring waters—check the label to learn more about the water source. Also note that many bottled spring waters lack fluoride, which may be a concern if small children will be drinking this water exclusively. It is a good idea to discuss this issue with your dentist.

It's easy to add flavor to water—imagination is the only limit. Add lemon, lime, or cucumber slices to a pitcher of water (wash the skin first and consider using organic, unwaxed produce). Rinsed mint leaves are another refreshing addition to water, whether used alone or together with the citrus or cucumber. A squeeze of citrus or a splash of juice livens up water, and a drop of orange flower or rose flower water lends an exotic, aromatic twist.

Even small portions of juice are typically high in carbohydrate, but juice fans can freeze their favorite fruity beverages in ice trays, and add a couple of cubes to water. This tactic delivers a longer-lasting, concentrated shot of flavor to water without overdoing the carbohydrate content.

Icing decaffeinated green or herbal tea is another fantastic way to flavor water. Follow the instructions on the tea box or add 4–6 tea bags to a heat-proof pitcher. (You may vary the number of tea bags depending on the size of the pitcher and your preferred tea strength.) Fill the pitcher halfway with boiling water and allow the tea bags to steep for 3–5 minutes. Remove the tea bags and squeeze them over the pitcher before discarding them. Add a generous amount of ice and fill the pitcher with cold water. Refrigerate until cold and enjoy. Try to skip (or at least scale back on) adding sugars and artificial sweeteners—a person's taste for sweet beverages often diminishes as he gets used to drinking water or flavored water served *au naturel*.

There are an increasing number of flavored waters—both still and sparkling—on the market as well. However, many have natural or artificial sweeteners added, so check the labels before you buy.

Still having trouble consuming enough water? Don't forget that foods with a high water content will help meet your needs. Try low-sodium soups or munch on cucumbers, salad greens, or melon.

Precautions:
Though difficult to accomplish, it *is* possible to drink too much water, which can lead to water intoxication, a potentially fatal condition characterized by electrolyte imbalances. Elite athletes are among those most at risk, although people new to intense, lengthy exercise may inadvertently overhydrate themselves as well by drinking copious amounts of water in response to profuse sweating. After obtaining clearance to exercise from a doctor, people embarking on intense physical training programs should talk to a registered dietitian with an expertise in sports nutrition regarding fluid needs and safe, appropriate hydration. A certified personal trainer can help safely adjust the intensity of an exercise regimen.

Infants are also extremely vulnerable to water intoxication. Under most circumstances, they should not be fed water—human breast milk (or properly mixed infant formula) supplies all the water they need. In unusual circumstances, such as a heat wave, consult a pediatrician. Generally speaking, infants should not be fed more than 1 ounce of supplemental water at a time, and no more than 4 ounces in a day.

Do not drink carbonated beverages, including sparkling water or seltzer, if you have undergone gastric bypass or Lap-Band surgery.

People who have been prescribed medical fluid restriction should consult a registered dietitan for meal and fluid planning assistance.

WHOLE-GRAIN BREAD

Serving size: 1 1-ounce slice

Per serving:
Calories:. 70
Carbohydrate: . . . . 13 g
Protein:. 4 g
Fat:. . . . . 1 g
Saturated fat: . . . . 0 g
Cholesterol: . . . . 0 mg
Sodium:. . . . . 160 mg
Fiber:. . . . . 3 g
Calcium: . . . . 40 mg

Note: Values are for commercially prepared whole wheat bread. Nutrient composition may vary by brand or with homemade recipes.

Good source of:

fiber, antioxidants, protein, carbohydrate, iron, B vitamins, selenium, folic acid

Description:

A foodstuff with such significance that it has been dubbed "the staff of life," bread has been a staple in cultures worldwide since antiquity. Bread-making is an ingenious means of rendering grains edible, portable, and preservable (depending on the recipe, water content, and climate, various breads may be best the day they're made or may last for months). Whether flat or leavened, breads may be made from a host of different grains, though the time-consuming nature of baking homemade bread has rendered the practice something of a lost art.

Bread's elemental nature makes it one of the ultimate comfort foods, and personal bread preferences are often rooted in childhood memories. Unfortunately, for many people growing up in the United States, formative bread experiences often involve sliced, prepackaged white bread.

That's a shame from both health and culinary standpoints. Squishy breads made of refined flours bear virtually no resemblance to freshly baked, crusty-on-the-outside, chewy-on-the-inside loaves of bread. The good news is that a wide variety of high-quality, whole-grain breads are becoming increasingly available. The USDA Dietary Guidelines for Americans, updated in 2005, now specifically emphasize the importance of choosing whole grains. That change, along with consumers' increasing awareness of the health benefits of whole grains, has helped motivate food manufacturers to bring more whole-grain options to the market.

Health benefits:

It has been a rocky road for bread over the past several years. Adherents to the Atkins Diet and other low-carbohydrate regimens strove to avoid the staple food that was virtually vilified by their adopted diets. While the developers of some of these diets have softened their anticarbohydrate stances and may even acknowledge the importance of so-called "good carbohydrates," the damage has been done. Many people still believe that bread and other carbohydrate sources should be kept off-limits, or that "light" or "low-carbohydrate" breads are superior to regular bread.

It is time to set the record straight. Carbohydrates provide the preferred source of fuel for our bodies, and whole grains should be a cornerstone of a health-promoting diet. Whole-grain breads are an accessible, convenient means of meeting the USDA's recommendation that we eat at least three servings of whole grain daily. The key to reaping the benefits of whole grain is to use those servings to replace servings of refined grain products (rather than adding to them). Moreover, replacing *more* than three servings of refined grain with whole grain magnifies whole grain's health-protecting effects.

What is so special about whole grains? Population studies suggest that diets rich in whole grains have a protective effect against diabetes, cancer, heart disease, and obesity. Conversely, higher rates of insulin resistance, diabetes, and obesity have been found among populations that favor white bread.

Whole grains are rich in fiber, vitamins, minerals, antioxidants, and other phytochemicals. Together, these components appear to play a role in everything from improving blood lipid levels and insulin sensitivity to fighting high blood pressure and reducing inflammation. Ultimately, that translates into a lower risk of heart disease, stroke, certain cancers, and diabetes development or progression.

The fiber and protein in whole grains contributes to feelings of fullness, which in turn may help with weight loss or management. Whole grains are also more texturally satisfying—unlike soft, homogeneously-textured, refined-grain products, whole-grain breads actually require chewing. That factor can help people to eat more slowly and respond better to feelings of fullness.

In a study published in 2006 in *The American Journal of Clinical Nutrition*, researchers reported that whole grain intake appeared to be associated with decreased risk of periodontitis (gum disease). Interestingly, there are links between gum disease and heart disease, so the findings in this study may point to additional cardioprotective benefits.

Selection tips:
Switching to whole-grain bread opens up a new world of flavor varieties. Whole wheat bread may be the most familiar option to most people, but there are also whole-grain oat, rye, pumpernickel, barley, and spelt breads. Multigrain breads are another option, and they vary in texture and flavor depending on the variety and proportion of grains used.

People who are accustomed to soft white breads might prefer to start with the softer whole-grain breads that are readily available in supermarkets and health-food stores. Fans of artisanal breads should have little trouble transitioning to whole-grain sourdough *boules* (round loaves) or multigrain *baguettes* (long, thin loaves). Specialty bakeries, gourmet shops, and farmers markets are often good sources of handcrafted whole-grain breads.

Taste around, especially if you don't care for the first whole-grain bread you try. Brands vary in quality, and some people simply find they prefer the flavor of one grain to another.

Check the expiration dates on packages, too. Freshness is an important factor when it comes to the flavor and texture of bread. In some supermarkets, the demand for whole-grain bread may be low and the bread may sit on the shelf longer than is ideal. If that's the case in your market, or if variety is lacking, try buying whole-grain breads at a health-food store, where the turnover tends to be more rapid and the options more varied.

Be sure to read labels carefully, since there are a surprising number of refined-flour breads masquerading as wholesome choices. Don't be fooled by the words "wheat bread," or even "100% wheat bread." Unless the ingredients list specifies whole wheat, that "100% wheat" bread is simply made from refined white flour.

Color is not always a reliable indicator of whole-grain status either. While true whole-grain breads tend to have a darker color than those made from refined flour, many refined-grain breads are made brown through the addition of caramel color or molasses.

Food labels must list ingredients in weight order, so the most predominant ingredients are listed first. Choose breads that list whole grains among the first few ingredients. Check the total amount of fiber per serving, too. If there is truly a significant amount of whole grain in the bread, there will usually be at least 3 grams of fiber per slice, if not more.

Fortunately, food labeling is becoming more transparent. Look for the Whole Grains Council's yellow and black stamp to help identify products that contain a significant amount of whole grain. Products labeled "8 grams or more per serving" provide at least half a serving of whole grain, while those stamped "16 grams or more per serving" provide at least one whole serving of whole grain.

Storage tips:
Prepackaged bread should be stored at room temperature, sealed in its original wrapper. It should keep for several days if purchased before the "sell by" date.

People who live in hot and humid climates should consider storing bread in the freezer to prevent mold growth. Freezing bread is also a good tactic for people who do not use bread rapidly enough to enjoy it before it goes stale.

Freeze presliced bread in its original package for up to three months. Remove and defrost individual slices as needed.

Do not store bread in the refrigerator, as this alters its texture and drastically reduces its shelf life.

Fresh, crusty breads are best eaten the day they are baked, and tend to go stale quite rapidly. Day-old bread can often be salvaged by toasting it, or by misting the crust with water, wrapping the bread loosely with foil, and warming it in a hot oven for 5–10 minutes.

Preparation tips:
Toast and sandwiches are nice, but expanding one's bread recipe repertoire is far more interesting. Sneak in some whole grain and thicken soups or sauces by adding a slice or two of whole-grain bread before pureeing the recipe.

Add flair to salads with homemade croutons—toss cubes of a crusty whole-grain bread with olive oil. Season with garlic or herbs if desired, spread on a cookie sheet, and bake at 425°F. Toss the bread cubes occasionally and bake until they are evenly browned (about 5–10 minutes), taking care not to burn them. Allow the croutons to cool and add to salad or *gazpacho* (a vegetable soup that is served cold).

Alternatively, instead of using bread to garnish a salad, feature it as a major ingredient. Created to make use of stale bread, Italian *panzanella* and Middle Eastern *fattoush* are salads that do just that, and both can easily be adapted to use whole-grain bread. Both panzanella and fattoush often have similar components, including cucumber, tomato, olives, herbs, and sometimes Feta. Panzanella is generally made with cubes of crusty bread and dressed in a balsamic or wine vinaigrette, while fattoush utilizes stale pita and lemon vinaigrette. Fresh bread can be used in either recipe, as long as it is toasted well first.

Use whole-grain bread in a favorite French toast recipe. Or, try a *strata* for a savory brunch option. Line a baking dish or casserole with sliced or cubed whole-grain bread. Add vegetables, herbs, and cheese (a combination of frozen spinach, chopped tomatoes, and Feta works well), and top with another layer of bread. Pour beaten eggs thinned with a bit of milk or soy milk (à la French toast) over the strata, and bake in a 350°F oven until set and lightly browned, about 45 minutes to one hour.

For an especially rewarding experience, bake your own whole-grain bread. Interested in bread baking but new to the process or short on time? Try making whole-grain pizza dough, which only needs to rise once and requires less kneading than regular bread dough. Rose Levy Beranbaum's *The Bread Bible* is a fantastic resource for novice and experienced bread bakers alike.

Precautions:
Beware of breads emblazoned with disingenuous "net carb," "effective carb," and "net impact carb" claims. To date, the U.S. Food and Drug Administration (FDA), which regulates food labeling, has not established legal definitions for carbohydrate-related labeling claims. Manufacturers have petitioned the FDA on this issue, but the FDA is still working to define terms. Canada, in the meantime, has outlawed misleading carbohydrate claims on food labels.

That hasn't stopped manufacturers in the United States, who hope to capitalize on the popularity of low-carbohydrate diet regimens by using phrases like "net carbs" on their packages. These manufacturers imply (and often state outright) that their products will not raise blood glucose levels the way other carbohydrate-rich foods do.

Typically, manufacturers of foods that make these claims add fiber, gums, or sugar alcohols to the bread recipes and subtract the resulting number of grams of fiber per serving from the total grams of carbohydrate per serving to arrive at the "net carb" number. There are no scientific studies supporting this tactic or the validity of net carb claims. Well-controlled studies that examine individual foods, each of the manufacturers' various additions, and the impacts of the different resulting products on blood glucose levels in a wide segment of the population (including people with and without diabetes) would be necessary before any such claims could be validated or applied.

Consider the example of tortillas that bear a net carb claim. The package states that one tortilla contains 15 grams of carbohydrate, but only five net carbs. If the claim is correct, a consumer with diabetes who uses insulin or a drug that promotes insulin secretion may not consume enough carbohydrate to avoid hypoglycemia (low blood glucose) after a meal. On the flip side, if the claim is bogus but the consumer only counts the advertised net carbs and eats extra tortillas, he may consume too much carbohydrate, resulting in high blood glucose levels. In either case, carbohydrate counting becomes unnecessarily complicated.

Beyond the issues of disingenuous labeling and shoddy science, most products engineered to carry "low net carb" claims simply don't taste very good. What's more, adding high amounts of fiber or gums often displaces important nutrients and may impede the absorption of those that are present.

If a product bears a carbohydrate claim on its label, doesn't appear to be full of additives, and is nutrient-dense, it may be fine to use—just look at the total carbohydrate to get a picture of how much a serving provides. Better yet, stick to whole-grain versions of the "real thing"—whether it's bread, wraps, crackers, or another carbohydrate-rich food.

People who prefer to avoid artificial sweeteners should be aware that at least one major, nationally available brand began adding sucralose to its breads when it jumped on the whole-grain bandwagon.

SOY YOGURT (*also called* CULTURED SOY)

Serving size: 6 ounces plain soy yogurt, Whole Soy & Company brand

Per serving:
Calories:. 150
Carbohydrate: . . . . 27 g
Protein:. . . . . 6 g
Fat:. . . . . 3 g
Saturated fat: . . . . 0 g
Cholesterol: . . . . 0 mg
Sodium:. . . . . 25 mg
Fiber:. . . . . 2 g
Calcium: . . . . 333 mg

Note: The nutrient content of soy yogurt varies by brand and flavor, so check the label for the most accurate nutrition information.

Good source of:

probiotics, calcium, protein, soy isoflavones, fiber

Description:

Research on the health benefits of soy, an increasing interest in soy products, and the growth of companies catering to vegetarians or accommodating those with food allergies and intolerances have paved the way for soy yogurts.

Manufacturers use the same process they would to make dairy yogurt, only they introduce probiotic bacterial cultures into soy milk instead.

Because there is no lactose in soy milk to feed the probiotics, soy yogurt manufacturers typically add some sugar to nourish the friendly bacteria.

The nutrition profiles of soy and dairy yogurts are similar, but soy yogurts have less sodium, no cholesterol, no lactose, and the bonus of soy protein and isoflavones. They also contain heart-healthy mono- and polyunsaturated fat, rather than the saturated fat present in full-fat and low-fat dairy yogurts.

Health benefits:

Soy yogurts boast the health benefits of probiotics, including improved digestive health, enhanced immune function, and optimal digestion of certain nutrients.

A recent study in the journal *Applied and Environmental Microbiology* found that *Lactobacillus bulgaricus* and *Streptococcus thermophilus,* the two main cultures in commercial yogurt, can survive transit through the human intestinal tract. This finding supports the probability that the cultures remain alive, active, and able to exert benefits in the human body even after the yogurt has been digested.

Probiotics consumed via foods like soy yogurt help populate the intestinal tract with friendly bacteria and help crowd out pathogenic, or disease-causing bacteria. For this reason, people who must take antibiotics, which wipe out both bad and good bacteria, are often advised to eat yogurt to repopulate the gut with "good guys" and to prevent the diarrhea that antibiotic use can trigger.

Probiotics may also help fight infections in their own right. By adhering to the lining of the intestinal and urinary tracts, they may help prevent disease-causing bacteria from taking hold. Probiotics may also be helpful in the prevention and treatment of yeast infections. Some studies have suggested that probiotics may have anticancer effects as well. Numerous studies have demonstrated the usefulness of probiotics in lessening the duration, severity, or frequency of diarrhea.

Previously, people with dairy allergies or lactose intolerance may not have been able to benefit from the health-promoting effects of probiotics via yogurt consumption. Now, with the wider availability of soy yogurts, they can.

The isoflavones in soy yogurts may confer additional benefits, including helping to reduce the symptoms of perimenopause and menopause. Soy isoflavones may also help fight certain cancers, including breast, endometrial, prostate, and colon cancer, although more research is needed to confirm these effects.

Soy yogurt may help promote heart health by improving blood lipid levels, reducing blood pressure, and helping the arteries remain elastic. While many studies on soy and cholesterol have looked at benefits for people with abnormal cholesterol levels, a 2003 study conducted in Portugal found that soy yogurt significantly increased the HDL ("good") cholesterol levels in men with normal blood lipid levels.

Since 1999, the FDA has allowed manufacturers to include the following health claim on the labels of foods that contain at least 6.25 grams of soy protein: "25 grams of soy protein a day, as part of a diet low in saturated fat and cholesterol, may reduce the risk of heart disease. One serving of [name of food] contains _ grams of soy protein."

Some soy yogurts contain enough soy protein to feature this health claim.

Excessive animal protein intake is taxing to the kidneys, but studies have found that replacing it with sources of soy protein such as soy yogurt may help prevent kidney damage or slow its progression. People with diabetes are at higher risk for kidney disease, so choosing soy yogurt may be a smart move.

Contrary to popular belief, some studies have shown that high dairy consumption is associated with higher, not lower, rates of osteoporosis. Soy yogurt, on the other hand, may help promote bone health. Unlike animal protein, soy protein does not cause excessive calcium losses in the urine, and calcium-fortified soy yogurts do provide a readily absorbable calcium source.

Most soy yogurts are free of casein, whey, and gluten; they are also lower in potassium, sodium, and phosphorus than cow's milk yogurts. For people on various special diets due to health conditions or allergies (other than soy allergies), soy yogurt may be a better choice than dairy yogurt.

Selection tips:
Soy yogurts are available in the dairy case of many supermarkets and most health-food stores. While the fruited versions of soy yogurts are typically lower in sugar than dairy yogurts, this can vary by brand and flavor, so read labels carefully.

Look for soy yogurt in containers that specifically state that the contents contain "live and active cultures" to ensure the presence of beneficial probiotics. Some companies include additional strains of live active cultures to boost the probiotic benefits of their product.

Check the "sell by" or expiration date, and select soy yogurt that displays a date as far from the current date as possible. Take a peek at the thermometer in the dairy case to make sure that the market keeps its refrigerator cold enough—between 35°F and 40°F.

Remember that any fat in soy yogurt is of the beneficial mono- and polyunsaturated types, so it isn't necessary to seek out fat-free soy yogurt.

Storage tips:
Soy yogurt is perishable and must be kept in the refrigerator. For best quality and optimal safety, use soy yogurt prior to its "sell by" or expiration date.

Preparation tips:
Use soy yogurt as you would dairy yogurt. Enjoy it as is, layer it with granola and fruit for a breakfast parfait, or try a spoonful in place of whipped cream with berries and a whole-grain waffle.

Plain soy yogurt is a great base for dips or sauces—mix it with herbs and spices, or use it to make a lactose-free, vegan version of *tzatziki* or *raita*.

Use a dollop of soy yogurt to garnish soups, or stir it into mashed potatoes to lend the spuds creaminess without lots of added fat.

While baking will destroy the beneficial probiotics in soy yogurt, it can be used in place of sour cream to reduce fat content or to adapt recipes for those with dairy allergies.

Precautions:
Certain antibiotics are rendered less effective when taken at the same time as (or in close proximity to) calcium-fortified products or calcium supplements. This can compromise treatment and contribute to the development of antibiotic resistant strains of bacteria. While the probiotics in soy yogurt can help mitigate the intestinal upset and diarrhea sometimes associated with antibiotic use, it is critical to ask a pharmacist if the antibiotic prescribed is compatible with the brand you've chosen. The calcium content of soy yogurts varies, so have the label available to show the pharmacist. If it has too much calcium, consider taking a probiotic supplement such as Culturelle (*Lactobacillus* GG).

While it is generally thought that the isoflavones in soy are safe and may even be beneficial in fighting cancer, people being treated for estrogen-dependent cancers should discuss soy yogurt consumption with their medical team.

According to the independent Pew Initiative on Food and Biotechnology, by 2004, nearly 85% of soybeans planted in the United States in 2004 were genetically engineered varieties.

People who are concerned about the application of genetic engineering technologies to foodstuffs should seek out organic soy yogurt.

Serving size: 1 eight-ounce container of plain, low-fat yogurt

Per serving:
Calories:. 143
Carbohydrate: . . . . 16 g
Protein:. . . . . 12 g
Fat:. . . . . 4 g
Saturated fat: . . . . 2 g
Cholesterol: . . . . 14 mg
Sodium:. . . . . 159 mg
Fiber:. . . . . 0 g
Calcium: . . . . 415 mg

Note: Keep in mind—especially when counting carbohydrates or measuring yogurt from a large container for recipes—that a typical eight-ounce container of yogurt contains slightly less than eight ounces. Read the label to determine if the nutrient values listed are for a particular quantity expressed in ounces, or "per container."

Good source of:

probiotics, calcium, protein, potassium, phosphorus, selenium, B vitamins

Description:

Yogurt is a thick, fermented dairy product made by introducing bacterial cultures into milk. The first yogurts were probably happy accidents in which friendly bacteria from the environment mingled with goat or sheep milk. The biological process that ensued raised the acidity of the milk, helping to turn it thick and creamy, preserve it, and give it a tangy flavor. Deliberate yogurt crafting followed and has occurred for thousands of years in Central Asia, India, and Europe.

It wasn't until the 1900's that yogurt production became industrialized. Russian biologist and Nobel prize winner Elie Metchnikoff believed that the frequent yogurt consumption by Bulgarian peasants contributed to their unusually long life spans, and devoted the last decade of his own life to studying the lactic-acid–producing bacteria that turn milk into yogurt. He identified and isolated two cultures, *Lactobacillus bulgaricus* and *Streptococcus thermophilus*, that are always present in modern yogurt.

Entrepreneur Isaac Carasso used these cultures—and carried on Metchnikoff's mission of promoting yogurt's health benefits—when he founded a small yogurt outfit in Spain called Danone in 1919. The business eventually grew to become the Dannon Company, one of the largest yogurt producers in the United States and a major player in terms of introducing Americans to yogurt.

Yogurt manufacturers are wise to the fact that most Americans like sweet stuff and have flooded the market with a tremendous amount of fruity, over-sweetened yogurts. It takes some careful label-reading to steer clear of desserts masquerading as yogurt. Fortunately, more traditional European yogurts, with their characteristic tangy or sour flavors, are increasingly available. There are also some American yogurt makers turning out great plain and fruited yogurts with less sugar and a wider range of probiotics (the friendly bacterial cultures that turn milk into yogurt).

Health benefits:

Many health benefits have been associated with regular yogurt consumption, and virtually all appear to be associated with the presence of probiotics.

A recent study in the journal *Applied and Environmental Microbiology* found that *Lactobacillus bulgaricus* and *Streptococcus thermophilus*, the two main cultures in commercial yogurt, survived transit through the human intestinal tract. This finding supports the probability that probiotic cultures remain alive, active, and able to exert benefits in the human body even after the yogurt has been digested.

Studies have demonstrated that probiotics like those found in yogurt play an important role in gastrointestinal health and immunity. They also help optimize the digestion of certain nutrients, which further enhances immune function and overall health.

Probiotics consumed via foods like yogurt help populate the intestinal tract with friendly bacteria and help crowd out pathogenic, or disease-causing, bacteria. For this reason, people who must take antibiotics, which wipe out both bad and good bacteria, are often advised to eat yogurt to repopulate the gut with "good guys" and to prevent the diarrhea that antibiotic use can trigger.

Probiotics may also help fight infection in their own right. By adhering to the lining of the intestinal and urinary tracts, they may help prevent disease-causing bacteria from taking hold. Probiotics may also be helpful in the prevention and treatment of yeast infections. Some studies have suggested that probiotics may have anticancer effects as well.

A study published in 2006 in *The Turkish Journal of Pediatrics* found that yogurt helped alleviate moderate acute diarrhea and decrease the length of hospitalization in small children with moderate dehydration.

In a study published in *The American Journal of Clinical Nutrition* in 2006, researchers reported that yogurt containing *Lactobacillus acidophilus* and *Bifidobacterium lactis* cultures increased the effectiveness of therapy for *Helicobacter pylori* (the bacteria that causes peptic ulcers) infection in milk-tolerant individuals. Standard therapy involving a type of drug called a proton pump inhibitor and two antibiotics had failed to eradicate the infection in the 138 study subjects, who were randomly assigned to receive a fourth drug or a fourth drug, plus yogurt. Even among people with antibiotic-resistant *H. pylori*—which is particularly difficult to treat—those in the yogurt group experienced a significantly higher rate of *H. pylori* eradication. Because *H. pylori* infection constitutes a major risk factor for esophageal and gastric cancers, the results of this study were especially promising.

Probiotics digest lactose, so some people who are lactose intolerant find that they can enjoy yogurt without gastrointestinal distress. Milk-based yogurt is also an excellent source of calcium and protein.

Selection tips:

Look for yogurt in containers that specifically state that the contents contain "live and active cultures." According to FDA regulations, manufacturers can't call their product yogurt unless it is made with active cultures. But some manufacturers subject the yogurt to heat treatment after making it, which kills the cultures. That robs the yogurt of the potential health benefits that live cultures provide.

Some yogurt companies include additional strains of live active cultures to boost the probiotic benefits of their product. One notable brand is Stonyfield Farm, which adds four additional yogurt cultures, and is the only U.S. company to include *Lactobacillus reuteri*. Studies have shown that among other benefits, *L. reuteri* inhibits the growth of several dangerous pathogens, including *Salmonella*, *E. coli*, *Staphylococcus*, and *Listeria*.

The company also adds inulin, a fiber that aids calcium absorption, to its yogurt.

Stonyfield Farm is one of several companies that opposes the use of recombinant bovine growth hormone (rBGH), which can increase rates of mastitis (an udder infection), the subsequent antibiotic use, and lameness, and decrease life expectancy in cattle that receive it. Artificial growth hormone usage also contributes to an already significant milk surplus, which drives dairy prices down and has devastating implications for the livelihoods of small dairy farmers.

Read labels carefully if you prefer to avoid artificial sweeteners. Thanks to the naturally occurring lactose, or milk sugar, in yogurt, an eight-ounce container of plain yogurt typically contains between 13 and 15 grams of carbohydrate. Once manufacturers add fruit and sugar to their yogurts, those numbers can soar. So, to please an increasingly carbohydrate-conscious yet sweet-loving public, several major yogurt manufacturers use artificial sweeteners in their yogurts. These yogurts still contain about 13 grams of sugar that occur naturally in the yogurt. In contrast, regular fruited yogurts sweetened with sugar might contain as much as 45 grams of carbohydrate, much of which comes from the added sugars.

Check the "sell by" or expiration date and select yogurt that displays a date as far from the current date as possible. Take a peek at the thermometer in the dairy case to make sure that the market keeps its refrigerator cold enough—between 35°F and 40°F.

Low-fat and fat-free yogurts are the best choices for heart health and possibly weight management. Full-fat yogurts are high in total and saturated fat.

Storage tips:
Yogurt is perishable and must be kept in the refrigerator. For best quality and optimal safety, use yogurt prior to its "sell by" or expiration date.

Preparation tips:
Have you ever opened a container of yogurt, seen a clear, watery substance on top, and poured the liquid down the drain? Next time, stir it in—that's the whey, which has health benefits of its own. Whey appears to optimize the immune function and promote healing, so it's definitely worth keeping!

Most Americans eat fruit-flavored and presweetened yogurt for breakfast or as a snack. A far better option is to buy plain unsweetened yogurt and add chopped or mashed fresh fruit to it. Even with the addition of a teaspoon of maple syrup, honey, or sugar, home-assembled fruited yogurt will be far higher in fiber, nutrients, and antioxidants and lower in sugar than the commercial yogurts. It's also totally customizable—serve up kiwi-banana yogurt one day and blackberry-nectarine yogurt the next.

Try cereal with yogurt for a more easily digested, probiotic-rich alternative to milk.

Yogurt is great with savory foods, too. Mix it with shredded, drained cucumber and a generous amount of chopped garlic to make *tzatziki,* a delicious, cooling Greek yogurt dip. Add mint, cayenne, or curry (with or without cucumber) for variations on *raita,* an Indian condiment.

Yogurt is fantastic in marinades—its acidity helps tenderize protein—and it's a great replacement for sour cream in recipes.

Yogurt cheese, which is simple to make at home and very versatile, is an excellent alternative to high-fat cream cheese. Line a colander set inside a bowl with cheesecloth, a clean tea towel, or even layers of paper towels. Add plain yogurt to the colander, cover well, and set in the refrigerator for several hours or overnight. Much of the liquid whey will drain out, and you'll be left with yogurt cheese. Spread plain yogurt cheese on toast or fold in herbs, dried fruit, or nuts to make flavored versions. Yogurt cheese also works well in cheesecake recipes. As for the whey that drains off, throw it into a smoothie to reap its immune-enhancing benefits!

The friendly bacteria in yogurt won't survive cooking or baking, but from a culinary standpoint, yogurt is still a great ingredient for baked goods, especially when used as a replacement for high-fat cream cheese or sour cream.

Precautions:

Some studies have found an association between dairy consumption and increased breast, ovarian, and prostate cancer risk. People with a personal or family history of these cancers should discuss their dairy intake with a health-care professional. A registered dietitian can help ensure you are getting adequate calcium without raising cancer risk. Nondairy calcium sources and supplements are among the options.

Certain antibiotics are rendered less effective when taken at the same time as (or in close proximity to) dairy products or calcium supplements. This can compromise treatment and contribute to the development of antibiotic-resistant strains of bacteria. While yogurt can help mitigate the intestinal upset and diarrhea sometimes associated with antibiotic use, it is critical to ask a pharmacist if the antibiotic prescribed is compatible with dairy. If it is not, consider taking a probiotic supplement, such as Culturelle (*Lactobacillus* GG), instead.

Yogurt is rich in potassium. People on potassium-restricted diets should consult a registered dietitian or doctor before eating yogurt.

Do not feed dairy products to babies under one year of age, as this can increase their risk of developing allergies or damage to the gastrointestinal tract. Some health experts feel that yogurt can safely be fed to babies over nine months of age, particularly if the baby was exclusively breastfed. Discuss your infant's individual situation with a registered dietitian or pediatrician before introducing yogurt, and be sure to seek out products without artificial sweeteners and preferably those produced without artificial growth hormones.

People who are concerned about the use of artificial growth hormones or antibiotic overuse in dairy cattle should choose organic yogurt.

EGGS

Serving size: 1 whole large egg

Per serving:

Calories:	74
Carbohydrate:	0 g
Protein:	6 g
Fat:	5 g
Saturated fat:	2 g
Monounsaturated fat:	2 g
Polyunsaturated fat:	1 g
Omega-3 fatty acids:	0 g
Cholesterol:	212 mg
Sodium:	70 mg
Fiber:	0 g
Calcium:	26 mg

Good source of:

protein, vitamin A, vitamin D, vitamin B_{12}, riboflavin, pantothenic acid, iron, selenium, choline, lutein, zeaxanthin

Description:

Eggs are an essential part of a female bird's reproductive system. Meant to protect and nourish baby birds, the egg has long been a staple of human diets thanks to its nutrient-dense contents. Although there are many types of edible eggs, including goose, duck, and quail, it's the chicken egg that tends to get all of the attention in the United States. Beyond breakfast, they are ubiquitous in baked goods, where they serve as both leavening agents and binders.

For several years, eggs got quite a bit of bad publicity, thanks to the high cholesterol content of the yellow yolk. Many people shunned eggs out of fear that they would cause high cholesterol and heart disease. But it turns out that cholesterol is only part of the story when it comes to heart health. Saturated fat and *trans* fat appear to be more important when it comes to raising blood cholesterol levels.

In most cases, saturated fat and cholesterol come packaged together in animal foods. But although there is a hefty dose of cholesterol in eggs, there is relatively little saturated fat—less than 2 grams—in an egg. By comparison, 3 ounces of choice sirloin has 83 grams of cholesterol and more than 19 grams of fat, almost 8 grams of which are saturated. (Keeping in mind that most people eat at least 6 ounces of steak, those numbers must be doubled.)

That's not to say it's wise to eat dozens of whole eggs per week. But they are a better choice among animal sources of protein when eaten in moderation.

Health benefits:

Many of us think of eggs solely as a protein source, but they are rich in many nutrients. They contain vitamins, minerals, and even unsaturated fats, as well as the antioxidants lutein and zeaxanthin.

It's actually the yolk of the egg that contains nearly all of the egg's nutrients. The fat-soluble vitamins A and D are present in the yolk. Conveniently, the fat that facilitates the absorption of those nutrients is packaged in the yolk as well. Vitamin A is important for vision, immune function, bone growth, and cell differentiation. Vitamin D is essential to bone health and the maintenance of calcium and phosphorus balance in the blood.

Egg yolks are an excellent source of the essential nutrient choline. Important in the synthesis of cell membranes, choline is also vital to cell signaling, or communication between cells. Choline plays a role in neurotransmission, helping to ensure muscle control and memory function. Pregnant and nursing mothers who like eggs should also consider eating the yolks, which help ensure that they'll get adequate choline, an essential nutrient for fetal and infant brain and nervous system development. Choline also helps the body to metabolize fat and cholesterol, and it helps keep fat from accumulating in the liver.

The lutein and zeaxanthin in eggs might help prevent macular degeneration.

Selection tips:
Purchase only grade AA or grade A eggs from a refrigerated case. Open the carton and check to make sure that none of the eggs are cracked or dirty. Most recipes call for large eggs, so stick to those for optimal results.

Choosing brown or white eggs is a matter of preference. The color of the shell is determined by the breed of the hen. Although brown eggs have thicker shells, they have the same nutrient profile as white eggs.

Shoppers who are concerned about the overuse of antibiotics in animal production should select organic eggs or those specifically labeled as antibiotic-free. The U.S. Department of Agriculture does not allow the use of hormones in raising chickens, so all eggs should be hormone-free.

Storage tips:
Refrigerate eggs in their carton in the coldest part of the refrigerator immediately after purchase. Do not store eggs in the refrigerator door—it's not cold enough to protect against bacterial growth.

As long as they are purchased before the date stamped on the carton, eggs can be kept in the refrigerator for three to five weeks. Keep in mind that the date on graded eggs is four weeks after the eggs were packed, so the further away the date is at the time of purchase, the fresher the eggs.

Hard-boiled eggs can be stored in the refrigerator for up to seven days.

Dishes made from eggs, such as casseroles, can be refrigerated for up to three days but must be reheated to 165°F before being eaten.

Eggs can be frozen for later use but must be removed from their shells first. Lightly beat whole eggs or egg whites and store in a well-sealed container in the freezer for up to one year.

Preparation tips:
Wash your hands, utensils, bowls, and work surfaces with hot, soapy water before and after handling raw eggs. Keep other foods—especially those that will be eaten raw, like salads—away from raw eggs.

Break each egg into a separate dish before adding it to a recipe or skillet. That way, if you encounter a bad egg, the entire recipe won't be ruined.

Cook eggs thoroughly so that the whites are opaque and the yolks are completely firm. Runny eggs or those prepared "sunny-side up" are not recommended because they carry a higher risk of transmitting food-borne illness.

Eggs might be common, but they needn't be ho-hum. Spice up the morning with a breakfast burrito—scramble an egg with onion, spinach, and black beans and roll into a whole wheat tortilla with tomato salsa. Or try an omelet made with one whole egg and one or two egg whites. Add veggies, herbs, and a little low-fat cheese, if desired. Serve with fruit salad or multigrain toast.

Use eggs to make buckwheat crepes and wrap them around ratatouille or roasted vegetables. Try quiches, frittatas, or soufflés for brunch or a light dinner.

Eggs are an essential part of most baked good recipes. From a food chemistry perspective, leaving out most of the eggs or using a substitute can compromise the texture or overall quality of the final product. *Eating Well* and *Cooking Light* magazines are good sources for well-tested recipes for baked goods that have fewer eggs, or a mix of whole eggs and egg whites, and that take the guesswork out of reducing the cholesterol content of recipes that rely on eggs.

Precautions:
To reduce the risk of food-borne illness, including salmonella, do not eat raw or undercooked eggs or taste uncooked foods containing eggs.

There is no longer a firm recommendation about how many whole eggs one may safely eat in a week. People with normal cholesterol levels can probably eat up to one whole egg per day without experiencing unwanted effects on total cholesterol or low-density lipoprotein (LDL, "bad") cholesterol levels—as long as other cholesterol-containing foods are kept to a minimum. In other words, if there's meat on the menu at another meal, it's probably wisest to skip the egg, or at least the yolk, that day. Also don't forget that eggs are present in many baked goods, casseroles, and even sauces or mayonnaise.

Remember, too, that although eggs can usually be included as part of a health-promoting diet, poorly chosen preparation methods and accompaniments can quickly overshadow any benefit from eggs. A three-egg and cheese omelet (using whole eggs), cooked in butter and served with bacon or sausage, fried potatoes, and buttered white toast spells disaster for one's health. On the other hand, an omelet made with one whole egg, one or more egg whites, and vegetables, cooked in a tiny bit of oil or cooking spray, served with a tofu "sausage" and multigrain toast is a fine and healthful breakfast.

The question of whole eggs is less clear-cut for those with *dyslipidemia,* which is a potentially harmful change in the amount of lipids in the blood. One to three whole eggs per week might be fine, but it's best to consult with a registered dietitian to determine the safest level of egg consumption. The extent of high cholesterol, which lipids are elevated, and which cholesterol-lowering medicines an individual takes (if any) should all be considered.

Serving size: 1 large egg

Per serving:

Calories:. 70
Carbohydrate: . . . . 0 g
Protein:. 6 g
Fat:. . . . . 4 g
Saturated fat: . . . . 1 g
Monounsaturated fat: . . . . 2 g
Polyunsaturated fat:. . . . . 1 g
Omega-3 fatty acids: . . . . . > 100 mg
Docosahexaenoic
    acid(DHA): . . . . > 50 mg
Eicosapentaenoic
    acid (EPA): . . . . 2 mg
Cholesterol: . . . . 180 mg
Sodium:. . . . . 60 mg
Fiber:. 0 g
Calcium: . . . . 25 mg

Note: Nutrition values are for the nationally available Eggland's Best brand of omega-3–fortified eggs. Nutrient values will vary, especially for omega-3 content, depending on the brand of egg and the feed used.

Good source of:

protein, omega-3 fatty acids, vitamin A, vitamin D, vitamin B_{12}, riboflavin, pantothenic acid, iron, selenium, choline, lutein, zeaxanthin

Description:

The health benefits of omega-3 fatty acids are deservedly getting increasing attention, yet many people find getting adequate omega-3's a challenge. Some egg farmers realized that they could boost the omega-3 content of eggs by changing the feed they offer their hens. For those who are allergic to (or dislike) fish, walnuts, or other omega-3-rich foods, fortified eggs are another option.

Health benefits:

Omega-3 fatty acids benefit cardiovascular health by helping to keep the arteries supple and elastic and by improving the lipid profile.

Omega-3's have anti-inflammatory properties, which are important for preventing or delaying progression of inflammatory conditions such as diabetes, heart disease, inflammatory bowel disease, and arthritis.

Adequate omega-3 intake is important for pregnant and nursing women because the fatty acids are vital to fetal and infant brain and eye development. Omega-3's might also help prevent postpartum depression.

Although cholesterol, nutrient, and omega-3 content varies among omega-3–fortified eggs, one nationally available brand, called Eggland's Best, is lower in cholesterol and saturated fat and higher in lutein, vitamin E, and iodine than regular eggs.

As with all eggs, those that are omega-3-fortified are good sources of protein, vitamins, minerals, and the antioxidants lutein and zeaxanthin.

Fat-soluble vitamins A and D are present in the yolk, together with the fat that facilitates their absorption. Vitamin A is important for vision, immune function, bone growth, and cell differentiation. Vitamin D is essential to bone health and the maintenance of calcium and phosphorus balance in the blood.

Egg yolks are also an excellent source of the essential nutrient choline. Important in the synthesis of cell membranes, choline is also vital to cell signaling, or communication between cells. Choline plays a role in neurotransmission, helping to ensure muscle control and memory function. Pregnant and nursing mothers who like eggs should consider keeping the yolks to help ensure that they'll get adequate choline, an essential nutrient for fetal and infant brain and nervous system development. Choline also helps the body to metabolize fat and cholesterol, and it helps keep fat from accumulating in the liver.

The lutein and zeaxanthin in eggs might help prevent macular degeneration.

Selection tips:
Purchase only grade AA or grade A eggs from a refrigerated case. Open the carton and check to make sure that none of the eggs are cracked or dirty. Most recipes call for large eggs, so stick to those for optimal results.

Choosing brown or white eggs is a matter of personal preference. The color of the shell is determined by the breed of the hen. Although brown eggs have thicker shells, they have the same nutrient profile as white eggs.

Those concerned about the overuse of antibiotics in animal production should select organic eggs or those specifically labeled as antibiotic-free. The U.S. Department of Agriculture does not allow the use of hormones in raising chickens, so all eggs should be hormone-free.

In the case of omega-3–fortified eggs, it's a good idea to do a little homework and find out more about the source of the omega-3's added to the hen feed. Some farmers feed their hens flax or add canola oil to the feed. Others feed their hens fish meal or fish oil, a more dubious practice because hens do not naturally eat fish. Depending on the source, fish meal might be contaminated with heavy metals or other environmental contaminants. Lacto-ovo vegetarians will also likely prefer eggs from hens that were fed vegetarian feed.

Storage tips:
Refrigerate eggs in their carton in the coldest part of the refrigerator immediately after purchase. Do not store eggs in the refrigerator door—it's not cold enough to protect against bacterial growth.

As long as they are purchased before the date stamped on the carton, eggs can be kept in the refrigerator for three to five weeks. Keep in mind that the date on graded eggs is four weeks after the eggs were packed, so the further away the date is at the time of purchase, the fresher the eggs.

Hard-boiled eggs can be stored in the refrigerator for up to seven days.

Dishes made from eggs, such as casseroles, can be refrigerated for up to three days but must be reheated to 165°F before being eaten.

Eggs can be frozen for later use but must be removed from their shells first. Lightly beat whole eggs or egg whites and store in a well-sealed container in the freezer for up to one year.

Preparation tips:
Wash your hands, utensils, bowls, and work surfaces with hot, soapy water before and after handling raw eggs. Keep other foods—especially those that will be eaten raw, like salads—away from raw eggs.

Break each egg into a separate dish before adding it to a recipe or skillet. That way, if you encounter a bad egg, the entire recipe won't be ruined.

Cook eggs thoroughly, so that the whites are opaque and the yolks are completely firm. Runny eggs or those prepared "sunny-side up" are not recommended because they carry a higher risk of transmitting food-borne illness.

Eggs might be common, but they needn't be ho-hum. Spice up the morning with a breakfast burrito—scramble an egg with onion, spinach, and black beans and roll into a whole wheat tortilla with tomato salsa. Or try an omelet made with one whole egg and one or two egg whites. Add veggies, herbs, and a little low-fat cheese, if desired. Serve with fruit salad or multigrain toast.

Use eggs to make buckwheat crepes and wrap them around ratatouille or roasted vegetables. Try quiches, frittatas, or soufflés for brunch or a light dinner.

Eggs are an essential part of most baked good recipes. From a food chemistry perspective, leaving out most of the eggs or using a substitute can compromise the texture or overall quality of the final product. *Eating Well* and *Cooking Light* magazines are good sources for well-tested baked-good recipes that have fewer eggs, or a mix of whole eggs and egg whites, and that take the guesswork out of reducing the cholesterol content of recipes that rely on eggs.

Precautions:
To reduce the risk of food-borne illness, including salmonella, do not eat raw or undercooked eggs or taste uncooked foods containing eggs.

There is no longer a firm recommendation about how many whole eggs one may safely eat in a week. Those with normal cholesterol levels can probably eat up to one whole egg per day without experiencing unwanted effects on cholesterol or LDL levels—as long as other cholesterol-containing foods are kept to a minimum. In other words, if there's meat on the menu at another meal, it's probably wisest to skip the egg, or at least the yolk that day. Also don't forget that eggs are present in many baked goods, casseroles, and even sauces or mayonnaise.

Remember, too, that although eggs can usually be included as part of a health-promoting diet, poorly chosen preparation methods and accompaniments can quickly overshadow any benefit from eggs. A three-egg and cheese omelet (using whole eggs), cooked in butter and served with bacon or sausage, fried potatoes, and buttered white toast spells disaster for one's health. On the other hand, an omelet made with one whole egg, egg whites and vegetables, cooked in a tiny bit of oil or cooking spray, served with a tofu "sausage" and multigrain toast is a fine and healthful breakfast.

The question of whole eggs is less clear-cut for those with *dyslipidemia*, which is a potentially harmful change in the amount of lipids in the blood. One to three whole eggs per week might be fine, but it's best to consult with a registered dietitian to determine the safest level of egg consumption. The extent of high cholesterol, which lipids are elevated, and which cholesterol-lowering medicines an individual takes (if any) should all be considered.

SALMON

Serving size: 3 ounces wild salmon, cooked

Per serving:

Calories:. 155
Carbohydrate: . . . . 0 g
Protein:. . . . . 22 g
Fat:. . . . . 7 g
Saturated fat: . . . . 1 g
Monounsaturated fat: . . . . 2 g
Polyunsaturated fat:. . . . . 3 g
Omega-3 fatty acids:. . . . . 2 g
Docosahexaenoic
    acid (DHA): . . . . 1 g
Eicosapentaenoic
    acid (EPA): . . . . 1 g
Cholesterol: . . . . 60 mg
Sodium:. . . . . 48 mg
Fiber:. . . . . 0 g
Calcium: . . . . 13 mg

Good source of:

protein, omega-3 fatty acids (including DHA & EPA), carotenoids, copper, selenium, phosphorus, potassium, vitamin B_{12}, niacin, thiamine, riboflavin

Description:

Salmon are silver-skinned, coral-fleshed fish that start and end their lives in fresh water and spend the interim in the ocean. There are several species of salmon, though only one—the aptly named Atlantic salmon—lives in Atlantic waters. Ironically, wild Atlantic salmon, unlike their Pacific counterparts, do not die after the first time they spawn, but are nearly extinct due to pollution and overfishing. Because of its endangered status, the Atlantic salmon on the market today is farmed (and the majority of it is farmed on the Pacific coast, where the Atlantic salmon species does not naturally occur).

The many species of Pacific salmon are available wild, thanks in part to regulated, sustainable fishing practices and the banning of salmon farming in Alaska. The most prized and widely consumed are chinook, sockeye, and coho salmon. Pink salmon are a small species with soft flesh that is commonly canned but rarely eaten fresh.

Chinook, also known as king salmon, are the largest of the Pacific salmon species, growing up to 120 pounds. Chinooks have firm, bright orange flesh that is high in omega-3 fatty acids.

Sockeye salmon are commonly canned, but the fresh fish are much desired by salmon aficionados thanks to their flavorful red flesh and brief season.

Coho salmon are a smaller species with a milder flavor than the chinook or sockeye salmon. They are also lower in fat, so their reddish-orange flesh is a bit drier.

Health benefits:

Among the most touted health benefits of salmon is the abundance of omega-3 fatty acids in the fish. From a practical standpoint, omega-3's act as a sort of antifreeze for fish that have to swim their way through icy waters. When we consume their flesh, we reap the benefits.

Omega-3 fatty acids benefit cardiovascular health by helping to keep the arteries supple and elastic and by improving the lipid profile.

Omega-3's have anti-inflammatory properties, which are important for preventing or delaying progression of inflammatory conditions such as diabetes, heart disease, inflammatory bowel disease, and arthritis.

Wild salmon owes its orange color to antioxidant carotenoids, which are naturally abundant in the fish flesh thanks to a diet of krill and tiny shrimp. (Farmed salmon are essentially "dyed"—they get their pigment through carotenoids added to their feed.)

And fish really is "brain food"! Omega-3's, particularly docosahexaenoic acid (DHA), are abundant in human brain and eye tissues. Studies have found that those who consume DHA-rich foods regularly have lower incidences of neurodegenerative diseases.

Pregnant and nursing women who love salmon and who make a point of enjoying wild salmon (avoid farmed salmon, which is high in environmental contaminants) will boost their infant's supply of omega-3's, which are vital to brain development. Omega-3's might also help prevent postpartum depression.

Selection tips:
Fresh fish are highly perishable and should be selected with care from a reputable fishmonger or market. If the shop itself smells bad, chances are the fish is, too. Make sure the fish is kept on clean ice and that there's no evidence of pooling water under the fish. Preparation counters should look clean, too.

Whole fish should have bright red gills, and the eyes should be clear, shiny, and convex. The skin and scales should be well-attached, and the flesh should be firm. If pressure from a finger leaves an indent in the flesh, the fish is no longer fresh. Slimy skin is another indication that the fish is past its prime. Finally, fish should smell fresh—never "fishy."

Fillets should be firm, with intact, consistently colored, moist flesh.

Increasingly, wild salmon are flash-frozen at sea, so it is possible to enjoy them after the season ends. Some stores sell partially frozen, or thawed, previously frozen fish. Looks-wise and taste-wise, not many can tell the difference between fresh fish and fish that was flash-frozen on boats and then thawed in the store. It must be labeled as previously frozen, however, because it is more perishable than fresh fish.

Frozen fish should be frozen solid and sealed in airtight packaging. It should show no evidence of freezer burn, ice crystals, or frost.

Storage tips:
Keep fresh or previously frozen fish cold at all times, and use it as soon after purchase as possible. Take fish home from the store in an insulated bag, or ask the help behind the fish counter for a separate bag of ice to keep near the fish while you transport it home.

Fresh, raw fish can be stored in the coldest part of the refrigerator for a maximum of one to two days.

Thawed, previously frozen fish must be cooked before it can be refrozen.

Salmon that was purchased frozen can be stored in the freezer for up to eight months (check the package label for specifics). Most home freezers are not cold enough to freeze fresh fish without compromising its texture. However, if a freezer thermometer indicates that your freezer is at or below 0°F and you have more salmon than you can use, you can rinse salmon portions in cold water and wrap them in heavy-duty foil or freezer bags. Be sure to press all the air out of the bags. Freeze individual portions in a single layer in the freezer to ensure that they freeze quickly. Use within one to two months.

Once the fish is cooked, it can be stored in the refrigerator for two to three days. Cooking the fish in acidic ingredients such as lemon juice, lime juice, or wine might extend the refrigerator shelf life by another day or two, depending on the temperature of the refrigerator and how fresh the fish was when it was purchased. Of course, if the fish smells or tastes "off," discard the leftovers.

Preparation tips:

For optimum safety, frozen salmon should be defrosted in the refrigerator. It can also be defrosted under cold, running water while it is still packaged in plastic. Do not defrost under hot water or on a countertop, as this raises the risk of bacterial growth (and might compromise the texture of the fish).

When it comes to preparation, salmon is one of the most versatile fish available. It can be poached, baked, or steamed and has a firm enough texture to handle grilling, sautéing, and pan-searing. Salmon has a distinctive flavor that shines when the fish is simply prepared, but it is equally wonderful with flavorful marinades or assertive spice rubs. Because salmon has a remarkable affinity for a wide range of herbs, spices, and flavor principles, it is one of the best fish choices for those who enjoy experimenting with ethnic cuisines.

Try poached salmon with *tzatziki* (cucumber and yogurt salad) or a yogurt-dill sauce. For an elegant presentation, bake salmon in parchment packets with julienned vegetables and a splash of white wine. Roast it over a bed of lemon slices and herbs, or treat it to a spice rub and grill or bake.

Try adding sautéed or baked salmon to curries, or use it in fish soups. Marinate salmon in chili pepper, lime juice, and olive oil, then grill and serve with tortillas, fresh salsa, black beans, and guacamole. Cube salmon and bake or grill it on kabobs. Use chopped salmon for fish burgers, or serve salmon over salad greens.

For crowd-pleasing hors d'oeuvres, marinate salmon cubes in reduced-sodium soy sauce and maple syrup. Drain the cubes and coat with fresh, coarsely ground black pepper. Place the cubes on a parchment-paper–lined cookie sheet, and bake at 450°F for 3–5 minutes or until cooked through. Skewer salmon on toothpicks, place the cubes on a platter, and serve.

Take a cue from the Japanese and have some grilled salmon for breakfast with miso soup and pickled vegetables. Or for an elegant brunch entrée that is the height of simplicity, bake a whole side of salmon, and serve warm or chilled with a blueberry and yellow pepper salsa.

Precautions:

Consuming raw or undercooked salmon is not recommended as this can raise the risk of food-borne illness or parasitic infection.

From health, safety, and environmental standpoints, wild salmon is a far better choice than farmed. Farmed salmon are dosed heavily with antibiotics, which may contribute to the development of dangerous antibiotic-resistant strains of bacteria. Environmental toxins, including PCBs and dioxins—two probable human carcinogens—have been found in high concentrations in farmed salmon. Farmed salmon are deliberately "fattened up," which might exacerbate the bioaccumulation of these contaminants.

Farmed salmon are higher in calories and saturated fat but approximately 35% lower in omega-3 fatty acids than wild salmon.

Current salmon farming practices can be devastating to delicate coastal ecosystems and to wild salmon stocks as well.

Wild Atlantic salmon is nearly extinct, and almost all Atlantic salmon on the market today is farmed. Alaska does not allow fish farming, which provides some assurance that fish specifically labeled as Alaskan is likely to be wild. In the summer months, during the wild salmon run, salmon labeled "wild" probably is. However, thanks to the markup in price that wild salmon commands, unscrupulous supermarkets and fishmongers have been known to sell farmed salmon as wild. If there seems to be an abundance of fresh wild salmon in the winter off-season, ask questions and think twice before purchasing it. Tip-offs that allegedly wild salmon isn't include paler, fattier, softer flesh (farmed salmon is dyed to look like its wild counterpart).

SALMON, CANNED

Serving size: 3 ounces sockeye salmon, canned, without salt, drained, with bones

Per serving:
Calories:. 130
Carbohydrate: . . . . 0 g
Protein:. 17 g
Fat:. . . . . 6 g
Saturated fat: . . . . 1 g
Monounsaturated fat: . . . . 2 g
Polyunsaturated fat:. . . . . 2 g
Omega-3 fatty acids:. . . . . 1 g
Docosahexaenoic
    acid (DHA): . . . . 1 g
Eicosapentaenoic
    acid (EPA): . . . . 1 g
Cholesterol: . . . . 37 mg
Sodium:. . . . . 64 mg
Fiber:. . . . . 0 g
Calcium: . . . . 203 mg

Good source of:

protein, calcium, omega-3 fatty acids (including DHA & EPA), carotenoids, selenium, vitamin B_{12}, niacin, phosphorus, potassium

Description:

Canned salmon is a convenient, inexpensive pantry staple. Several varieties of wild salmon are canned, so it's a great option in the winter months, when fresh wild salmon is unavailable (and when stores often sell thawed, previously frozen wild salmon at a markup, or, worse yet, pass off farmed salmon as wild).

Among the species most commonly canned are the softer pink salmon, coho salmon, and the firm, deep red-orange, sockeye salmon.

Health benefits:

Canned salmon is rich in omega-3 fatty acids, which benefit cardiovascular health by helping to keep the arteries supple and elastic and improving the lipid (blood fats) profile.

Omega-3's have anti-inflammatory properties, which are important for preventing or delaying progression of inflammatory conditions such as diabetes, heart disease, inflammatory bowel disease, and arthritis.

One of the omega-3's abundant in salmon, docosahexaenoic acid (DHA), might reduce the risk of neurodegenerative diseases. It is also an important nutrient for pregnant and nursing women, whose consumption of omega-3's boosts the supply of the fatty acids for their infant's brain and eye development. Omega-3's might also help prevent postpartum depression.

Because it is processed with the bones, canned salmon is an excellent source of calcium, which is essential to bone and muscle health and might help prevent colon cancer.

As a bonus, canned salmon is generally made from wild Pacific species, which tend to be far lower in environmental contaminants than farmed salmon.

Selection tips:
Purchase canned salmon only in undented cans that show no evidence of bulging, damage, or rust. Be sure to check the expiration date before purchase.

Storage tips:
Keep cans of salmon in a cool, dry place until ready for use and consume before the expiration date.

After opening, store any leftover canned salmon in a separate, well-covered container in the refrigerator for up to three days.

Preparation tips:
Top green salads with chunks of canned salmon. Mix the fish with a squeeze of lemon and pepper or a bit of fat-free mayonnaise and diced veggies to make salmon salad for sandwiches. Canned salmon also makes great fish cakes.

Precautions:
The bones in canned salmon are safe to eat and are a great source of calcium. However, to minimize any choking hazard, they should not be fed to small children or to those with chewing or swallowing difficulties.

SARDINES

Serving size: 1 can (3.75 ounces), packed in oil, drained, with bones

Per serving:
Calories: 191
Carbohydrate: . . . . 0 g
Protein: . . . . 23 g
Fat: . . . . 11 g
Saturated fat: . . . . 1 g
Monounsaturated fat: . . . . 4 g
Polyunsaturated fat: . . . . 5 g
Omega-3 fatty acids: . . . . 1 gram
Docosahexaenoic
     acid (DHA): . . . . 1 g
Eicosapentaenoic
     acid (EPA): 1g
Cholesterol: . . . . 131 mg
Sodium: . . . . 465 mg
Fiber: . . . . 0 g
Calcium: . . . . 351 mg

Good source of:
protein, calcium, omega-3 fatty acids, phosphorus, potassium, iron, zinc, selenium, niacin, vitamin B_{12}, vitamin D

Description:
Sardines are small silver-skinned fish that are related to herrings. There are several species of sardines, though the name is used generically to encompass them all. Sardines live in temperate waters and tend to travel in very large schools. They are featured in cuisines throughout the Mediterranean—especially in Spain, Portugal, Greece, and France—and in Norway. Sardines are delicious fresh, but they are quite perishable and are commonly canned, especially for export.

Canned sardines come in several varieties—they may be packed in water, oil (olive oil is most delicious and healthful), tomato sauce, or mustard sauce. Both salted and unsalted varieties are available for the oil-packed and water-packed options. Canning companies are even breaking from traditional preparations and launching new flavors such as pesto or garlic and red pepper-marinated sardines.

Health benefits:
Sardines are rich in omega-3 fatty acids, which benefit cardiovascular health by helping to keep the arteries supple and elastic and by improving the lipid profile.

Omega-3's have anti-inflammatory properties, which are important for preventing or delaying progression of inflammatory conditions such as diabetes, heart disease, inflammatory bowel disease, and arthritis.

Sardines have docosahexaenoic acid (DHA), a type of omega-3 fatty acid that might reduce the risk of neurodegenerative diseases. It is also an important nutrient for pregnant and nursing women, whose consumption of omega-3's boosts the supply of the fatty acids for their infant's brain and eye development. Omega-3's might also help prevent postpartum depression.

Thanks to the presence of soft, edible bones, canned sardines are an excellent source of calcium. They also contain an abundance of vitamin D, which, together with calcium, is essential to bone health.

Selection tips:
Buy only undented cans of sardines that show no evidence of bulging, damage, or rust. Be sure to check the expiration date before purchase.

Fresh sardines should have clear eyes and gills, their flesh should be firm, and they should have a pleasant, mild aroma.

Storage tips:
Store canned sardines in a cool, dry place and use before the expiration date marked on the package. Leftover canned sardines should be transferred to another container and stored, well covered, in the refrigerator for up to two days.

Gutted and well-wrapped, fresh sardines will keep in the refrigerator for up to two days, although they are best used as soon as possible after purchase.

Preparation tips:
Canned sardines can be eaten as is or with a squeeze of lemon. Serve them as part of a tapas platter with good olives and manchego cheese. Try them on rye crispbread, serve sardines over salad, or integrate them into pasta sauces. Mash sardines with mustard or horseradish and lemon, spread on whole-grain, rye, or pumpernickel bread, and top with sliced tomato, onion, and baby spinach or arugula.

If you are lucky enough to find fresh sardines, try grilling them. Be sure to wash the scaled and gutted fish in cold water before grilling.

Precautions:
Canned sardines are often high in sodium. If you are on a sodium-restricted diet or have high blood pressure, buy the no-salt-added varieties, or read the label carefully to determine if there is an acceptable portion of the salted sardines, and be sure to measure out the serving.

The bones in canned sardines are safe to eat and are a great source of calcium. However, to minimize any choking hazard, they should not be fed to small children or to those with chewing or swallowing difficulties.

AVOCADOS

Serving size: ⅕ avocado (2 tablespoons, or 1 ounce)

Per serving:
Calories:. 55
Carbohydrate:. . . . . 3 g
Protein: . . . . 1 g
Total fat: . . . . 5 g
Saturated fat:. . . . . 1 g
Trans fat: . . . . 0 g
Polyunsaturated fat: . . . . 1 g
Monounsaturated fat:. . . . . . . 3 g
Cholesterol: . . . . 0 mg
Sodium: . . . . 0 mg
Fiber: . . . . 3 g

Good source of:
folate, lutein, potassium, monounsaturated fat

Description:
Although typically consumed with savory dishes, the avocado is actually a fruit. Avocado trees are native to Mexico, Central America, and South America, where they have been eaten for centuries. The Aztecs considered avocados to be a powerful aphrodisiac, and archaeologists have found avocado seeds buried with mummies in Peru. Thanks to the bumpy, dark green skin on some varieties, avocados are sometimes called "alligator pears."

Although they were introduced to the United States in the late 1800's, avocados were still considered an obscure luxury item as late as the 1950's. It took until the 1970's for the Hass avocado, first cultivated in the 1930's by California postman Rudolph Hass, to surge to its current popularity. Nearly 90% of the U.S. avocado crop is grown in California, and the Hass—which typically weighs between 6 and 8 ounces—is the most commonly cultivated and consumed variety. Occasionally, larger, smooth-skinned varieties like the Bacon or Florida avocado are available in U.S. markets.

The greenish-yellow flesh of the avocado has a smooth, buttery texture and a mild, slightly nutty taste. Avocados are a good foil for spicy foods or tangy vinaigrettes and even work well in desserts.

Health benefits:
Avocados are nutritional powerhouses with multiple benefits. They are a rich source of lutein, an antioxidant that might help prevent macular degeneration, a common cause of age-related blindness. Avocados contain an abundance of folate, which is important throughout the life cycle. Folate helps prevent neural tube birth defects and heart disease and is vital to proper blood cell growth.

When used in place of saturated fat sources, the monounsaturated fat in avocados can help improve a person's lipid profile by lowering LDL ("bad") cholesterol and raising HDL ("good") cholesterol, while the beta-sitosterol in avocados can prevent the formation of cholesterol. Moreover, the fat and fiber in avocados can contribute to between-meal satisfaction without impairing blood glucose control. As an added plus, the fat in avocados helps the body absorb fat-soluble nutrients.

In a 2005 study, researchers at the University of California Los Angeles found that avocado extract (as opposed to pure lutein) appeared to significantly inhibit the growth of certain prostate cancer cells. This suggests that the various compounds in avocados might work together synergistically and that you can reap the biggest benefits by enjoying the fruit instead of taking isolated supplements.

Preparation tips:
Slice the avocado lengthwise around the seed, and then gently twist the halves apart. Remove the seed with a spoon before scooping the avocado flesh from the inedible skin. If you're not going to eat the avocado immediately, add 1 teaspoon of lemon juice for each sliced or mashed avocado to prevent browning. Place a sheet of plastic wrap directly on the surface of the avocado and refrigerate until ready to serve.

Avocados are most commonly eaten raw. Spread on multigrain toast, avocado is a great, heart-healthy alternative to butter. Diced avocado works well in salads and salsas, while the sliced or mashed fruit is delicious in sandwiches, wraps, and sushi. Pureed avocado makes an interesting addition to cold soups and smoothies.

Selection tips:
Look for heavy, dark-skinned, unbruised avocados that yield to gentle pressure. If purchasing avocados a few days before you intend to eat them, choose firmer fruits and ripen them at home.

Storage tips:
Avocados are unusual in that they are generally harvested prior to ripening and will ripen off the tree. Hard avocados will ripen in three to five days if allowed to sit at room temperature. You can speed the ripening process by placing the avocado in a paper bag or alongside another fruit that emits ethylene gas, such as a banana or an apple. Once ripe, uncut avocados should be stored in the refrigerator, where they will stay fresh for two to three days. Cut avocado is best eaten the day it is prepared, but it can be refrigerated for one to two days. Mashed avocado, mixed with 1 teaspoon of lemon juice per fruit, can be frozen for up to one year.

Precautions:
Avocados are rich sources of potassium, vitamin K, and tyramine. Those on potassium-restricted diets, warfarin therapy, or monoamine oxidase (MAO) inhibitors should talk to a doctor or registered dietitian before eating avocados.

Serving size: ¾ cup

Per serving:

Calories:	62
Carbohydrate:	16 g
Protein:	1 g
Fat:	0 g
Saturated fat:	0 g
Cholesterol:	0 g
Sodium:	1 mg
Fiber:	3 g
Calcium:	7 mg

Good source of:

vitamin A, vitamin C, potassium, folate, anthocyanins

Description:

Blueberries are one of only three fruits native to North America (Concord grapes and cranberries are the others). Wild blueberry shrubs grow in forests and bogs and were valued tremendously by Native Americans, who used the various parts of the plant for food, medicine, and dye. Tribal elders deemed "star berries" (so-called because of the blueberries star-shaped calyx) a gift from the Great Spirit.

In the early 1900's, attempts were made to domesticate the wild blueberries, which led to the eventual development of today's cultivated blueberries. North America remains the world's largest producer of both wild and cultivated blueberries. The growing season for blueberries runs from April to October, which makes those months the best time of year to enjoy the berries.

Health benefits:

In a 2004 study published in the *Journal of Agricultural and Food Chemistry,* wild blueberries ranked highest in antioxidant capacity among over 20 fruits tested. Be aware that although its producers and promoters also refer to the cultivated blueberry as the "improved" blueberry, research shows that the wild blueberry boasts higher antioxidant activity than its cultivated counterpart. Blueberries also possess anti-inflammatory properties.

The various components in blueberries appear to inhibit cancer growth at the initiation, promotion, and proliferation stages. They might also help reduce cholesterol and improve heart health. Blueberries have been shown to help prevent urinary tract infections by preventing the adhesion of bacteria to cells lining the urinary tract.

Among the blueberry's most publicized potential health benefits is protection against neurodegenerative diseases such as Alzheimer disease. So far, most research in this arena has been gathered through in vitro (laboratory) and animal studies, so it is not yet known how results apply to the human brain. In a U.S. Department of Agriculture (USDA) study, however, rodents supplemented with blueberry extract did have improved navigational and motor skills.

Rumor has it that during World War II, British pilots ate bilberries, a European cousin of blueberries, to improve their night vision. While there is doubt about the veracity of this story and no well-designed studies confirm this claim, the anthocyanins in blueberries might help prevent eye fatigue and protect against age-related changes in the eye, such as macular degeneration.

Anecdotally, blueberries were once regarded as a folk-medicine remedy for morning sickness; some pregnant women today report that they can tolerate blueberries—especially when eaten frozen—if they are feeling queasy.

Selection tips:
Look for blueberries that are firm and deeply colored. A light bloom (or powdery coating) on the surface is normal. Avoid berries that look wet, shriveled, or crushed or that show evidence of mold.

Dried blueberries are a relative novelty in modern markets, but the concept is an old one—the Pilgrims learned to dry the berries from their Native American neighbors. Look for dried blueberries that are deeply colored and feel pliable.

Storage tips:
Store blueberries unwashed in the refrigerator for up to three days. Remove any crushed or moldy berries before storing. Rinse well before eating.

Blueberries freeze very well. Remove damaged or moldy berries, wash and dry them, and store them in an airtight container in the freezer for several months. Alternatively, spread sorted, unwashed blueberries in a single layer on a cookie sheet. Freeze until firm, then transfer to an airtight container and return to the freezer. Be sure to wash these berries before use. Frozen blueberries can be added directly to recipes without defrosting.

Dried blueberries will keep in a cool, dry place for up to 12 months. Refrigerate dried blueberries for optimal freshness.

Preparation tips:
Although blueberries are commonly eaten with breakfast, in desserts, or in baked goods, they also make an unexpected—and delicious—accent to savory dishes. In fact, Native Americans historically used dried blueberries in the preparation of preserved dried venison, soups, and stews.

Puree blueberries into a favorite balsamic vinaigrette recipe, incorporate them into wine-based sauces, or add them to salsas and chutneys to serve alongside roasted game, such as duck. For a sweet departure from blueberry baked goods, try a cold fruit soup or blueberry sorbet.

Precautions:
Whole blueberries may pose a choking hazard and should not be offered to small children or to people with swallowing disorders. It should be safe, however, to offer blueberries that have been mashed first.

CHERRIES

Serving size: ¾ cup cherries with pits, or about 13 cherries

Per serving:

Calories:	55
Carbohydrate:	15 g
Protein:	1 g
Fat:	0 g
Saturated fat:	0 g
Cholesterol:	0 g
Sodium:	0 mg
Fiber:	2 g
Calcium:	11 mg

Good source of:

vitamin C, fiber, potassium, anthocyanins

Description:

Cherries come from a class of fruits known as drupes (or "stone fruits"), which boast plump flesh surrounding a hard, seed-protecting "stone." For a plant, drupe fruits are an evolutionary boon. Animals are attracted to the bright fruits; when they eat them, they help transport—and sow—the seeds, which stay viable, packaged in their undigestible stones. Scientists speculate that cherry-loving birds helped transport the fruits from Asia all along their migratory patterns, so cherries now grow throughout the world.

French settlers in what is now the midwestern United States included cherry trees in their gardens. The first cherry orchard was planted by a Presbyterian minister in Michigan in the 1850's, but commercial production in the United States didn't occur until the late 1800's. Michigan grows close to 75% of the U.S. cherry crop and even hosts a national cherry festival.

Cherries come in many varieties, but most are classed as either "sweet" or "sour." Two of the more popular varieties are the dark, red-fleshed Bing and the tart, gold and red-hued Montmorency.

Health benefits:

The quercetin in cherries, a type of antioxidant flavonoid, might contribute to reduced risk of heart attack and stroke. Anthocyanins, which give cherries their red color, are another antioxidant especially abundant in the unprocessed fruits. Anthocyanins possess anti-inflammatory properties that appear to rival those of aspirin or COX-2 inhibitors (drugs used to treat arthritis). Anecdotal evidence suggests that eating tart cherries might help mitigate the pain of inflammatory conditions such as arthritis and gout.

Selection tips:

Look for firm, glossy cherries without soft spots. The stems should look fresh.

Storage tips:
Store cherries in a plastic bag in the refrigerator for up to three days.

Cherries also freeze well. They can be frozen with their pits left in, but they will be easier to use straight from the freezer if you take the time to pit them before freezing. Lay cherries in a single layer on a cookie sheet and freeze until firm. Transfer them to an airtight container and return to the freezer.

Dried cherries should look plump and feel pliable. They can be stored for several months in a cool, dry place and will keep best in the refrigerator.

Preparation tips:
Rinse cherries well. Serve them whole or stem and pit them to add to recipes. A cherry pitter makes quick work of this task.

Alternatively, cut cherries in half with a paring knife and remove the stone.

Add cherries to cereal, smoothies, or whole-grain pancakes. Spread multigrain toast with almond butter and sliced fresh cherries.

Halved fresh cherries are a great addition to rice pilaf or couscous. Tart or sour cherry sauces or salsas are a great accent to game or salmon.

Precautions:
The Environmental Working Group, a non-profit environmental organization, recommends purchasing organic cherries because it found significant pesticide contamination on 91% of the cherry samples it tested. The group also noted that most cherries were contaminated with more than one pesticide.

GRAPEFRUIT

Serving size: ½ large grapefruit

Per serving:
Calories:.....................53
Carbohydrate:..............13 g
Protein:....................1 g
Fat:........................0 g
Saturated fat:................0 g
Cholesterol:...............0 mg
Sodium:...................0 mg
Fiber:......................2 g
Calcium:..................20 mg

Good source of:
vitamin C, bioflavonoids

Description:
Grapefruits are a hybrid of the pomelo and the sweet orange. Exactly where and how grapefruits originated is unclear, although they were found in Barbados in the 1750's. They made their way to other Caribbean islands and were allegedly dubbed "grapefruit" in the early 1800's by a Jamaican farmer who noted that they grew in clusters like grapes.

Today, Florida, Texas, and California have joined the ranks of top grapefruit producers.

Health benefits:
Grapefruits are great sources of vitamin C, which in addition to boasting plenty of antioxidant activity, is essential to proper immune function. Vitamin C is important for collagen production and helps maintain the integrity of body tissues, including the skin, gums, and capillaries. It also is vital to wound healing.

The bioflavonoids in grapefruits potentiate the action of vitamin C and have health-promoting functions of their own. Research has shown that bioflavonoids appear to promote heart health and reduce the risk of cancer. A 2006 study published in the *Journal of Agricultural and Food Chemistry* found that grapefruit consumption significantly lowered total cholesterol, LDL cholesterol (the "bad" cholesterol), and particularly triglycerides among study subjects as compared to a control group. Moreover, researchers concluded that red grapefruits were more beneficial than blond grapefruits, owing in part to their higher antioxidant capacity.

You can reap the greatest health benefits by eating the fruit rather than by drinking the juice. Vitamin C is less stable once fruits or vegetables are cut. Because juices are subject to processing and tend to sit on grocery shelves longer, vitamin C might be less present or less potent. In addition, some of the beneficial components of grapefruits, such as the white pith that adheres to the surface of the peeled sections, the pulp sacs, and fiber, are generally absent from the juice.

Finally, remember that you'll get a considerably smaller portion of juice for the same amount of carbohydrate, as compared to a portion of actual fruit.

Selection tips:
Look for uniformly shaped, firm grapefruits that are heavy for their size. They should have no soft spots or traces of mold. Grapefruit skin might vary in color. White or blond grapefruits generally have yellow skins, while pink or red grapefruit rinds might range from yellow with a pinkish or reddish blush to a more uniform salmon color. All three varieties might have a greenish tint. This can occur if nights were warm before the fruits were harvested, or so-called "regreening" can occur in the spring, when maturing fruits get an extra dose of chlorophyll from trees that are simultaneously nourishing new citrus blossoms.

Storage tips:
Grapefruits can be stored in any cool, dry place, although they'll last longest in the refrigerator. Do not store in airtight bags or containers because trapped moisture can encourage mold growth.

Preparation tips:
You can peel and eat a grapefruit as you would an orange. Alternatively, to serve grapefruit halves, start by slicing in half along the grapefruit's "equator." Using a paring or grapefruit knife, slip the knife between the fruit and its skin and peel all around the circumference of the grapefruit. Next, slip the knife between the membranes and the fruit (as close to the membrane as possible). This frees the fruit from the membranes so sections can be eaten easily with a spoon, straight from the rind.

Grapefruits work as well beyond breakfast. Their tart astringency makes them a great complement to seafood. Grapefruits also pair well with avocado and fennel—try all three in a composed or tossed salad.

Precautions:
Grapefruit juice or grapefruit can interact with certain drugs and might lead to potentially toxic levels of these medicines in the bloodstream. This occurs because substances in grapefruit inhibit the breakdown of certain drugs in the intestinal tract, with the result that more active drug remains in your system. Not all drugs are a problem, but most calcium channel blockers (such as nifedipine [brand name Procardia] and felodipine [Plendil]), sedatives such as alprazolam (Xanax), and certain HIV medicines are commonly affected. Talk to a doctor or pharmacist to check the compatibility of your medicines with grapefruit.

Serving size: 1 large kiwi, peeled

Per serving:
Calories:.....................56
Carbohydrate: ....13 g
Protein:....................1 g
Fat:........................1 g
Saturated fat: ....0 g
Cholesterol: ....0 mg
Sodium:...................3 mg
Fiber:.....................3 g
Calcium: ....31 mg

Good source of:

vitamin C, fiber, potassium, vitamin A, vitamin E, magnesium, antioxidants

Description:

Kiwifruits, which originally hailed from China and are also known as Chinese gooseberries, spread with the aid of missionaries to New Zealand and California in the early 1900's.

The fruits were still rather obscure in the United States in the 1960's, when a woman named Frieda Caplan, who founded one of the most powerful specialty produce companies in the country, began importing the furry little fruits from New Zealand. She is also credited with dubbing the fruits "kiwis," after New Zealand's similar-looking flightless bird.

In the late 1970's and early 1980's, French chefs started shaking up the culinary world with *nouvelle cuisine*—and because they were so fond of the unusual-looking kiwi, they raised the fruit's profile while they did it.

Once the exotic fruit hit diners' radar, it wasn't long before the kiwi's popularity surged. Around the same time, growers in California embraced the kiwi; now the United States ranks among the world's top kiwi producers.

The small oval fruits are quite adorable. They have a fuzzy brown outer skin and slippery, bright-green flesh that's studded with lots of tiny, edible black seeds surrounding a white, edible core. Kiwis have a sweet-tart flavor that some liken to a cross between a strawberry and a banana.

New Zealand growers are also reacquainting consumers with the kiwi's exotic side—they've recently begun marketing a yellow-fleshed, tropical-flavored kiwi that was developed through hybridization.

Health benefits:

Little kiwifruits pack a big nutritional punch. By weight, they rank highest among the most commonly eaten fruits for nutrient density.

Kiwis contain almost twice as much vitamin C as the same amount of oranges. Vitamin C is a powerful antioxidant and is important for wound healing, immunity, and the maintenance of skin and connective tissue.

As a rich source of lutein, kiwifruits help preserve the health of the eyes and may aid in prevention of macular degeneration, a leading cause of age-related blindness.

Kiwis are great for heart health, too. The potassium and magnesium they contain help regulate blood pressure, while the pectin and other fibers in kiwis help promote favorable blood lipid levels. In a study published in the journal *Platelets* in 2004, researchers found that when healthy study subjects consumed two to three kiwifruits per day, their triglyceride levels dropped. Platelets also became less "sticky," reducing the risk of clots.

Kiwis also show promising anticancer capacities. In a study published in the journal *Carcinogenesis* in 2003, researchers from the University of Oslo reported that kiwifruit consumption not only protected DNA from potentially carcinogenic oxidative damage, but that it also helped stimulate DNA repair. Researchers are now examining whether gold kiwis have the same DNA-repairing capabilities that the green kiwis possess.

Selection tips:
Look for firm, symmetrically-shaped kiwis. They will give slightly to light pressure when ripe but can be purchased when harder and left to ripen at room temperature for two to three days. Avoid kiwifruits with soft spots or wrinkly skins.

Gold kiwis are usually softer at the time of purchase than green kiwis because they are already ripe when they come to market. As a result, they have a shorter shelf life than green kiwis and should be eaten immediately or refrigerated for up to three days.

Storage tips:
Green kiwifruits can be stored unpeeled at room temperature for up to seven days or in the refrigerator for up to three weeks.

Preparation tips:
Peel the skin with a paring knife or vegetable peeler. Slice or dice the kiwi to add to recipes, or just eat out of hand. If you're keeping the kiwi all to yourself, you can just cut it in half and scoop the flesh out with a spoon.

The enzyme *actinidin* in kiwifruits breaks down protein. That makes kiwi a poor addition to gelatin, which may not solidify properly. Adding kiwifruits to milk or cream-based recipes like custard or pudding is tricky too, unless the recipe will be eaten within a couple of hours. A better strategy is to add the kiwis just before serving.

On the flip side, the enzymes in kiwis make them great tenderizers for protein foods, so they are an excellent addition to marinades. Just puree the fruits into the marinade recipe.

Try kiwis in smoothies, add them to yogurt, or serve them over buckwheat pancakes for a tropical twist at breakfast. Use kiwi chunks in fruit kebabs, or go savory and use them in salsas or salads.

Kiwis are also a fun addition to sushi rolls—try making your own maki at home by rolling brown rice, grilled fish, scallions, and kiwi in a sheet of nori (a type of seaweed). Slice into rolls, and serve with wasabi, pickled ginger, and reduced-sodium soy sauce.

Precautions:
Kiwifruits are a rich source of potassium. People on potassium-restricted diets should talk to a registered dietitian or doctor before consuming kiwis.

MANGOES

Serving size: ½ cup sliced

Per serving:
Calories:....................54
Carbohydrate: ....14 g
Protein:....................0 g
Fat:........................0 g
Saturated fat: ....0 g
Cholesterol: ....0 mg
Sodium:....................2 mg
Fiber:......................2 g
Calcium: ....8 mg

Good source of:

beta-carotene, fiber, potassium, vitamin C

Description:

Thanks to their tropical origins, mangoes retain an exotic allure in the United States, but they are a common staple in India and southeast Asia, where they've been cultivated for over 6,000 years. Today mangoes are also grown throughout the Americas and in Australia, Africa, and the Caribbean.

There are hundreds of varieties of mango, but the Tommy Atkins, which is sturdy enough to withstand transport, is the most commonly available in the United States. While it is not the lushest variety, a well-ripened Tommy Atkins mango can still be quite delicious.

Health benefits:

Studies suggest that, because of an abundance of antioxidants, mangoes appear to have anticancer properties and may protect against oxidative stress. Ripe mangoes are high in antioxidant plant chemicals called *polyphenols,* which may confer cardioprotective effects. The fiber in mangoes likely contributes to these potential cancer-preventing and heart-protecting properties.

Mangoes are also rich in beta-carotene, which is converted by the body into vitamin A and is a potent antioxidant in its own right. Vitamin A is vital to proper immune function, vision, and cell growth.

Despite the sweet flavor of ripe mangoes, the fruits have a low glycemic index, and a serving of mango has a low glycemic load.

Selection tips:

Choose firm, unbruised mangoes with unblemished, wrinkle-free skin. Ripe fruits will give to slight pressure and should have a pleasant aroma and feel heavy for their size.

Mango skins can range from yellow to deep red, depending on the variety of the mango and its stage of ripeness. Green-skinned mangoes are not yet ripe. They can, however, be used in savory salads or be allowed to ripen at home.

Tommy Atkins mangoes tend to have a plump, oblong shape and a somewhat fibrous flesh—particularly when they are underripe. When allowed to ripen properly, they take on a smoother, juicier texture and a more balanced, less acidic flavor.

Less tart and fibrous than other varieties, Champagne (or Ataulfo) mangoes are a small, flattish, oval variety with a light golden skin and a mild, sweet flavor.

Storage tips:

Unripe mangoes can be stored at room temperature for about a week. Speed the ripening process by placing the mangoes in a closed paper bag. Do not store unripe mangoes in the refrigerator, as this will retard the ripening process.

Ripe mangoes can be stored in the refrigerator for 1–2 weeks. Once peeled and cut, leftover mango can be stored in a well-sealed container for 2–3 days.

Peeled, cut mango can be frozen for use in smoothies or baked goods. To prevent frozen mango chunks from sticking together, place the cut mango on a parchment- or wax-paper–lined cookie sheet and freeze until solid. Transfer the frozen mango pieces to a freezer bag or airtight container and freeze for up to four months.

Preparation tips:

Mangos are extremely versatile. They are delicious raw or cooked and enhance both sweet and savory recipes. Unripe green mangos are edible, too, and are often used in Thai and Indian cuisines for salads.

Mango flesh can be slippery, and it is firmly attached to the large, flattish seed inside. One of the best ways to safely free the mango from the seed is to hold the unpeeled fruit vertically on a cutting board. Using a large, sharp knife, cut the wide side of the mango vertically along the seed. Repeat on the other side. You should have two large oval halves and a seed surrounded by a "halo" of mango flesh along its edges. Remove the fruit remaining on the seed

and peel off the strip of skin that surrounds it with a paring knife. To remove the flesh from the mango halves, score the flesh side of the mango vertically and horizontally, taking care not to cut through the skin. Push the halves inside out, then cut the cubes from the skin. Or simply peel the skin off each half with a paring knife and slice the mango as desired.

Perk up a winter breakfast with a tropical twist by adding cubed mango and ginger to oatmeal. Stir diced or pureed mango into yogurt, or blend it into a smoothie or Indian lassi drink.

Take a spicy cue from South American, Mexican, or West Indian cuisines and snack on mango slices dipped in chili powder or hot sauce. Or trade ho-hum condiments for some exotic flavor in sandwiches and wraps with a homemade mango chutney.

Diced fresh mango makes a fantastic salsa addition—try combining it with diced peppers, red onion, tomatoes, lime juice, and olive oil. Use mango salsa atop grilled fish, or serve it as a party snack with baked blue corn tortilla chips.

Add mango to sushi rolls, salads, or stir-fries, or use an unripe mango for a savory Thai salad. Peel and shred the mango and toss with hot pepper, shallots, chopped cilantro, lime juice, and reduced-sodium soy sauce.

Sliced mango makes an elegant, impromptu dessert tossed with lime juice and chopped, crystallized ginger. Or use pureed mango as a sauce for angel food cake and berries.

Precautions:

Mangoes are related to poison ivy, and their skins and sap contain a compound that causes dermatitis (inflammation of the skin) in some people. People who are susceptible to this reaction can try rinsing the mango before cutting it (which is also advisable from a food safety perspective) or having someone else peel the mango.

People who are allergic to cashews or latex may experience a cross-allergy with mangoes and vice-versa. People who are affected by food allergies should talk to an allergist or registered dietitian before introducing mangoes into the diet.

Mangoes are a good source of potassium. People who are on potassium-restricted diets should talk to a registered dietitian or doctor before adding mangoes to the diet.

POMEGRANATES

Serving size: ½ pomegranate

Per serving:
Calories:. 80
Carbohydrate: . . . . 18 g
Protein:. . . . . 1 g
Fat:. . . . . 1 g
Saturated fat: . . . . 0 g
Cholesterol: . . . . 0 g
Sodium:. . . . . 3 mg
Fiber:. 0 g

Good source of:
potassium, vitamin C, polyphenols, tannins

Description:
Pomegranates have enjoyed one of the longest histories of cultivation, possibly beginning around 4000 B.C. The first attempts to domesticate the pomegranate probably occurred in Persia (now Iran) or Turkey, but they were valued tremendously throughout the Fertile Crescent (a historical region in the Middle East).

Pomegranate motifs and references show up in many of the world's early religions, attesting to the fruit's importance. Buddhism regards the pomegranate as one of three blessed fruits. Pomegranates are counted among the "Seven Species" important in ancient Israel and were included in the offering of first fruits brought each year to the Temple in Jerusalem. To ancient and modern Jews alike, the seeds of the pomegranate symbolize the *mitzvoth*, or divine commandments. The Koran describes pomegranates as a feature of paradisiacal gardens. And the recently discovered *Gospel of Judas* appears to have been written in pomegranate juice-based ink.

Many cultures regarded pomegranates as symbolic of fertility and abundance—the Chinese, for example, historically decorated bridal chambers with the fruits. That pomegranates appear in numerous significant artworks, including Botticelli's "Madonna of the Pomegranate," is further testament to the fruit's status.

Health benefits:
Pomegranates have long been regarded as medicinal. Among other uses, they were a popular treatment for digestive ills in areas as diverse as ancient Egypt and Greece (Hippocrates was an advocate) and in Sri

Lanka. The coats of arms of both the British Medical Association and the Royal College of Midwives feature pomegranates.

Pomegranates are rich in polyphenol antioxidants, including anthocyanins and tannins. These point to probable anticancer and cardioprotective benefits. The journal *Clinical Nutrition* published a small 2003 study conducted in Haifa, Israel, in which 19 people with narrowing or blockage of the carotid arteries (the arteries supplying the brain) supplemented their normal diets with pomegranate juice or a placebo. Study subjects were followed for one year; half of the group was followed for three years. In the first year, the condition of the control group, which did not take the juice, worsened significantly, while the study group benefited from up to a 30% degree decrease in carotid intima-media thickness, an important measure of atherosclerosis. Their antioxidant status jumped significantly and oxidative stress decreased, as did systolic blood pressure. Although further improvements were not seen after the first year, the results nonetheless indicate benefits for those with atherosclerosis.

Both Ayurvedic (South Asian) and Unani (Graeco-Arabic) medicine use pomegranates in the treatment of diabetes. Researchers are now attempting to learn if pomegranates help control blood glucose and by means of what mechanism.

Selection tips:
Choose large, unbruised pomegranates that feel heavy for their size. The color of the leathery, inedible skin can vary from light reddish-yellow to deep, intense red. Either is fine, but avoid pallid-looking pomegranates or those that are wrinkled.

Storage tips:
Whole fresh pomegranates can be kept at room temperature for one to two weeks or in the drawer of the refrigerator for a month, and sometimes longer.

Pomegranate arils, the ruby-colored edible seeds, will keep in an airtight container in the refrigerator for up to three days.

Arils also freeze very well. They will keep in a plastic bag in the freezer for up to one year. Because pomegranates have relatively short availability—typically from October to January—freezing the arils is a great way to enjoy the fruits year-round.

Preparation tips:
Separating the seeds from the skin and the inedible membranes can be messy, especially if you slice through the entire pomegranate—the juice does stain.

There is an easy technique for removing the seeds with minimal mess. Cut off the flower (or "crown") end of the pomegranate. You should be able to see where the membranes separate the seeds. With a paring knife, cut through the skin, taking care not to go so deep that you hit the seeds.

Fill a large bowl with cool water. Submerge the pomegranate under water, and gently pull apart the sections along the scored lines. Pull away the thin whitish membrane covering the aril bunches and gently detach the arils from the skin. The arils will drop to the bottom of the bowl, while the skin and membranes will float. Scoop out the skin and membranes, discard, and drain the arils.

Pomegranate arils can be eaten straight from the fruit. Some people prefer to eat only the fleshy red part of the aril, while others enjoy the crunch and slightly bitter taste of the tiny white seed in the center.

The arils are quite beautiful, and, when tossed over salads or used as a garnish, they can really elevate the look of a dish.

Pomegranates have an affinity for Middle Eastern and Mediterranean flavors. Try using the arils in couscous or rice dishes, or sprinkled over Middle Eastern-inspired chicken recipes, or as a garnish on hummus or baba ganoush.

The arils are a nice mix-in for yogurt and are an interesting addition to baked goods such as quick breads and muffins. They even work well in pancake or waffle batter.

Precautions:
Pomegranates are a rich source of potassium. People on potassium-restricted diets should consult a registered dietitian or doctor before eating pomegranates.

Pomegranate arils are a choking hazard and should not be fed to small children or to people with swallowing disorders.

PRUNES (*also called* DRIED PLUMS)

Serving size: 5 prunes

Per serving:
Calories:. 101
Carbohydrate: . . . . 27 g
Protein:. . . . . 1 g
Fat:. . . . . 0 g
Saturated fat: . . . . 0 g
Cholesterol: . . . . 0 mg
Sodium:. . . . . 1 mg
Fiber:. . . . . 3 g
Calcium: . . . . 18 mg

Good source of:

beta-carotene, vitamin K, vitamin A, potassium, copper, zinc, fiber

Description:
Prunes are the dried version of certain plum varieties. (Not all plums can be turned into prunes.) Prunes are thought to have originated in Western Asia, though France is now known for producing some of the world's finest prunes. Since the mid-1800's, the prized French Prune d'Agen has also grown in the United States thanks to the efforts of California orchardist and French native Louis Pellier.

Prunes are important in European and Middle Eastern cuisines, where they are used in both sweet and savory dishes.

In 2001, as part of an effort to bolster prune consumption in the United States, the FDA approved a name change request by the then-California Prune Board (now the California Dried Plum Board) allowing use of the name "dried plums" in place of "prunes."

The rationale for the change had much to do with marketing. "Prune" connoted a dark, shriveled constipation cure that just didn't sound that enticing to consumers. Plums, on the other hand, are generally recognized as luscious fruits. Calling prunes what they actually are—dried plums—seemed like a far better way to encourage people to eat them.

No matter what you call them, prunes are incredibly nutrient-dense. They are loaded with fiber and have a sophisticated flavor that's perfect for satisfying the craving for a little something sweet and chewy.

Health benefits:
Prunes have among the highest levels of antioxidant activity of any fruit. These

include high levels of phenolic compounds which appear to help protect heart health by preventing oxidation of LDL cholesterol. (The potassium in prunes also promotes heart and general health and decreases risk of stroke by keeping blood pressure in check). The abundant antioxidants in prunes may also play a role in cancer prevention.

The phenolic and flavonoid compounds in prunes may play a role in the fruits' apparent impact on bone formation. In a study published in the *Journal of Women's Health & Gender-Based Medicine* in 2002, researchers reported that two important markers of bone formation rose significantly in postmenopausal women who consumed about 12 prunes daily for three months. That suggests that regular prune consumption may help preserve bone strength, or help prevent osteoporosis.

Researchers had an unexpected finding as well—the women in the study did not make room for the addition of dried fruit in their diets by reducing calories elsewhere, though they were instructed to do so. Despite the fact that they ended up eating approximately 400 extra calories per day, the women did not gain weight during the study. The researchers speculate that this may have to do with the high fiber content of prunes.

Though they pack a sweet punch, prunes actually have a low glycemic index of 29. The glycemic load for a serving that weighs 60 grams is 10, which is also categorized as low. Moreover, the standard serving of five prunes weighs approximately 40 grams. So people who stick to the smaller portion will likely experience a lesser impact on blood glucose levels.

Selection tips:
Prunes are sold with or without their pits. The latter are easiest to use in recipes. Pitted prunes are also a good option for small children, since prunes that still have their pits represent a choking hazard.

Look for plump, unblemished prunes that are black, shiny, and relatively soft. They should be in well-sealed packages.

Storage tips:
Store prunes in an airtight container in a cool, dry place for up to six months. It is fine to keep prunes at room temperature, though they will last longer when stored in the refrigerator.

Preparation tips:
Prunes are fantastic eaten out of hand, and together with nuts they make a delicious accompaniment to cheese plates.

They are an unexpected but welcome addition to smoothies, and they lend chewy sweetness to hot and cold cereals.

Prunes lend great depth to savory dishes. Try them in Moroccan tagine dishes or with roasted meats. Try prunes in salads—they are especially good over baby greens with orange slices, walnuts, and red onions. Chopped prunes are also wonderful in pilafs—try them in whole wheat couscous with pine nuts and lemon zest.

Chopped prunes might sound like an obvious addition to baked goods, but there's a stealthy way to sneak in their goodness *and* cut the fat in cookies and cakes, too. Just replace about half of the fat in the recipe with an equal amount of prune puree. There are commercially produced prune purees on the market (you can even use prune baby food), but it is easy and cost-effective to make your own. Place 1⅓ cups of pitted prunes (about eight ounces, or 24 prunes) and six tablespoons of warm water in a food processor or blender. Puree until smooth. The recipe makes one cup of prune puree. Leftover prune puree can be stored, well-covered, in the refrigerator for four to five days. Use it in baked goods, stir it into plain yogurt, or spread it on multi-grain toast.

For a simple Mediterranean-inspired, antioxidant-rich confection, press whole almonds into the hollows of prunes. Serve on a pretty platter, or place them in cellophane bags tied with ribbon and send them home with dinner party guests.

Precautions:
Prunes are a rich source of potassium. People on potassium-restricted diets should consult a registered dietitian or doctor before eating prunes.

Prunes are an excellent source of vitamin K. People who take blood-thinning drugs such as warfarin (Coumadin) should consult a doctor or registered dietitian before adding prunes to their diet. People who consumed prunes regularly prior to the initiation of blood-thinning drug therapy should be able to continue eating them, provided that their daily intake of vitamin K remains consistent. Talk to your prescribing doctor for further information.

STRAWBERRIES

Serving size: 1 cup, or about 12 medium berries

Per serving:
Calories:. 46
Carbohydrate: . . . . 11 g
Protein:. . . . . 1 g
Fat:. . . . . 0 g
Saturated fat: . . . . 0 g
Cholesterol: . . . . 0 mg
Sodium:. . . . . 1 mg
Fiber:. . . . . 3 g
Calcium: . . . . 23 mg

Good source of:
vitamin C, potassium, fiber, folic acid, vitamin K

Description:
Botanically speaking, strawberries are an unusual fruit. The red flesh we enjoy is actually a vegetable, while the tiny achenes all over its surface, although commonly referred to as seeds, are actually the fruit component of the berry.

There are some 20 species and over 600 different varieties of strawberry plants worldwide. Tiny wild strawberries are especially prized, particularly in Europe, although most of the berries consumed in the United States are of the larger domesticated varieties.

Health benefits:
Strawberries are rich in ellagic acid, a phenolic compound that appears to have cancer-fighting capabilities. A recent study in the *Journal of Agriculture and Food Chemistry* found that quercetin, another phytochemical abundant in strawberries, also appears to have powerful anticancer effects. Other studies have found anti-inflammatory benefits from strawberries.

Strawberries have both a low glycemic index and are low in carbohydrate, which makes them a boon for those with diabetes. They are also rich in folate, which helps prevent neural tube birth defects and heart disease. The vitamin C in strawberries promotes healthy immune function, while the potassium protects against hypertension and is important to proper muscle function.

Selection tips:

Look for deeply and uniformly colored, well-shaped, firm, and shiny berries. Avoid wet or smashed strawberries or those with wilted stems. Take a look at the bottom of the container; too much wetness is a sign that the berries were handled roughly or that they are rotting.

It is also a good idea to smell the berries. Choose those that possess a distinctive berry aroma. No matter how beautiful they are, scentless berries will disappoint. Generally speaking, smaller berries are more flavorful than those that are overgrown, as are local strawberries grown in season. Organic berries tend to have a truer berry flavor; some tasters can detect an off-putting "chemical" taste in conventionally grown berries.

Storage tips:

Depending on their ripeness, strawberries will keep for two to five days in the refrigerator. Store them unwashed in their original container, and be sure to remove any damaged or moldy berries first.

Strawberries can be frozen. Sort out any damaged berries and lay the desirable berries in a single layer on a cookie sheet. Freeze until firm, and then transfer to an airtight container and return to the freezer.

Preparation tips:

Rinse strawberries well before eating. It is best to leave the green stem attached to prevent the berries from getting waterlogged; if desired, remove it before serving with a strawberry huller or a paring knife.

Strawberries have the best flavor and texture when eaten fresh. Add them to cereal, or use them to top multigrain pancakes or waffles. Rather than purchasing over-sweet-ened fruited yogurts, stir fresh strawberries into plain yogurt and sweeten with a teaspoon of maple syrup or honey, if you like. Try layering sliced strawberries over a peanut butter or almond butter sandwich in place of jam. Frozen berries are great in homemade smoothies and are much higher in fiber than juice if you crave a fruity drink.

Strawberries are also great in savory dishes. Try them in salads—they are especially nice with peppery greens like arugula. For a quick hors d'oeuvre, top crostini with goat cheese, sliced strawberries, and freshly cracked black pepper.

Strawberries also have an incredible affinity for balsamic vinegar, which intensifies their flavor. Macerate 3 to 4 cups of halved or sliced strawberries in a tablespoon or two of good-quality balsamic vinegar and a teaspoon of sugar. Serve with a dollop of mascarpone cheese, if desired. Or leave out the sugar and make a sauce with the berries and vinegar. Reduce over low heat, puree, and serve over chicken or alongside shellfish.

Precautions:

The Environmental Working Group (EWG) recommends purchasing organic strawberries based on government tests that found significant pesticide contamination on 90% of the strawberry samples tested. Thirty-six different pesticides were found on the berries, and most strawberries were contaminated with more than one pesticide. The three pesticides found most often included animal carcinogens and pesticides that cause hormonal, brain, and nervous system damage. Because strawberries are soft and porous, pesticide residues infiltrate the berries and can't simply be washed off.

WATERMELON

Serving size: 1¼ cup watermelon chunks

Per serving:
Calories:.....................57
Carbohydrate: ....14 g
Protein:.....................1 g
Fat:........................0 g
Saturated fat: ....0 g
Cholesterol: ....0 mg
Sodium:..................2 mg
Fiber:.....................1 g
Calcium:..................13 g

Good source of:

vitamin A, vitamin C, vitamin B$_6$, potassium, lycopene

Description:

Watermelons likely originated in Africa, although hundreds of varieties grow in warm climates throughout the world. Watermelons grow on vines and, as their appearance might suggest, are related to cucumbers and gourds such as pumpkins and butternut squash. Thanks to their sweetness (and the fact that they wear their seeds on the inside), they are generally classified as fruits.

Watermelons boast a remarkably high water content, hence their name. In countries where potable water is scarce, they can play an important role in helping people to stay safely hydrated. Watermelons come in many shapes and sizes, from the small, round, dark green "Sugar Babies" to large, oval melons with striped, thick rinds.

Health benefits:

Watermelons owe their red-colored flesh to lycopene and contain more of the antioxidant—about 7.5 to 10 milligrams per cup—than other fruits and vegetables tested to date. The vitamins C and A in a watermelon are important for proper immune function. Vitamin B$_6$ is vital to neurotransmitter production, which contributes to normal brain function.

For those who find it challenging to drink the quantity of water that is recommended each day, watermelons can help bridge the gap.

Selection tips:

Look for firm, symmetrically shaped melons that are heavy for their size. (Remember, water is heavy, and a ripe watermelon is 92% to 95% water!) Avoid melons that have soft spots or damaged rinds.

A light yellow area on the underside of the melon, on the other hand, *is* desirable. The presence of this "ground spot" means the melon was allowed to ripen properly, resting on the ground as it grew heavy, while still attached to the vine.

Tapping a watermelon with your knuckle to determine its ripeness does have some utility—you should hear a hollow-sounding thump, another indication that the melon has a high proportion of water.

When selecting precut watermelon, make sure it has been refrigerated and that the cut side is covered in plastic. The flesh of the melon should look firm. Refrigerate precut melon immediately and consume within 2 to 3 days.

Storage tips:
Whole, uncut watermelons prefer warmer temperatures and can be kept at room temperature for 7 to 10 days. Very cold temperatures can actually compromise the flavor and texture of an uncut watermelon. After cutting, however, the melon should be refrigerated and consumed within 3 to 4 days. Watermelons have too high a water content to freeze successfully for snacking, but they can be frozen as part of a sorbet or granita recipe.

Preparation tips:
Wash watermelons well before cutting. For informal events like barbeques, serve watermelon wedges. Simply cut the melon lengthwise into halves, then cut each half lengthwise (you should now have a quartered melon). Place the melon rind-side down on a cutting board. Slice off the curved end of the melon (the first 2 to 3 inches or so). Cut the melon vertically in even increments of about 1 inch; you should end up with plenty of triangle-shaped melon wedges, complete with rind "handles."

To cube a melon, start by cutting it in quarters, as described above. Make evenly spaced horizontal, then vertical cuts across the length and width of the melon quarter. Keep a large bowl handy for the melon cubes, which should come out effortlessly.

For a fancier presentation, try using a melon baller to scoop out melon spheres, or use cookie cutters to cut more unusual shapes for sliced melon (this is best tried with seedless watermelons).

Beyond their obvious uses in fruit salads, beverages, or sorbets, watermelons are an interesting foil for spicy or savory dishes. Try small crouton-size watermelon dices in a baby spinach salad. The natural sweetness and refreshing texture of watermelon is a great counterpoint to salty Feta cheese—try a composed salad of watermelon and Feta slices strewn with minced herbs and a drizzle of high-quality extra-virgin olive oil. Or use roughly chopped watermelon in salsas to accompany spicy shellfish or grilled chicken dishes.

Although most people eat only the watermelon flesh, some pickle the rind. In Israel, roasted, lightly salted watermelon seeds are a popular snack.

Precautions:
Be sure to wash the outside of melons well before cutting, or you risk carrying bacteria—which could cause food-borne illness—from the surface of the melon to the flesh.

GRAINS

BARLEY

Serving size: ½ cup pearled barley, cooked

Per serving:
Calories:. 97
Carbohydrate: . . . . 22 g
Protein:. . . . . 2 g
Fat:. . . . . 0 g
Saturated fat: . . . . 0 g
Cholesterol: . . . . 0 mg
Sodium:. . . . . 2 mg
Fiber:. 3 g
Calcium: . . . . 9 mg

Good source of:
soluble fiber, iron, selenium, niacin

Description:
Barley is one of the oldest known cereal grains and grows throughout the world. In Asia, Africa, and the Middle East, barley remains an important part of the human diet. However, the highly nutritious grain gets short shrift in most American diets. Over half the U.S. barley crop is used for animal feed, and most of the rest is grown to make the malt necessary for beer making.

Research is constantly affirming the importance of whole grains. Barley is especially versatile and approachable and is an excellent choice for some whole-grain experimentation. Barley comes in many forms. "Hulled" and "hull-less" barley undergo minimal processing to remove their inedible outer hull; both are considered whole grains. "Pearled" or "pearl" barley—the version most Americans are familiar with—has undergone repeated polishing, which strips it of its bran and endosperm, along with some of its micronutrients. Pearled barley is technically not considered a whole grain, although it does contain a significant amount of soluble fiber, and it's a far healthier food choice than refined grains. Pearled barley also takes less time to cook than hulled barley, so some might find it easier to integrate into the diet.

Health benefits:
A U.S. Department of Agriculture (USDA) study found that the soluble fiber in barley helped both men and women significantly lower elevated total and LDL ("bad") cholesterol levels.

A 2005 study published in *Plant Foods for Human Nutrition* demonstrated that in people both with and without diabetes, barley cereal induced much lower glycemic (blood-glucose-raising) and insulin responses than the oatmeal and meal replacement beverages to which it was compared.

The lipid-improving benefits and lower after-meal blood glucose levels related to consumption of whole grains such as barley were noted by a research team led by David Jenkins, a professor of nutrition and metabolism at the University of Toronto, who suggested in a 2003 study published in *The American Journal of Clinical Nutrition* that vegetarian diets might be useful in the prevention and treatment of diabetes.

Selection tips:
Pearl barley is readily available in most grocery stores. Hulled barley and barley flakes, grits, and flour are more often found in health-food stores.

Storage tips:
Store barley in an airtight container in a cool, dry place. Uncooked barley can be refrigerated or frozen to preserve freshness. Barley requires a relatively long cooking time, but it can be cooked ahead of time and refrigerated or frozen for later use. Cooked barley can be refrigerated for up to a week or frozen for up to three months.

Preparation tips:
Hulled barley should be soaked for several hours before cooking and typically requires a ratio of 3 or 4 cups of water or broth to each cup of barley. Pearl barley does not require soaking and generally requires a bit less water. Most recipes will indicate the proper amount of liquid to grain to ensure that all of the liquid is absorbed. It is also possible to cook barley as you would pasta— simply cook in a generous amount of water and drain once the barley is tender.

Pearl barley usually takes approximately 30 to 45 minutes to cook, while hulled barley can take at least an hour.

Barley has a pleasant, chewy texture and a mild nutty flavor. It can be served as a hot porridge-like breakfast cereal with fruit and nuts. Try adding a handful of cooked barley into pancake or muffin batter, or stir a spoonful of cooked barley into yogurt.

Add barley to chili or soup recipes to boost fiber content and enhance texture. Transform your favorite risotto recipe by using barley in place of Arborio rice. Serve it as a hot side dish with herbs and sautéed mushrooms during the cooler months. In the summer, try the grain as a base for a cool salad or light main dish: toss cooked barley with grilled vegetables and vinaigrette or with chopped dried fruit, nuts, lemon juice, and olive oil. Refrigerate until ready to serve. Cold barley salads are great served atop baby greens or alongside grilled or poached fish.

BROWN RICE

Serving size: ½ cup cooked long-grain brown rice

Per serving:
Calories:. 108
Carbohydrate: . . . . 22 g
Protein:. 3 g
Fat:. . . . . 1 g
Saturated fat: . . . . 0 g
Cholesterol: . . . . 0 mg
Sodium:. . . . . 5 mg
Fiber:. . . . . 2 g
Calcium: . . . . 10 mg

Good source of:
fiber, niacin, thiamine, magnesium, phosphorus, zinc, copper

Description:
Most white rice starts as brown rice, but the germ and endosperm—and most of the fiber and nutrients—are removed when the rice is refined and polished. So, just as there are many varieties of white rice, there are many varieties of brown rice, too. Whether your preference is for short-, medium-, or long-grain rice, or for Basmati, sushi, or jasmine rice, all of it is available in its unrefined, brown form!

In fact, there are whole-grain rice varieties that are not brown at all—adventuresome eaters will want to seek out the delicious red, black, and purple rice cultivars that were once reserved for emperors and royal courts.

Health benefits:
Whole-grain rice is rich in fiber, protein, and phytochemicals that help promote cardiovascular health through improved cholesterol and blood pressure levels. Diets rich in whole grains—including brown rice—have also been associated with reduced risk of certain cancers and diabetes.

People with diabetes who switch from white to brown rice typically see improvements in blood glucose control. Brown rice might also facilitate weight loss and weight management thanks to its satisfying high fiber content.

Rice is very easy to digest, rarely allergenic, and is gluten-free.

Selection tips:
Because there are many varieties of brown rice, personal preference may dictate which you favor. Start by finding the brown version of your favorite white rice. When purchasing brown rice in bulk, make sure to shop at a store with rapid stock turnover to ensure that you are purchasing fresh rice.

Storage tips:
Store whole-grain rice in an airtight container in a cool, dry, preferably dark place, away from any heat source.

Precooked brown rice can be kept in a well-covered container in the refrigerator for three to four days. It can also be frozen in small portions for later use. Freeze cooled, cooked rice in a well-sealed container for three to six months.

Preparation tips:
Cooking times and the amount of cooking liquid required for brown rice can vary by variety, so it's best to check package directions or a reliable cookbook. Generally speaking, the rice to liquid ratio is 1:2, so one cup of rice would require 2 cups of water or broth. Brown rice typically takes 45 to 50 minutes to cook.

Place rice and liquid in a saucepan and bring to a boil. Reduce the heat, cover, and simmer the rice until it is tender. Try to resist the urge to check the rice frequently, especially early in cooking, or the cooking liquid will dissipate as steam.

Brown rice is extremely versatile. It can be served plain as a side dish, embellished with herbs and spices, or mixed with other grains. Use it to stuff peppers, zucchini, mushroom caps, or rolled eggplant slices, and drizzle the vegetables with vinaigrette or top with tomato sauce. It's also a great addition to soups and a hearty base for stews.

Consider using brown rice as a base for a summertime cold rice salad—add chopped cucumbers, tomatoes, scallions, and peppers to chilled rice, toss with a lemon vinaigrette, and sprinkle with crumbled Feta or goat cheese. Or use chopped mango, avocado, and scallion, toss with a sesame-soy vinaigrette, and top with cubes of grilled tofu.

Cooked brown rice can be added to bread or baked goods recipes. Try cooking it with milk or soy milk to make a breakfast porridge. Or replace white rice with brown in rice pudding recipes.

MILLET

Serving size: ½ cup cooked

Per serving:

Calories:	104
Carbohydrate:	21 g
Protein:	3 g
Fat:	1 g
Saturated fat:	0 g
Cholesterol:	0 mg
Sodium:	2 mg
Fiber:	1 g
Calcium:	3 mg

Good source of:
niacin, magnesium

Description:
Millet is a tiny, round, prehistorically cultivated grain. Officially, "millet" refers to many species, including common millet, sorghum, and teff. However, these grains have their own identities, flavors, and uses.

The grain known simply as millet is a staple in India and is an important part of the diet in China, South America, and Eastern Europe. In the United States, however, it's mostly birds that benefit from the whole grain—millet is the round, buff-colored grain found in birdseed.

Health benefits:
Millet is gluten-free, so it can be eaten by those with celiac disease. It is a source of high-quality plant protein and is rich in fiber, magnesium, and B vitamins, all of which are important for promoting normal blood pressure and heart health.

A 2005 study published in *Diabetes Medicine* found that, among a small group of

Sudanese subjects with diabetes, millet produced lower post-meal blood glucose and insulin responses than meals composed of other grains.

Selection tips:
Look for millet in health-food stores or larger gourmet markets. When buying in bulk, shop at stores with high turnover to ensure a fresher grain.

Storage tips:
Store millet in an airtight container in a cool, dry, dark place. Properly stored, it will keep for several months.

Preparation tips:
Try toasting millet before cooking to enhance its nutty flavor: Add millet to a lightly oiled hot saucepan, and stir or toss lightly just until the grains turn golden. (Take care not to burn the millet.) Add water or broth and simmer until the grains are cooked, usually about 30 to 40 minutes. Plan to use about two cups of liquid per cup of millet.

Try making a breakfast porridge from cooked millet. Add the cooked grain to soups or pilafs or mix it into bread recipes.

Precautions:
Sort and rinse millet before cooking to remove any small pebbles or foreign matter.

Millet contains substances known to be goiterogenic. People with established thyroid disease should therefore discuss the safety of consuming millet with an endocrinologist or registered dietitian.

QUINOA

Serving size: ¼ cup dry, or approximately ½ cup cooked

Per serving:

Calories:	159
Carbohydrate:	29 g
Protein:	6 g
Fat:	2 g
Saturated fat:	0 g
Cholesterol:	0 mg
Sodium:	9 mg
Fiber:	3 g
Calcium:	26 mg

Good source of:
iron, magnesium, potassium, protein, fiber

Description:
Quinoa (pronounced *keen*-wa) is often touted as a veritable "supergrain," although technically quinoa "grains" are the seeds of a plant related to beets, Swiss chard, and spinach.

Cultivated for thousands of years in South America, quinoa was revered by the Incas. Today the Andean seed is enjoying a renaissance thanks to its impressive health profile and culinary versatility.

Despite its botanical classification, quinoa is generally regarded as a grain because it shares nutritional similarities with other staple grains. But quinoa surpasses other grains in the protein department—not only is it rich in the macronutrient, but also it's the only grain that is a complete protein—that is, one that contains all the essential amino acids. ("Essential" amino acids are those our bodies can't synthesize on their own and must therefore be supplied by the diet.)

Quinoa can be pink, orange, purple, red, or black, although virtually all of the quinoa consumed in the United States is a buff color. The tiny, disc-shaped seeds become almost translucent when cooked, and the white, ringlike germ surrounding the seeds can be seen. Cooked quinoa has a light, fluffy texture while retaining a little crunch and a nutty flavor that is enhanced by toasting.

Health benefits:

A 2005 study published in the *British Journal of Nutrition* found that study subjects reported less hunger and higher satiety (fullness) after eating quinoa. Furthermore, quinoa has a low glycemic index, meaning it raises blood glucose less than many other foods, and a typically consumed portion has a low glycemic load. These factors might have implications for both weight and blood glucose control.

A 2004 study published in the *European Journal of Nutrition* found that relative to other gluten-free foods tested, quinoa induced a lower blood glucose response among both subjects without celiac disease and those with celiac disease. Subjects' after-meal free fatty acid and triglyceride levels were also lower after eating quinoa than they were after consuming other foods. This further supports abundant research that has shown that eating whole grains promotes a favorable lipid profile.

As a gluten-free option, quinoa is an excellent choice for those with celiac disease.

Selection tips:

Quinoa is easy to find in health-food stores and gourmet markets. It is increasingly available in supermarkets, sometimes as a component of newer convenience wholegrain mixes.

Storage tips:

Store quinoa in an airtight container in a cool, dry place, away from any heat source. Quinoa flour can be stored in an airtight container in the refrigerator for three to six months.

Great uses for quinoa abound, so it is worth cooking extra and storing it in a covered container in the refrigerator for three to four days to be added to recipes throughout the week.

Cooked quinoa can also be frozen in small portions. Place cooked, cooled quinoa in well-covered containers and freeze for up to several months for later use.

Preparation tips:

Quinoa seeds should be rinsed before use because they are covered by saponin, a soaplike substance that is a natural deterrent to pests and tastes bitter to humans.

Quinoa cooks quickly, in about 15 to 20 minutes. Try toasting the quinoa in a bit of oil before simmering to intensify its nutty flavor. Use two cups of water or broth for each cup of quinoa.

Serve hot quinoa as a side dish in place of rice or couscous. Quinoa works well when tossed with beans, lentils, or chopped nuts and dried fruits, and it complements other grains beautifully in pilafs. For a fancier presentation, mold quinoa—whether plain or enhanced with additions—into timbales.

Use quinoa as a base for vegetarian main dishes, topped with roasted or stir-fried vegetables, chili, or stew. Fold cooked quinoa into bread, muffins, or grain-based veggie burger recipes, or add it to soups. Wrap quinoa and julienned vegetables in lettuce leaves for quick summer rolls, or use it— along with vegetables and grilled tofu, fish, or chicken— to fill sandwich wraps or whole wheat pita.

Quinoa makes a comforting hot cereal when cooked with milk or soymilk. Quinoa can even enhance desserts—use it in place of rice to make a nourishing, protein-rich pudding.

Serving size: ⅓ cup whole-grain sorghum, cooked

Per serving:
Calories:. 215
Carbohydrate: . . . . 47 g
Protein:. . . . . 7 g
Fat:. . . . . 2 g
Saturated fat: . . . . 0 g
Cholesterol: . . . . 0 mg
Sodium:. . . . . 4 mg
Fiber:. 4 g
Calcium: . . . . 18 mg

Good source of:

iron, niacin, protein, lactobacilli

Description:
Although the grain is rarely seen on American tables, sorghum is among the world's most widely cultivated cereal crops. The drought-resistant grain is a staple in African diets and is widely consumed in India, China, Australia, parts of the Caribbean, and Latin America.

Because sorghum is gluten-free, it's an excellent whole grain choice for those with celiac disease or others who must abstain from gluten.

Sorghum is sometimes called millet or "milo." It should not be confused with Nestlé Milo, a chocolate malted milk powder high in added sugar that is marketed as an energy drink. Nor is it the same as sweet sorghum, a syrupy sweetener also called "sorghum molasses."

Health benefits:
Sorghum is rich in phytochemicals, including tannins, phenolic acids, anthocyanins, and plant stanols. A 2004 study published in *Phytochemistry* noted that these phytochemicals are associated with decreased risk of cardiovascular disease, cancer, and obesity, and urged further research into sorghum's potential health benefits for humans.

Studies have found lower rates of esophageal cancer among those who regularly consume sorghum. And in 2005 the journal *Medical Hypotheses* published an article in which the author noted that esophageal cancer rates have risen among black South Africans as they've replaced sorghum with maize.

Sorghum is also a good source of lactobacilli, "friendly" bacteria that help promote gastrointestinal health and proper immune function.

Selection tips:
You can find whole-grain sorghum and sorghum flour in health-food stores or on Web sites catering to those who must follow

a gluten-free diet due to celiac disease or other conditions.

Storage tips:
Sorghum will keep in an airtight container in a cool, dry place for several months.

Preparation tips:
Sort out any foreign matter and rinse the sorghum grains. Soak sorghum in a generous amount of water overnight in a large bowl in the refrigerator. To cook, use 3 cups of liquid per cup of whole-grain sorghum. Simmer for 45 to 60 minutes, or until the sorghum is tender.

Use the cooked grains as a gluten-free alternative to barley, couscous, or pasta or mix it into grain pilafs. Experiment with sorghum in recipes for veggie burgers or grain croquettes. Try sorghum flour in flat-bread or other recipes for baked goods.

You can even pop sorghum like popcorn. Place the (unsoaked) grains in a saucepan with oil. Cover and place the pan over medium heat. When the sorghum starts to pop, shake the pan over the heat; remove it from the heat when the popping slows. Be careful when removing the lid—the steam inside the pot will be quite hot. Drizzle the popped sorghum with olive oil and herbs or spices if desired and enjoy.

Precautions:
Sorghum is quite nutritious and is an excellent whole grain option. It is rich in carbohydrate, however, so do pay attention to portion size. Of course, because it is so fiber-rich and satisfyingly chewy, odds are that even a small portion of sorghum will feel sufficient.

TEFF

Serving size: ¼ cup

Per serving:
Calories:. 160
Carbohydrate: . . . . 32 g
Protein:. . . . . .5 g
Fat:. . . . . .1 g
Saturated fat: . . . . .0 g
Cholesterol: . . . . .0 mg
Sodium:. . . . . .5 mg
Fiber:. .6 g
Calcium: . . . . .97 mg

Good source of:
iron, calcium, fiber

Description:
Teff is a tiny, spherical type of millet that is a staple in the Ethiopian and Eritrean diets. It is a key ingredient in *injera,* a spongy flatbread that is both a centerpiece of the cuisine and a utensil for eating stew-like dishes.

The grains might range in color from white to red to dark brown and have a subtly sweet, nutty flavor. The ivory variety has a milder taste than the dark brown grain.

Teff grains are too tiny to refine so they are always whole grain.

Health benefits:
Teff is gluten-free, which makes it appropriate for those with celiac disease. It is an excellent source of iron and calcium, minerals vital to bone health and muscle function. Cup-for-cup, teff has about 100 milligrams (mg) more calcium than milk; even a modest ¼-cup portion of teff provides 97 mg of calcium.

Because it is so fiber-rich, teff might help promote blood glucose control. Studies conducted in Israel found that diabetes rates among Ethiopian immigrants were remarkably low upon arrival but that after acculturation to an Israeli diet (which often involved replacing teff with wheat flour), glucose intolerance and diabetes rates neared those of the general Israeli population.

Selection tips:
Teff is available in both grain and flour forms at health-food stores and over the Internet (try www.bobsredmill.com or www.teffco.com).

Storage tips:
Store teff in a cool, dry place in an airtight container for up to several months.

Preparation tips:
Teff cooks far more quickly than most whole grains and is very versatile. It requires no presoaking or rinsing—just use 3 cups of water or stock for each cup of teff and simmer for approximately 20 minutes.

Try lightly toasting teff before simmering to enhance the nutty flavor of the grains. Add the grains to a saucepan with a bit of oil and stir constantly over low heat until lightly browned, taking care not to burn them. Add the cooking liquid, stir, and simmer over low heat until cooked.

Cook teff as you would porridge or polenta, or use it in pilafs with other grains. Although the lack of gluten prevents teff flour from rising, it works well in flatbreads, pie crusts, and cookie recipes.

WILD RICE

Serving size: ½ cup, cooked

Per serving:
Calories:. 83
Carbohydrate: . . . . .18 g
Protein:. . . . . .3 g
Fat:. . . . . .0 g
Saturated fat: . . . . .0 g
Cholesterol: . . . . 0 mg
Sodium:. . . . . .5 mg
Fiber:. .2 g
Calcium: . . . . .2 mg

Good source of:
fiber, protein, phosphorus, zinc, copper

Description:
Wild rice is actually the seed of an aquatic marsh plant. Historically, it was a staple of the Native American tribes in the Great Lakes region, who hand-harvested the seeds by beating the grassy stalks, on which they grow, and catching the seeds in their canoes. Certain tribes, like the Ojibwe (also called the Chippewa), consider the rice sacred, and there are ceremonial aspects to the harvest.

The traditional manner of harvesting wild rice is very labor-intensive, and yields are typically low, in part because the plant requires very particular growing conditions and is remarkably sensitive to climactic or environmental changes. As a result, commercially grown and harvested wild rice has become increasingly mechanized. Wild rice is commercially cultivated in Minnesota and California.

Wild rice is green when it is harvested. It takes on its distinctive glossy blackish brown appearance after it is dried, threshed, and winnowed.

Health benefits:

Although botanically speaking wild rice is not a grain, it is classed among whole grains because of its similar structure and nutrient profile. Wild rice is higher in fiber and protein than most other grains, and it is particularly rich in lysine, an essential amino acid.

As with other whole grains, wild rice consumption likely promotes a favorable lipid profile, normal blood pressure, healthy weight, and reduced risk of certain cancers and diabetes.

Wild rice is a good source of phosphorus, which is essential to DNA, RNA, bone, and phospholipid structure, as well as to cellular energy transport. The zinc in wild rice is vital to immune function.

Wild rice is gluten-free, so it can be enjoyed by those with celiac disease, or gluten intolerance.

Selection tips:

Wild rice is available in most supermarkets as well as in gourmet shops and health-food stores. If buying wild rice in bulk, purchase it from a store with frequent turnover.

Storage tips:

Store uncooked wild rice in an airtight container in a cool, dry place. It will keep indefinitely when properly stored.

Cut down on midweek meal preparation time by storing cooked, drained wild rice in a well-covered container in the refrigerator, where it will keep for one to two weeks.

For further convenience, cooked, drained wild rice can be frozen for later use. Place small portions in individual containers and freeze the wild rice for up to several months.

Preparation tips:

Clean wild rice thoroughly before cooking. Place it in a large bowl filled with cool water.

Swish the water around with clean hands, then allow the rice to rest for a moment before pouring off the water. Repeat the process if necessary.

The cooking time for wild rice depends on where it was grown and how it was processed, so follow the preparation directions on the package. Generally speaking, for each cup of wild rice, use 3 cups of water or broth.

Wild rice can take anywhere from 30 to 60 minutes to cook. The kernels will expand and split, but if they've begun to curl or become mushy, they're overcooked.

The distinctive nutty taste and chewy grain of wild rice is a nice counterpoint to softer, blander grains, so it's often used in pilafs. Wild rice can also stand on its own as a side dish. It has a wonderful affinity for earthy mushrooms—try tossing wild rice with sautéed shiitakes, criminis, and oyster mushrooms, or mound wild rice into a roasted portobello mushroom cap. Or try adding chopped, roasted vegetables into wild rice, toss with a vinaigrette, and serve warm. Dried fruit and toasted nut-studded wild rice is another nice option.

Wild rice also makes elegant cold grain salads. Try adding seeded, diced cucumbers, carrots, radish, or scallions, and toss with a rice vinegar-based vinaigrette.

Cooked wild rice also adds texture and fiber to bread and muffin recipes.

Precautions:

If possible, avoid wild rice from northern Wisconsin, particularly if you consume it often. A 2000 study conducted by U.S. Geological Survey researchers found elevated levels of the heavy metals, arsenic and lead, in wild rice samples from that area.

ALMONDS

Serving size: 1 ounce whole, natural almonds (about 23 nuts)

Per serving:
Calories:. 164
Carbohydrate: . . . . 6 g
Protein:. . . . . 6 g
Fat: . . . . 14 g
Saturated fat: . . . . 1 g
Monounsaturated fat: . . . . 9 g
Polyunsaturated fat:. . . . . 4 g
Phytosterols: . . . . 34 mg
Cholesterol: . . . . 0 mg
Sodium:. . . . . 0 mg
Fiber:. . . . . 3 g
Calcium: . . . . 70 mg

Good source of:
vitamin E, alpha-tocopherol, phosphorus, calcium, riboflavin, niacin

Description:
Although it is unclear whether almonds originated in the Middle East or in Asia, we do know that they have been cultivated since antiquity. Almonds are mentioned in the Bible and several other ancient texts. Silk Road traders and explorers carried almonds and helped spread their cultivation through the Mediterranean to Spain, Italy, Morocco, Greece, and Israel. They were important as food, medicine, and fertility symbols to the ancient Greeks and Romans.

In the 1700's, Franciscan padres brought almonds to their missions in California from Spain, although the temperature-sensitive trees didn't thrive at first. Only when planted inland did almond trees begin to do well in California; today the state is one of the world's largest almond producers and exporters, with over 500,000 acres of almonds in cultivation.

Almonds are actually the seeds of the almond tree and are related to peaches. This kinship is most evident in the resemblance of baby almonds, which have a fuzzy green hull, to immature peaches.

Health benefits:
In a 2002 study published in *Circulation*, Dr. David Jenkins and a team of researchers found that both men and women who ate about 1 ounce of almonds each day (a small handful, or about 23 almonds) lowered their LDL ("bad") cholesterol by 4.4%. Even more significant, for subjects who ate 2 ounces per day, LDL cholesterol dropped 9.4%, suggesting that the LDL-lowering effect is dose-dependent. Best of all, study subjects maintained their weights, even with higher almond consumption.

In numerous other studies, almonds have been shown to reduce total cholesterol, and triglycerides as well, while raising HDL ("good") cholesterol. The plant sterols in almonds might play a role in their cholesterol-lowering prowess.

This is further evidence that recommendations to follow very-low-fat diets for weight loss, weight management, or cholesterol reduction may be misguided. It is true that saturated fat intake should be kept to a minimum and that *trans* fat should be eliminated from the diet. But missing out on cardioprotective fats such as those found in almonds would be a mistake. The fat in almonds helps aid the absorption of the fat-soluble vitamin E they contain. In addition, almonds are rich in protein and fiber. Fat, protein, and fiber all contribute to feelings of fullness when eating, which in turn helps prevent overeating, and all three help promote stable blood glucose levels.

Two small studies found improvements in weight and blood glucose control among people with diabetes or metabolic syndrome when almonds were added to their diets.

Anecdotally, research suggests that thanks to the cell walls in almonds, humans do not digest all of the fat they contain. It seems we get just enough to reap significant benefit but not so much that we gain weight.

Almonds are a rich source of alpha-tocopherol, a particularly potent form of the antioxidant vitamin E. They are also rich in calcium and phosphorus, two minerals that are vital for bone health.

Selection tips:

When buying almonds in the shell, look for ones with undamaged shells.

Shelled almonds—whether whole, blanched, sliced, chopped, slivered, or ground—should be sold in well-sealed packages, preferably with an expiration date. If buying almonds in bulk, choose a store that stocks high-quality foodstuffs and has a rapid supply turnover to better ensure that the almonds are fresh.

If you are lucky enough to find fresh baby almonds, a delicacy in Middle Eastern cul-

tures, look for those with uniformly pale green, fuzzy outer hulls.

Storage tips:

Whole almonds in their shells will keep at room temperature, but shelled almonds are more perishable. They can be refrigerated for up to six months, or frozen for up to a year. In both cases they should be kept in a well-sealed container or plastic bag.

Baby almonds are much more perishable and should be refrigerated and eaten within a couple of days.

Preparation tips:

Uses for almonds abound. They're great eaten out of hand or alongside a bit of cheese and fresh or dried fruit. They are excellent complements to virtually any ethnic cuisine imaginable and work in both savory and sweet dishes.

Sprinkle almonds in hot or cold cereal or yogurt or try almond milk in coffee or tea.

Add toasted, slivered almonds to salads. Sauté slivered or sliced almonds with string beans, spinach, or asparagus, or use whole almonds in stir-fries.

Replace some of the breadcrumbs in baked or oven-fried chicken or fish recipes with ground or chopped toasted almonds.

Ground almonds enrich baked goods and raise their nutritional profile; try substituting ½ to 1 cup of ground almonds for an equal amount of flour in your favorite recipe.

Spread almond butter on multigrain toast, crackers, or sliced apple. If you can't find almond butter in the store, you can make your own by blending or food-processing whole almonds with a drizzle of oil (try almond oil), and, if desired, a pinch of salt and sugar.

To toast almonds, preheat the oven to 350°F, place the nuts in a single layer on a cookie sheet, and bake, stirring periodically, until the almonds are golden. Be sure to keep an eye on them—they can go from nicely toasted to burnt in a matter of seconds! Remove almonds from the oven and transfer to a container to cool.

Alternatively, you can toast almonds in a skillet. This method works especially well for slivered almonds. Place a skillet over medium heat and add the almonds. (You can add a little bit of oil to the pan, if you wish.) Toss or stir the almonds constantly until toasted and then remove from the pan to cool.

Precautions:
People who have been diagnosed with an allergy to peanuts (ground nuts) or any tree nut should consider avoiding all tree nuts, including almonds.

Small children should not be offered almonds, due to risk of both choking hazard and potential allergenicity. Talk to a pediatrician or registered dietitian before introducing nuts into children's diets.

PISTACHIOS

Serving size: 1 ounce (49 whole pistachios, dry-roasted with salt)

Per serving:
Calories: 160
Carbohydrate: . . . . 8 g
Protein: . . . . 6 g
Fat: . . . . 13 g
Saturated fat: . . . . 2 g
Polyunsaturated fat: . . . . 4 g
Monounsaturated fat: . . . . 7 g
Cholesterol: . . . . 0 mg
Sodium: . . . . 115 mg
Fiber: . . . . 3 g

Good source of:
fiber, vitamin B_6, thiamine, phosphorus, copper, phytosterols, potassium, lutein

Description:
The pistachio tree is indigenous to Asia and Asia Minor, and the seeds (pistachio nuts) were part of the human diet at least as early as 7000 B.C. They were introduced to the Mediterranean from Syria in the first century B.C. Pistachio trees are quite drought-resistant, thrive in arid areas, and live and produce clusters of edible nuts for hundreds of years, making them valuable throughout the Middle East and in other pistachio-growing regions with challenging climates or topography.

Pistachios weren't grown commercially in the United States until 1976; today, however, California's pistachio industry is booming, with over 100,000 acres in cultivation.

Health benefits:
The thiamine in pistachios is important for carbohydrate metabolism, while the vitamin B6 they contain helps the body produce insulin, hemoglobin, and antibodies.

A 2004 study evaluating data from the Nurses' Health Study found that women who consumed at least five ounces of nuts per week had significantly reduced risk of cholecystectomy (gallbladder removal).

Pistachios are also rich in disease-fighting antioxidants, including lutein.

Selection tips:
Before pistachios were grown in the United States, imported dyed pistachios were the

norm. The finger-staining bright red dye wasn't meant to mimic the pistachio shell's natural color (Although when pistachios are ready for harvest, an outer hull, which is soaked off during processing, takes on a rosy hue.); it was there to hide blemishes on shells that received rough handling during harvesting, and to help draw attention to the nuts, which were sold from vending machines.

Look for natural pistachios with light tan shells surrounding green nuts. (The green color of pistachios is natural; chlorophyll is responsible for that.)

Storage tips:
Pistachios will absorb water from the air, so to ensure that they stay crunchy, keep them in an airtight container. They'll remain the freshest in the refrigerator, where they can be stored for six months, or in the freezer, where they can be kept for up to a year.

Preparation tips:
Shelling pistachios is quite easy. The shells naturally split open as the nuts mature, so they can be pried open by hand. If you chance across a totally unsplit pistachio shell, it's likely to contain an immature nut and should be discarded. If a shell is partially open and the nut inside looks enticing, try using half a pistachio shell as a "key"—insert the shell into the opening and twist, and the shell should split the rest of the way with little effort.

As might be expected, pistachios are an excellent accompaniment to Middle Eastern foods. They are also used in Asian and Indian cuisines, particularly with vegetable and rice dishes. Add whole pistachios to couscous or grain dishes. Try ground or chopped pistachios in stuffing or use them to replace some of the breadcrumbs in savory toppings or breading. Pistachios are also a nice accent in baked goods or served with cheese and dried fruit.

Precautions:
People who have been diagnosed with an allergy to peanuts (ground nuts) or any tree nut should consider avoiding all tree nuts, including pistachios.

Small children should not be offered pistachios, due to risk of both choking hazard and potential allergenicity. Talk to a pediatrician or registered dietitian before introducing nuts into children's diets.

Serving size: 1 ounce (14 unsalted, unroasted halves)

Per serving:
Calories:. 190
Carbohydrate: . . . . 4 g
Protein:. 4 g
Fat: . . . . 18 g
Saturated fat: . . . . 2 g
Monounsaturated fat: . . . . 3 g
Polyunsaturated fat:. . . . . 13 g
Linolenic acid (omega-3): . . . . . 3 g
Cholesterol: . . . . 0 mg
Sodium:. . . . . trace
Fiber:. . . . . 2 g

Good source of:

omega-3 fatty acids, melatonin, magnesium, copper, manganese, phytosterols

Description:

The walnut tree and the nuts it produces have been valued since antiquity. Beyond their cultivation for food and medicinal purposes, walnut trees have also provided oil for light and wood for building, among other uses. There are several varieties of this impressive tree. "English" or "royal" walnuts likely originated in Europe and Asia. The trees grow to anywhere from 30 to 80 feet tall and can live for 200 to 400 years. Black and white walnuts are indigenous to North America and grow on trees that reach a soaring 100 to 130 feet.

The archaeological record in France—where petrified roasted walnut shells were uncovered—shows evidence of walnut consumption in the Neolithic (New Stone Age) period. Walnuts were important in Mesopotamia and figured prominently in Greek mythology. Roman culture likewise revered the walnut; Roman invaders helped reintroduce the walnut tree, which might have been wiped out from the region during the glacial period, to northern Europe.

Walnuts were first produced commercially in the United States in the mid-to-late 1800's. Today, the California walnut industry supplies virtually all of the walnuts in the United States and exports about two-thirds of the world supply.

Health benefits:

Walnuts are unusual among tree nuts in that they are an excellent source of polyunsaturated omega-3 fatty acids. A 2005 Australian study published in the *Journal of the American Dietetic Association* found that for people with Type 2 Diabetes, eating one ounce of walnuts per day helped to raise the percentage of heart-healthy fats in the diet while lowering the percentage of saturated fat.

Melatonin, an antioxidant found in walnuts, helps improve the body's response to oxidative stress by scavenging free-radicals. The body's melatonin production decreases as we age, while free-radical damage increases. In a 2005 study published in *Nutrition*, researchers found not only that walnuts contain a significant amount of melatonin, but also that it is well absorbed and utilized. This might confer disease-fighting benefits, particularly against cancer, cardiovascular disease, and possibly neurodegenerative diseases associated with aging, such as Alzheimer disease and Parkinson disease. Researchers speculate that it is not the melatonin alone that fights disease, but the interaction between the walnut's many health-promoting components (including omega-3 fatty acids and melatonin) that is important.

Selection tips:

Walnuts sold in the shell should feel heavy for their size and should have uncracked shells. Those that are "full" of walnut are best. Give the shell a little shake; it shouldn't rattle much.

Shelled walnuts should be firm and crunchy. If you can't taste a sample, feel them, and reject walnuts that are soft or look shriveled. If you are purchasing prepackaged walnuts, check for an expiration date.

Storage tips:

While they are still in their shells, walnuts will keep for two to three months in a cool, dry place. Shelled walnuts are more perishable. They should be refrigerated in an airtight container for up to six months or frozen for up to one year. If your walnuts have an "off" smell or a paint-like aroma, the oils they contain have gone rancid and the nuts should be discarded.

Preparation tips:

Walnuts are fantastic in salads—try adding the roasted nuts to an arugula and pear salad. For a composed salad or a quick hors d'oeuvre, place a bit of herbed goat cheese on endive spears, and top with chopped walnuts. They are a great addition to a cheese course, as well.

Add walnuts to stir-fries, use them in pesto or other sauces, add them to breading or stuffing, or mix them into grain dishes. They can be blended into smoothies (they are especially good with banana!) or added to recipes for baked goods. Ground walnuts can even be used to replace some of the flour in baked goods—start with a half cup and work up from there.

Roasting heightens the flavor of walnuts. Place them on a cookie sheet in a preheated 375°F oven for 8 to 10 minutes, stirring occasionally, until they've browned. Watch carefully to avoid burning the nuts. Remove the nuts from the oven, transfer to a container, and allow them to cool before using.

Incidentally, a nutcracker is the best and safest way to open walnuts in the shell. Place the nutcracker along the seam of the walnut to open them easily.

Precautions:

People who have been diagnosed with an allergy to peanuts (ground nuts) or any tree nut should consider avoiding all tree nuts, including walnuts.

Small children should not be offered walnuts, due to risk of both choking hazard and potential allergenicity. Talk to a pediatrician or registered dietitian before introducing nuts into children's diets.

CANOLA OIL

Serving size: 1 tablespoon

Per serving:
Calories:. 120
Carbohydrate: . . . . 0 g
Protein:. . . . . 0 g
Fat: . . . . 14 g
Saturated fat: . . . . 1 g
Monounsaturated fat: . . . . 9 g
Polyunsaturated fat:. . . . . 4 g
Omega-3 fatty acids:. . . . . 1 g
Cholesterol: . . . . 0 mg
Sodium:. . . . . 0 mg
Fiber:. 0 g
Calcium: . . . . 0 mg

Good source of:

monounsaturated fat, alpha-linolenic (omega-3) fatty acids, vitamin K

Description:

Canola oil is made from a cultivar of the rapeseed plant. Ordinary rapeseed is related to Brussels sprouts and mustard greens. In the past, rapeseed's greenish oil was used in oil lamps and as a lubricant in steam engines. It had limited use as a cooking oil, and the seed was used in animal feed, but it was poorly accepted by both humans and livestock due to the presence of bitter, sulfur-containing compounds called *glucosinolates*. Ordinary rapeseed also contains a high concentration of *erucic acid*, a fatty acid that is a suspected carcinogen if consumed in large quantity.

Through selective breeding beginning in the late 1960's (and, more recently, thorough gene splicing), Canadian scientists successfully developed low erucic acid, low-glucosinolate plants that they named "Canola," which stands for "Canadian Oil, Low Acid."

Health benefits:

Canola oil is a predominantly monounsaturated fat source. It also contains a generous dose of alpha-linolenic acid, an essential omega-3 fatty acid. Both the monounsaturated fat and omega-3 fatty acids in canola oil help protect cardiovascular health by improving lipid levels, keeping the arteries smooth and elastic, and preventing blood platelets from sticking together and forming clots. What's more, a small amount of the alpha-linolenic acid consumed through the diet is converted to eicosapentaenoic acid (EPA) and docosahexaenoic acid (DHA), two other omega-3 fatty acids that are key to optimal health.

Diets high in monounsaturated fat and low in saturated fat have been demonstrated to confer protection against the development of certain cancers, including breast cancer.

When it comes to diabetes, both monounsaturated fat and omega-3 fatty acids, when used in place of saturated fat sources, may help prevent diabetes complications, particularly heart disease and stroke.

Moderate-fat diets that emphasize monounsaturated fats like canola oil also tend to be better for long-term weight loss and weight management than low-fat diets.

Fat increases feelings of fullness and slows the rate at which food empties from the stomach. Studies have found that consuming moderate amounts of heart-healthy fat (about 30% of daily calories) helps diners eat fewer total calories at meals and between meals, and helps keep their blood glucose levels more stable as well.

For people who are overweight or obese, even a relatively small (5% to 10%) weight loss can significantly help reduce the risk of developing various chronic diseases, including high blood pressure, heart disease, cancer, and diabetes. What's more, for people with diabetes who need to lose weight, doing so can help them improve their blood glucose levels.

Selection tips:
If possible, buy expeller-pressed, organic canola oil. It can be pricier than ordinary canola oil, but buying expeller-pressed organic oil is the only way to ensure that the oil was not extracted with chemicals or exposed to synthetic pesticides.

Storage tips:
Canola oil should be stored in a well-sealed container in a cool, dry place for up to a year. To prevent rancidity, it can also be kept in the refrigerator. It may become cloudy or solidify slightly, but this will not affect its quality. The oil will return to its normal liquid state at room temperature.

Preparation tips:
Canola oil has a light, neutral flavor that makes it a great choice for delicately flavored recipes or baking.

Try canola oil in light citrus vinaigrettes. It is a great replacement for predominantly polyunsaturated fats such as vegetable, corn, and safflower oils, which do not provide as many health benefits.

Precautions:
One tablespoon of canola oil provides approximately 25% of the recommended daily allowance of vitamin K, which can interact with certain drugs. People who take blood-thinning drugs such as warfarin (brand name Coumadin) should discuss the use of canola oil with their doctor or registered dietitian.

Canola oil should not be used for very high-heat cooking techniques, which can alter the structure of the fatty acids. If the oil starts to smell "off," discard it and start over with fresh oil at a lower heat.

Do not attempt to bottle garlic-infused, fresh-herb–infused, or citrus-peel–infused canola oil at home. Doing so can promote the growth of the deadly bacteria *Clostridium botulinum,* which produces the toxin that causes botulism. Stick to commercially prepared infused oils to ensure safety.

OLIVE OIL

Serving size: 1 tablespoon

Per serving:
Calories:. 120
Carbohydrate: . . . . 0 g
Protein:. 0 g
Fat: . . . . 14 g
Monounsaturated fat:. . . . . . . 10 g
Polyunsaturated fat:. . . . . 2 g
Saturated fat: . . . . 2 g
Cholesterol: . . . . 0 mg
Sodium:. . . . . 0 mg
Fiber:. 0 g
Calcium: . . . . 0 mg

Good source of:

monounsaturated fat, antioxidants, phyto-sterols, oleocanthal

Description:

A cornerstone of the Mediterranean diet for eons, olive oil is among the healthiest—and most health-promoting—fats in the world. Beyond its use as a foodstuff, olive oil has long been used in religious rituals, as medicine, in cosmetic products, and as a fuel source.

Olives have been grown throughout the Mediterranean region and in North Africa since antiquity; now they are also cultivated in the United States and Australia.

While Italian olive oil has a certain cachet among consumers, there are also excellent olive oils produced in Spain, Greece, Israel, Turkey, Morocco, Portugal, Tunisia, and France. Small artisanal producers in the United States and Australia are also turning out some very respectable olive oils.

Health benefits:

A tremendous amount of research has found that the traditional Mediterranean eating pattern is one of the healthiest in the world. Large population studies have found that people who consume a traditional Mediterranean diet—which emphasizes vegetables, whole grains, fruits, and a moderate amount of fat that comes from predominately monounsaturated sources like olive oil and nuts—have significantly lower rates of heart disease, high blood pressure, stroke, diabetes, obesity, certain cancers, and some forms of age-related dementia.

Other studies have found that people who replace the saturated fat sources that are standard in the Western diet with olive oil do experience improved blood pressure and blood lipid levels. Switching fat sources may also confer protection against the development or progression of diabetes, breast and colon cancer, and obesity.

Numerous studies have documented the anti-inflammatory effects of olive oil, which appear to provide some protection against chronic diseases. Now, researchers from the Monell Chemical Senses Center may have honed in on one of the compounds in olive oil that contributes to this effect.

Monell biologist Gary Beauchamp, Ph.D., was attending a conference in Italy, when, during an olive oil tasting, he observed the same stinging sensation at the back of his throat that ibuprofen produced. Back at Monell, Beauchamp and his colleagues identified a substance that they dubbed *oleocanthal,* which displayed the same anti-inflammatory mechanism as ibuprofen. In an article published in the scientific journal *Nature* in 2005, the researchers suggested that this component may be responsible for some of the cardioprotective and anticancer activity of extra-virgin olive oil.

Contrary to popular belief, moderate-fat diets that emphasize monounsaturated fats like olive oil tend to be better for long-term weight loss and management than low-fat diets. Fat increases feelings of fullness and slows the rate at which food empties from the stomach. Studies have found that consuming moderate amounts of heart-healthy fat (about 30% of daily calories) helps diners eat fewer total calories at meals and between meals, and helps keep their blood glucose levels more stable as well.

For people who are overweight or obese, even a relatively small (5% to 10%) weight loss can significantly help reduce their risk of developing various chronic conditions, including high blood pressure, heart disease, cancer, and diabetes. What's more, for people with diabetes who need to lose weight, doing so can help them improve their blood glucose levels. Using an antioxidant-rich, anti-inflammatory, highly monounsaturated fat like olive oil may also help prevent complications associated with diabetes.

Selection tips:

Extra-virgin olive oil is the most flavorful and least processed of all olive oils. Extracted during the first pressing of the olives, extra-virgin olive oil is prized for its quality. Depending on the variety and origin of the olives and the pressing technique, the oil can range from golden to green and may even have some sediment from the fruits. As with wine, extra-virgin olive oil is often described in terms of its fragrance and flavor notes. For example, the oils may be fruity, herbal, grassy, bitter, or peppery.

According to strict standards set by the International Olive Oil Council (IOOC), extra-virgin olive oil must have an acidity of less than 0.8%.

Unfortunately, when shopping for olive oils in the United States, it's easy to get duped unless you read the bottle carefully. The United States is not a member of the IOOC, and the USDA uses its own set of standards, established in 1948, for grading olive oil. The USDA does not recognize IOOC classifications such as "extra-virgin" and "virgin," and some companies use disingenuous labeling practices to make consumers think they're buying unadulterated extra-virgin olive oil, when in fact they're not. Sometimes a mix of vegetable and olive oils is sold as pure olive oil; other times the olives have been subjected to chemical oil extraction. Often, cheap olive oil is imported from Tunisia or Libya, but bottled in Italy, and labeled "imported from Italy."

To ensure that you're getting what you pay for—including the health benefits associated with extra-virgin olive oil—look for bottles that specifically say "first cold pressed extra-virgin olive oil." Check to see if the acidity level and production date are listed, too, as further assurance that you are getting the real thing. If the label bears the seal of the IOOC or the California Olive Oil Council (COOC, an independent trade group) you've got reliable certification that the oil in the bottle is worth buying.

Storage tips:

Store olive oil in a well-sealed container in a cool, dark place. The antioxidants in extra-virgin olive oil help protect it against the oxidation that turns fat rancid, so it can be kept at room temperature, especially if it will be used within a couple of months of opening.

To extend the shelf life of the oil, it can also be stored in the refrigerator. This tends to cause some of the oil to harden into waxy, white beads. These are harmless, and once the oil returns to room temperature, it will resume its normal liquid state.

Preparation tips:
Toss vegetables in olive oil before roasting or grilling them.

Whisk olive oil with balsamic vinegar, Dijon mustard, fresh-squeezed lemon juice, garlic, and freshly-cracked black pepper for a simple, zippy vinaigrette. Use your imagination and try complementing olive oil with different vinegars, herbs, spices, and citrus juices to create dressings for salads and grain pilafs.

Brush whole fish with olive oil, stuff the cavity with herbs and lemon slices, and grill for a Mediterranean-style meal. Or try the same approach with baked or broiled fish fillets.

For a simple appetizer, slice good-quality Feta cheese and serve it with whole olives and a bit of olive oil. Or drizzle hummus or pureed soups with a deeply-colored extra-virgin olive oil for an elegant finish.

Believe it or not, olive oil—even the strongly flavored extra-virgin variety—works well in baking. It lends a subtle flavor to cakes, biscotti, and cookies and is especially nice in recipes that showcase nuts, apples, or chocolate.

Host an olive oil tasting party. Have guests bring bottles of extra-virgin olive oil (you can even assign each guest a country of origin for their oil). Provide crusty whole-grain bread, crudités, and grilled vegetable spears for dipping. Give guests notepads and pens to record their reflections, discuss the oils, and vote on a favorite. Give whoever provided the winning oil a cookbook on Mediterranean cuisine.

Precautions:
Do not attempt to bottle garlic-infused, fresh-herb–infused, or citrus-peel–infused olive oil at home. Doing so can promote the growth of the deadly bacteria *Clostridium botulinum*, which produces the toxin that causes botulism. If you'd like to serve flavored olive oils for dipping, stick to commercially prepared oils, or pour plain extra-virgin olive oil over chopped garlic, herbs, or citrus zest just before serving (refrigerate for up to a few hours if necessary), and discard any leftovers.

Take care with infused oils in restaurants, too. It's probably best to steer clear of any small bottles of oil on the table that contain herbs or garlic. If the waiter brings a dish of herbs and pours oil over them in front of you, the oil is fine to eat.

SESAME OIL

Serving size: 1 tablespoon

Per serving:
Calories:...................120
Carbohydrate:..............0 g
Protein:...................0 g
Fat:......................14 g
Saturated fat:..............2 g
Monounsaturated fat:........5 g
Polyunsaturated fat:.........6 g
Cholesterol:..............0 mg
Sodium:...................0 mg
Fiber:.....................0 g
Calcium:..................0 mg

Good source of:
plant sterols, lignans, monounsaturated fat, polyunsaturated fat.

Description:
The tiny sesame seed has been used since antiquity to produce sesame oil for food and cosmetic use. Sesame oil is important in Middle Eastern, Indian, and East Asian cuisines. Both regular and toasted sesame oils are available; the latter has a more intense sesame flavor and a deeper color. With its fairly high smoke point of about 420°F, sesame oil can be used successfully for higher-heat preparation methods like stir-frying.

Health benefits:
In a study conducted in India and published in the scientific journal *Clinica Chimica Acta* in 2005, researchers found that people with high blood pressure who replaced other cooking oils with sesame oil for two months experienced significant improvements in blood pressure, blood lipid, and antioxidant levels in the blood. All study subjects were taking the calcium channel blocker nifedipine (brand name Procardia), and three oils were tested against a nifedipine-only control group. Only the sesame oil group experienced dramatic improvements.

It appears that *sesamin*, a type of *lignan* (a chemical compound with antioxidant effects) present in sesame oil contributes to the calcium channel blocking effect, helping to reduce blood pressure. It may also block cholesterol absorption, thereby improving blood lipid levels. The mono- and polyunsaturated fats and plant sterols present in sesame oil also have a favorable effect on blood lipids.

Other studies have found possible cancer-inhibiting effects from sesame seeds and oil.

Another study found that rats with induced diabetes who were fed sesame oil had improvements in blood glucose, glycosolated hemoglobin (HbA_{1c}), and antioxidant levels. If and how the results of this study can be applied to humans remains to be seen, but it is an interesting finding, nonetheless.

Selection tips:
Whether you're buying refined, unrefined, or toasted sesame oil, look for expeller-pressed sesame oil to ensure that the sesame seeds' naturally occurring lignans and plant sterols remain intact. Expeller-pressed oils also have superior flavor.

Refined sesame oil has the highest smoke point, so it can be used for high-heat applications like frying. It also has the mildest sesame flavor, so it is a good choice for baking.

Unrefined sesame oil has a more distinctive sesame flavor. While it shouldn't be used at extremely high heat, it still has a fairly high smoke point and is well suited to stir-frying and sautéing. Its flavor is also a good complement to nut-based baked-goods recipes.

Toasted sesame oil is darker in color and has a much more pronounced sesame flavor than other sesame oils. It is best used for finishing dishes (adding a small amount of oil to the dish right before serving) and it also works well in marinades and sauces.

Storage tips:
Thanks to the presence of sesamin, sesame oil is fairly stable and less prone to rancidity than many other oils. Unopened, it will keep in a cool, dry, preferably dark place for at least a year.

Despite its stability, once opened, it is best to keep sesame oil in the refrigerator for optimal freshness. Refrigerated, refined sesame oil can be kept for up to one year. Unrefined oil should be used within six months.

Preparation tips:
Sesame oil is fantastic in Asian-inspired marinades and sauces. Try whisking together toasted sesame oil, rice vinegar, minced ginger, garlic, and tamari (a type of soy sauce), and use the sauce to marinate tofu or chicken.

Whisk together sesame oil, fresh-squeezed lime or orange juice, rice or wine vinegar, grated ginger, and reduced-sodium soy sauce, and serve over baby greens or spinach, topped with slivered almonds.

For a quick peanut sauce, blend peanut butter, sesame oil, ginger, garlic, chili pepper flakes, reduced-sodium soy sauce, and rice vinegar, and thin with a bit of hot water. Allow the flavors to blend in the refrigerator, then serve over noodles with tofu or chicken and vegetables, or use as a dipping sauce.

Drizzle sesame oil on hummus or baba gannoush, or use it for dipping toasted pita. Try sesame oil in baking or in homemade granola recipes.

Precautions:
Do not attempt to bottle garlic-infused, fresh-herb–infused, or citrus-peel–infused sesame oil at home. This can promote the growth of the deadly bacteria *Clostridium botulinum,* which produces the toxin that causes botulism. Stick to commercially prepared infused oils to ensure safety.

WALNUT OIL

Serving size: 1 tablespoon

Per serving:

Calories:. 120
Carbohydrate: . . . . 0 g
Protein:. . . . . 0 g
Fat: . . . . 14 g
Saturated fat: . . . . 1 g
Monounsaturated fat: . . . . 3 g
Polyunsaturated fat:. . . . . 9 g
Omega-3 fatty acids:. . . . . 1 g
Cholesterol: . . . . 0 mg
Sodium:. . . . . 0 mg
Fiber:. 0 g
Calcium: . . . . 0 mg

Good source of:

polyunsaturated fat, alpha-linolenic acid

Description:

Walnut oil was once highly appreciated by Renaissance masters for its paint-thinning properties. Its distinctive flavor also makes it a prized culinary oil, especially in France and Italy, where much of it is produced.

Health benefits:

Walnut oil contains predominantly polyunsaturated fats. A decent percentage of these are omega-3 fatty acids, in the form of alpha-linolenic acid.

Walnut oil can contribute to improved cardiovascular health by helping to keep the arteries supple and elastic. It can also play a role in improving blood lipid levels by lowering LDL ("bad") cholesterol and triglycerides, and by raising HDL ("good") cholesterol.

The omega-3 fatty acids in walnut oil have anti-inflammatory properties, which are important for preventing or delaying progression of inflammatory conditions such as diabetes, heart disease, inflammatory bowel disease, and arthritis.

Adequate omega-3 intake is important for pregnant and nursing women, as the fatty acids are vital to fetal and infant brain and eye development. Small studies have shown that omega-3's may also help prevent postpartum depression.

Selection tips:

Choose expeller-pressed or cold-pressed walnut oil. Bottles labeled "100% pure walnut oil" are a good bet; bottles labeled "refined" may be diluted with other oils. Cold-pressed walnut oil tends to be the most flavorful, and it retains more of the walnuts' naturally occurring antioxidant and anti-inflammatory compounds.

Use regular, untoasted walnut oil for baking or for lighter recipes like vinaigrettes. Toasted walnut oil has a more intense, nutty flavor that can be a great accent for vegetables and grains.

Storage tips:
Store unopened walnut oil in a cool, dry, preferably dark place for up to 10 months. Once opened, walnut oil should be refrigerated and used within 6 months.

Preparation tips:
Walnut oil is an excellent choice for drizzling over vegetables—it is especially nice with string beans, haricots verts, artichokes, and asparagus. It also enhances the natural nuttiness of whole-grain dishes.

Walnut oil has a great affinity for goat cheese—try marinating slices of goat cheese in the refrigerator with walnut oil and herbs. Serve with good, crusty multigrain bread, radish slices, and chopped tomatoes.

Use walnut oil to sauté baby spinach, or whisk walnut oil into a vinaigrette and serve over baby greens.

Try using walnut oil in your favorite pesto recipe in place of olive oil (swap walnuts for the pine nuts, too).

Or puree roasted red peppers, walnuts, garlic, a bit of walnut oil, and whole-grain bread crumbs if desired, and use the resulting mixture as a dip for crudités or as a sauce for baked or grilled fish or pasta.

Walnut oil is wonderful in baked goods, too. Substitute it for other vegetable oils in your favorite recipes. Walnut oil is an especially good choice for recipes that feature nuts, apples, pears, or chocolate.

Precautions:
When cooking with walnut oil, avoid high-heat cooking techniques, which can alter the structure of the fatty acids. If the oil begins to smoke or to smell "off," discard the oil, lower the heat, and begin again with fresh oil.

Do not attempt to bottle walnut oil infused with garlic, herbs, or citrus peel at home. Doing so can promote the growth of the deadly bacteria *Clostridium botulinum*, which produces the toxin that causes botulism. Stick to commercially prepared infused oils to ensure safety.

SOY PRODUCTS AND MEAT ALTERNATIVES

EDAMAME

Serving size: ½ cup (beans only)

Per serving:
Calories:. 127
Carbohydrate: . . . . 10 g
Protein:. 11 g
Fat:. . . . . 6 g
Saturated fat: . . . . 1 g
Cholesterol: . . . . 0 mg
Sodium:. . . . . 13 mg
Fiber:. . . . . 4 g
Calcium: . . . . 130 mg

Good source of:
protein, fiber, calcium, soy isoflavones, essential fatty acids

Description:
Edamame are young soybeans that are harvested while still green. They grow in fuzzy pods that are about 2 inches long. The pod itself is inedible, but part of the fun of edamame is pulling the beans out of the boiled pods with one's teeth. Protein-rich edamame have been an important part of the diet throughout Asia for thousands of years. They are ubiquitous in Japanese bars, where they are served alongside beer—a far healthier option than potato chips!

Health benefits:
Soybeans are rich in isoflavones, a class of phytoestrogens, or plant estrogens, which might have a beneficial effect on health. It has been observed that Japanese and Chi-

nese women who regularly consume soy foods have lower rates of menopausal symptoms and breast cancer. These observations have sparked a multitude of studies. The full picture on soy foods and women's health is still developing, but much research supports the hypothesis that soy foods might help mitigate symptoms associated with perimenopause and menopause, preserve bone health, and protect against breast cancer or inhibit its growth.

Isoflavone phytoestrogens can attach to human estrogen receptors, where they exert a weak estrogenic effect. This might effectively block a woman's natural estrogen from attaching to those same receptors, where it would exert a far stronger effect.

Men aren't left out of the picture when it comes to soy and health. Soy foods might help reduce prostate and colon cancer risks. Soy protein might also help protect the cardiovascular health of both men and women by improving lipid profiles, reducing blood pressure, and helping the arteries remain elastic. Since 2002 the Food and Drug Administration has allowed manufacturers to include the following health claim on food labels: "25 grams of soy protein a day, as part of a diet low in saturated fats and cholesterol, may reduce the risk of heart disease."

Studies about soy and other health claims remain inconclusive, but that might reflect the fact that they were of varying lengths and that many studies have looked only at the effects of isolated isoflavones or isolated soy protein in widely varying doses rather than examining whole soy foods.

The best—and safest—strategy for reaping the possible benefits of soybeans is to stick to whole soy foods and to try to emulate the dietary habits of those who seem to have benefited from regular consumption. Most Japanese adults consume 35 to 40 milligrams of soy isoflavones from soy foods per day. That translates to one to two servings of a soy food such as edamame, tofu, or soy milk.

Selection tips:
Edamame are available year-round in the freezer section of many supermarkets and health-food stores and are a mainstay in Asian markets. Frozen edamame are available both in the pod and shelled.

Increasingly, edamame are grown in the United States. Those who live near a farmer's market might be lucky enough to find fresh edamame in the late summer and early fall. Look for bright green, unblemished pods.

Storage tips:
Keep frozen edamame in the freezer until ready for use. Fresh edamame are best when used immediately, but they can be refrigerated for up to two days or frozen for several months.

Preparation tips:
There's no need to thaw frozen edamame before cooking—simply dump them into a pot of boiling water and cook for 4 to 5 minutes. (Fresh edamame might take only 2 to 3 minutes to cook.) Drain the edamame and rinse.

Whole edamame in their pods can be sprinkled lightly with coarse sea salt if desired.

Serve edamame in their pods as a snack or informal appetizer. Shelled edamame are a fantastic addition to salads or mixed into grains. Add them to stir-fries or soups. Try making a dip with pureed, cooked edamame—if you need inspiration, try using them in place of the chickpeas in a favorite hummus recipe or use them to replace some of the beans in a white bean spread.

Precautions:
Whole soy foods such as edamame are nutritious, healthy choices that might offer additional health benefits beyond basic nutrition. However, isolated soy isoflavone supplements or so-called "functional" foods made with soy are not recommended because they might exert too strong an estrogenic effect.

Those undergoing treatment for estrogen-dependent cancers should discuss soy consumption with their medical team.

According to the independent Pew Initiative on Food and Biotechnology, 85% of soybeans planted in the United States in 2004 were genetically engineered varieties. Those concerned about the application of genetic engineering technologies to foodstuffs should seek out certified organic soybeans and soy products.

MISO

Serving size: 1 tablespoon

Per serving:
Calories:.....................34
Carbohydrate: ....5 g
Protein:.....................2 g
Fat:.........................1 g
Saturated fat: ....0 g
Cholesterol: ....0 mg
Sodium:.................641 mg
Fiber:.......................1 g
Calcium: ....10 mg

Good source of:
antioxidants, iron, zinc, selenium

Description:
Miso is a fermented, aged, pastelike condiment made from soybeans, salt, and a mold culture. It may include grains such as barley, millet, or rice. As with cheese or wine, miso is a complex "live" food (unless or until it is pasteurized), and producers strive to cultivate special flavor qualities and color when making it by carefully considering grain additions or fermenting times. Miso is typically salty, but it might have sweet notes as well. The flavor can range from mild to quite intense.

Miso has been eaten in Japan for thousands of years and remains a cornerstone of the cuisine and culture. Although Americans might enjoy miso soup as an appetizer only when dining out, many Japanese begin each day with miso soup.

Health benefits:
Because it's made from soybeans, miso might confer the same benefits as other soy products, including reduced risk of heart disease and certain cancers. According to traditional Chinese medicine, miso is beneficial to digestion.

Selection tips:
Miso is often packaged in plastic tubs or bags and can usually be found in the refrigerator section of health-food stores, gourmet shops, Asian markets, and some supermarkets. Light miso is well suited to soups, salad dressings, and fish dishes. Dark miso, which has a more intense flavor, is better suited to heartier bean dishes, winter root vegetables, and heavier meats.

Storage tips:
Miso is perishable, so it should be stored in the refrigerator, where it will keep for several months. Light miso can be refrigerated for approximately nine months, while dark miso can be stored for about one year. Check the package for specific storage times, as this can vary by variety. Look for miso with an expiration date printed on the container, and avoid miso that has added MSG.

Preparation tips:
Miso is traditionally used as a flavoring for soup—stir one tablespoon of miso into hot water for the simplest version. For more depth, add miso to dashi, a simple broth made with sea vegetable kombu and bonito flakes. Many health-food stores carry instant powdered dashi.

Miso can be whisked into vinaigrettes or sauces or can be added to marinades for fish or tofu.

Precautions:
Miso is high in sodium, so it should be used sparingly, particularly by those who have high blood pressure. When including miso in a meal, take care to keep the rest of the served foods low in sodium.

SEITAN

Serving size: 3 ounces

Per serving:

Calories:. 90
Carbohydrate: . . . . 3 g
Protein:. . . . . 18 g
Fat:. . . . . 1 g
Saturated fat: . . . . 0 g
Cholesterol: . . . . 0 mg
Sodium:. . . . . 380 mg
Fiber:. . . . . 1 g
Calcium: . . . . 0 mg

Good source of:
protein

Description:
Seitan is wheat gluten that has been cooked in a dashi, or broth, that usually contains soy sauce, the sea vegetable kombu, and ginger. It's a popular foodstuff in the macrobiotic diet and Buddhist cuisine, and it's often used as a meat analog in vegetarian restaurants.

Gluten has a characteristic strength and a chewy texture, and innovative chefs and food manufacturers have turned out some very convincing seitan-based vegetarian "chicken" and "duck." Some even call seitan "wheat meat" because its texture is so akin to that of animal protein.

Health benefits:
Numerous studies have found strong links between the consumption of animal protein and various chronic diseases, including cardiovascular disease and cancer. Most Americans eat two to three times the recommended amount of protein, and much of it comes from animal sources.

Conversely, vegetarian diets have been associated with reduced risk of chronic diseases, including cancer, heart disease, diabetes, and osteoporosis. Some studies have also found that vegetarian diets can have a therapeutic effect on these disease states.

Replacing some of the animal protein in the diet with vegetarian protein sources is a smart move and one that will help bring individual protein consumption more in line with dietary guidelines for Americans.

Seitan is a great choice for those experimenting with vegetarian meals because it has a satisfying texture and flavor and works well in recipes that call for chicken or red meat.

Selection tips:
Seitan can be purchased at health-food stores and some supermarkets. It should be refrigerated.

Storage tips:
Store seitan in the refrigerator for up to a week. Once opened, use the remainder of the package within a few days.

Preparation tips:
Seitan is best when it is added to recipes near the end of cooking. Heat it through, but try not to subject it to long cooking times unless specified in a recipe. Use seitan in stir-fries or stews. Try it on a "steak" sandwich with lettuce and tomatoes, or roll it up in a wrap with lots of veggies and sliced avocado.

Precautions:
Seitan is not appropriate for those with celiac disease or wheat allergies. Those on a protein-restricted diet should be able to enjoy seitan but should discuss its inclusion in meal plans with a registered dietitian, as it is very protein-rich.

TEMPEH

Serving size: 3 ounces

Per serving:
Calories:. 147
Carbohydrate: . . . . 7 g
Protein:. . . . . 14 g
Fat:. . . . . 9 g
Saturated fat: . . . . 2 g
Cholesterol: . . . . 0 mg
Sodium:. . . . . 10 mg
Fiber:. . . . . 7 g
Calcium: . . . . 72 mg

Note: Nutrient values and serving size vary by brand, style, and flavor. Check package labels for the most accurate information.

Good source of:
protein, fiber, B vitamins, calcium, iron, phosphorus, potassium, probiotics, phytochemicals

Description:
Tempeh, a cultured soybean cake, likely originated in Indonesia. It's made of cooked, hulled soybeans that have been inoculated with a mold culture. Sometimes grains are added for additional flavor and texture. As the tempeh incubates, the flavor develops and the cakes become more solid. The culture and fermentation process also makes the soybeans more digestible.

Tempeh has mushroomy and nutty flavor nuances and a meaty texture.

Health benefits:
Tempeh is an excellent source of protein and fiber and contains heart-healthy fat and phytochemicals from soybeans. As a cultured food, it's also an excellent source of probiotics, or the friendly bacteria that promote digestive health and proper immune function.

Studies have found that probiotics appear to inhibit *Helicobacter pylori*—a bacteria that has been implicated in ulcers, gastroesophageal reflux disease (GERD), and certain gastrointestinal cancers—from colonizing or adhering in the gastrointestinal tract. Researchers hypothesize that probiotics might even help treat existing *H. pylori* infection and might also help fight other disease-causing bacteria in the gastrointestinal tract. Similarly, probiotics seem to protect the urinary tract from bacterial infection.

Selection tips:

Tempeh is available in both pasteurized and unpasteurized versions. Pasteurized tempeh can be found in the refrigerator section of health-food stores and some supermarkets.

Unpasteurized tempeh can be found in the freezer section. Unpasteurized tempeh has a more complex taste and texture than the pasteurized version and absorbs marinades better.

Increasingly, it's possible to find precooked, flavored, or marinated tempeh. These are usually found in the refrigerator section.

Blocks of tempeh should feel solid. There should be no evidence of colored molds (that is, green, red, or orange), which indicate spoilage.

However, like the rind on a cheese, the whitish appearance of tempeh is normal—this is the culture, which is both safe and edible.

Storage tips:

Frozen, packaged tempeh will keep for up to one year in the freezer. Once defrosted, it will keep for three to four weeks in the refrigerator if it is well wrapped. (To ensure food safety, always defrost food in the refrigerator, rather than on a countertop.) Tempeh that has already been marinated and cooked will keep for up to ten days in the refrigerator if it is well wrapped.

Preparation tips:

The ultimate texture of tempeh is dependant on the preparation and cooking methods used. Sliced thin and sautéed or stir-fried, tempeh takes on a chewier, meaty texture, while marinated, braised, or baked tempeh is more succulent.

Thanks to its own nutty flavor, tempeh pairs well with nut-based sauces. Try it in a vegetable stir-fry and serve it over brown rice or buckwheat soba with peanut sauce. Tempeh also works well in tacos or fajitas and is a great addition to curry recipes.

For party hors d'oeuvres, serve baked tempeh cubes with a coconut-cilantro dipping sauce. Or let tempeh make an appearance at your next barbeque. Alternate tempeh cubes and vegetables on kebab skewers, marinate, and grill.

Serving size: ½ cup

Per serving:
Calories:. 88
Carbohydrate: . . . . 2 g
Protein:. . . . . 10 g
Fat:. . . . . 5 g
Saturated fat: . . . . 1 g
Monounsaturated fat: . . . . 2 g
Polyunsaturated fat:. . . . . 2 g
Cholesterol: . . . . 0 mg
Sodium:. . . . . 15 mg
Fiber:. . . . . 1 g
Calcium: . . . . 253 mg
(if prepared with calcium sulfate)

Good source of:

protein, calcium, iron, copper, phytoestrogens, omega-3 fatty acids

Description:

Tofu, which is also known as *doufu* (dow-fu) or soybean curd, is a protein-rich foodstuff made from soy milk. The process is essentially like cheesemaking (without the aging or fermentation)—hot soy milk is coagulated, and the curds are separated out and pressed into cakes of tofu.

Traditionally, tofu was coagulated with nigari, or distilled, desalinated seawater. Nigari is abundant in minerals, most notably magnesium chloride. Today, most commercially prepared tofu is coagulated with calcium sulfate, sometimes with the addition of magnesium chloride. This adds to the mineral content of the finished tofu.

Tofu has a smooth, almost custard-like texture, and a fairly neutral flavor. (Fresh, handmade tofu has a more distinctive, though still mild, soybean flavor). Because its own flavor is so mild, tofu is an excellent canvas for a wide range of spices and herbs. It absorbs marinades readily and adapts beautifully to the flavor principles of many ethnic cuisines.

Tofu's exact origins are unclear, but it is known to have been important in ancient China and Japan. It has been consumed throughout Asia for thousands of years and treated to a myriad of preparations.

Health benefits:

Tofu is rich in protein, heart-healthy fats, calcium, and phytochemicals, including isoflavones. The calcium and magnesium in tofu are important to bone health.

Soy isoflavones from whole soy foods such as tofu might help mitigate the symptoms of perimenopause and menopause and appear to help fight certain cancers, including breast, endometrial, prostate, and colon cancer.

Tofu might also help promote heart health by improving lipid profiles, reducing blood pressure, and helping the arteries remain elastic. Since 2002, the FDA has allowed manufacturers to include the following health claim on food labels: "25 grams of soy protein a day, as part of a diet low in saturated fats and cholesterol, may reduce the risk of heart disease." Just one half-cup serving of tofu contains 7 grams of soy protein, or slightly more than a quarter of the FDA recommendation.

Tofu is also a good source of anti-inflammatory omega-3 fatty acids. Adequate omega-3 intake might be beneficial in preventing, or helping to ease the symptoms of many inflammatory disease processes, including heart disease, arthritis, diabetes, inflammatory bowel disease (IBD), or irritable bowel syndrome (IBS).

Tofu might also benefit pregnant and nursing women, as adequate omega-3 intake is vital to fetal and infant brain development, and it has been associated with lower rates of maternal postpartum depression.

Tofu is gluten-free, so it can be enjoyed by those with celiac disease, or gluten intolerance.

Selection tips:

"Regular" tofu is available in soft, firm, and extra-firm versions (silken tofu is also available and is described below). Each lends itself to different preparations, so the first thing to consider is the recipe or intended use.

Soft tofu is good for blending into dressings, sauces, or soups or for adding into salads.

Firm tofu holds its shape well, so it can be sliced or cubed and can stand up to pan-frying, stir-frying, or baking.

Extra-firm tofu is the least delicate and the best bet for preparations that call for longer cooking times—like chilis, stews, or casseroles—or higher temperatures, such as grilling or broiling.

Personal preference is a factor, too—some like a stir-fry with firm tofu, while others like only extra-firm tofu.

Keep in mind that the firmness of tofu is related to how much water it contains—softer tofu has more, while firmer tofu has less. As a result, firmer tofu can absorb more marinade, especially if it is pressed first.

Look for tofu in the refrigerator section of supermarkets, health-food stores, and Asian markets. It's generally packaged in a solid block in a sealed plastic container filled with water. Avoid bulging packages, which suggest that the tofu is past its prime.

The water should be relatively clear, and the tofu should smell fresh, with a faint soybean scent. If the water is a bit cloudy but the tofu smells fresh, it should be fine. However, if the water looks cloudy and the tofu smells or tastes sour, it should definitely be discarded.

Commercially prepared tofu usually has an expiration or "best before" date that might be as long as two months after the production date. If tofu at your market typically seems to have a close expiration date, turnover might not be high and the tofu might not be optimally fresh.

Incidentally, as tofu consumption in the West increases, companies are simplifying preparation with preseasoned tofu and even prebaked, marinated, and ready-to-eat versions.

Storage tips:

Tofu should be stored in its unopened, original package until ready for use and eaten before its expiration or "best before" date. If the entire package is not needed, the remaining tofu can be stored in a clean, airtight container, covered in fresh water, for three to five days. Every other day, change the water. Discard the tofu if it develops an "off" odor.

Tofu can also be frozen (this works best with firm or extra-firm tofu). Freezing causes a remarkable change in tofu's texture and renders it even more receptive to marinades.

Simply put a whole, unopened package of tofu in the freezer. As it freezes, ice crystals form in the block of tofu, creating little pockets throughout. To ensure food safety, defrost the package in the refrigerator and drain. After defrosting, the tofu will have a spongier, chewier texture and a darker color that is often appealing to meat eaters.

Preparation tips:
Some cooks try to disguise tofu as a "meat," hiding it in lasagna or chili, for example. But tofu really shines when it gets respect and retains its identity. Tofu is also extremely versatile, so experimentation is often worthwhile.

As one might expect, tofu has an incredible affinity for pan-Asian flavoring principles such as ginger, soy sauce, lemongrass, or Chinese five-spice powder. It's also great in Thai or Indian curries or with coconut or peanut-based sauces.

Drain tofu before use. To maximize the amount of marinade the tofu will absorb, press it between clean dishtowels or paper towels with your hands or under a weighted plate. (This works best with firm or extra-firm tofu. Soft tofu might fall apart if pressed and, in any case, is meant to have a higher water content.)

Tofu can be sliced in large slabs, cubes, or triangles. It can be marinated or treated to a spice rub before cooking or sauced after preparation (or both).

Baking tofu pieces on a lightly oiled cookie sheet is a fairly foolproof way to brown it with minimal fuss. Turn the tofu pieces over midway through cooking to brown on both sides.

To achieve the delicate, crispy "skin" typical of deep-fried tofu without the added fat, try pressing the tofu and dredging the pieces lightly in cornstarch or in a mix of cornstarch and whole-grain pastry flour. Remember to measure the starch (and flour, if using) and to account for the carbohydrate it contains.

Place the dredged tofu pieces on a lightly oiled cookie sheet and bake at 400°F. After about 20 to 25 minutes, or when the tops of the tofu look dry and the bottoms are barely brown, flip the pieces with a spatula, and return to the oven for 10 to 15 minutes. The tofu pieces will shrink a bit. The tofu can be tossed into steamed or stir-fried vegetables or served on toothpicks as hors d'oeuvres with a dipping sauce. Or transfer the oven-fried tofu to a baking dish and pour on your favorite marinade. At this point it can be covered and returned to a 300°F oven. The crispiness will disappear, but the starch will thicken the marinade and the tofu will become chewier. Or place the covered dish in the refrigerator and enjoy the tofu cold after it has absorbed the marinade.

Try marinated, baked tofu in wraps or sandwiches, or add the pieces to salads or noodle dishes.

Tofu that has been frozen can be sliced or cubed and marinated. Previously frozen tofu will also be drier after thawing and draining, so it's ideal for crumbling into chili or tomato sauce.

Precautions:
Many health-food stores and Asian markets sell tofu in large, open, water-filled bins. Buying this tofu is not advisable, as the water is easily contaminated and the tofu can harbor dangerous bacteria. Stick to properly refrigerated, prepackaged tofu, and don't forget that tofu is perishable. Keep it refrigerated, use it before the expiration or "best before" date, and be sure to cook it properly.

Although it is generally thought that the phytoestrogens in tofu are safe and might even be beneficial in fighting cancer, those undergoing treatment for estrogen-dependent cancers should discuss tofu consumption with their medical team.

According to the independent Pew Initiative on Food and Biotechnology, 85% of soybeans planted in the United States in 2004 were genetically engineered varieties. Those concerned about the application of genetic engineering technologies to food-stuffs should seek out certified organic soybeans and soy products.

Serving size: 3 ounces, or ¼ package

Per serving:
Calories:.....................52
Carbohydrate:...............2 g
Protein:....................6 g
Fat:........................2 g
Saturated fat:...............0 g
Monounsaturated fat:.........0 g
Polyunsaturated fat:..........1 g
Cholesterol:...............0 mg
Sodium:..................30 mg
Fiber:.....................0 g
Calcium:.................27 mg

Good source of:
protein, isoflavones, iron, copper

Description:
Silken tofu was developed for the emperor and other denizens of the ancient Japanese royal court. It has an elegant texture that is far creamier and smoother than ordinary tofu. Like regular tofu, it ranges from soft to extra-firm.

Health benefits:
As with regular tofu, silken tofu contains protein, heart-healthy fats, phytochemicals, including isoflavones, and some calcium. Due to its higher water content, it is less nutrient-dense than ordinary tofu, but it appears to promote heart health and to display the similar cancer-fighting and anti-inflammatory qualities as regular tofu.

Silken tofu is an additional option for those who find that soy foods help alleviate symptoms of perimenopause and menopause, such as hot flashes.

Silken tofu is included among the soy products that may utilize the FDA health claim regarding soy and heart health on food labels stating "25 grams of soy protein a day, as part of a diet low in saturated fat and cholesterol, may reduce the risk of heart disease."

Silken tofu is gluten-free, so it can be enjoyed by those with celiac disease, or gluten intolerance. Thanks to its soft texture, high water content, and anti-inflammatory fats, silken tofu might benefit those with inflammatory bowel disease (IBD) or irritable bowel syndrome (IBS).

Selection tips:
Many supermarkets and health-food stores stock silken tofu. It's usually aseptically packed, so it might be on regular store shelves rather than in the refrigerated section. Sometimes it's refrigerated, although if it's unopened, it's generally shelf stable without refrigeration. Check the package to be sure.

Look for silken tofu in undamaged boxes

and check the expiration date before purchase.

Storage tips:
Most silken tofu found in the United States is packaged in aseptic, shelf-stable boxes. It generally has a shelf life of one year as long as it is unopened.

Once silken tofu is opened, it becomes very perishable. Any unused portion should be placed in an airtight container and refrigerated for a maximum of two to three days. Unlike regular tofu, it should not be covered in water for storage.

As with "regular" tofu, silken tofu can be frozen, but it should not be frozen in its aseptic packaging. Transfer silken tofu to an airtight container before freezing for up to 60 days.

Preparation tips:
Unlike regular tofu, which should always be properly cooked before being eaten due to food safety issues, aseptically packaged silken tofu can be used without cooking.

Silken tofu purees beautifully. It can be used to bolster the protein and micronutrient value and impart a rich creaminess to smoothies, mousses, and puddings or to salad dressings, sauces, and soups.

A package of silken tofu blended with one cup of water and two tablespoons of lemon juice can even be used to replace eggs, yogurt, sour cream, or liquid dairy products in recipes. Five tablespoons of this blend is equivalent to one egg.

Try crumbling silken tofu to make a vegetarian, cholesterol-free version of egg salad, or scramble it as you would an egg.

Silken tofu can be cubed and served cold with grated ginger, scallions, and a drizzle of reduced-sodium soy sauce. Or add cubes of silken tofu to miso soup or soba salad.

Of course, silken tofu also works in cooked dishes. Try stir-frying or baking it.

Frozen silken tofu should be thawed in the refrigerator. Drain and pat dry with a clean dishtowel or paper towels before marinating and cooking as desired.

Precautions:
Although it is generally thought that the phytoestrogens in tofu are safe and might even be beneficial in fighting cancer, those undergoing treatment for estrogen-dependent cancers should discuss tofu consumption with their medical team.

According to the independent Pew Initiative on Food and Biotechnology, 85% of soybeans planted in the United States in 2004 were genetically engineered varieties. Those concerned about the application of genetic engineering technologies to foodstuffs should seek out certified organic soybeans and soy products.

ARTICHOKES

Serving size: 1 medium artichoke

Per serving:
Calories:.....................60
Carbohydrate:..............13 g
Protein:.....................4 g
Fat:........................0 g
Saturated fat:...............0 g
Cholesterol:..............0 mg
Sodium:..................114 g
Fiber:.....................7 g

Good source of:
fiber, potassium, vitamin K, lutein, folate

Description:
Artichokes are the edible flower bud of a Mediterranean plant related to the cardoon. Once the bud starts to open, the artichoke becomes inedible, so the prized buds are harvested early. Nearly all of the world's artichokes are grown in Italy, Spain, and France, where they are an important component of those countries' cuisines. In recent years growers in the United States, predominantly in California, have had success growing artichokes.

Large globe artichokes and baby artichokes are most commonly available in American markets, though it is sometimes possible to find other varieties—including purple artichokes—at farmer's markets and specialty gourmet shops.

The tender heart of the artichoke, which hides beneath a thistle-like choke and is protected by the bud's sharp-tipped leaves, is especially delectable. Though getting to the heart can be daunting, the preparation is worth the effort, though some prefer to bypass the work and purchase frozen or pickled artichoke hearts.

Health benefits:
Several studies have found that artichoke leaves or their extract appear to ease indigestion; one study also found that the extract may even help reduce the frequency and severity of bouts of irritable bowel syndrome.

Artichokes contain prebiotics, which help nourish the friendly bacteria in the gastrointestinal tract. This is important for both gastrointestinal health and general immune function. Fiber-rich artichokes also appear to have lipid-lowering capabilities, and they are antioxidant rich, which may point to potential cardioprotective benefits.

Selection tips:
Look for artichokes that are heavy for their size, with tight, closely packed leaves. The

shape of the artichoke and the color of the leaves will vary by variety, but brown discoloration at the tips of the leaves is not a good sign. Avoid artichokes with spreading leaves—they are past their prime. Be sure to turn the artichoke over to inspect the stem and avoid any with holes; there may be worms.

Storage tips:

Despite their armored appearance, fresh artichokes are actually fairly perishable. They should be refrigerated in a plastic bag and used within three to four days. Once cooked, the hearts can be frozen for later use.

Preparation tips:

Artichokes can be steamed whole, so that both the leaves and the heart (or artichoke bottom) can be enjoyed. Or, with more preparation in the kitchen, the tender artichoke bottoms can be freed from the bud, and prepared as desired.

Artichokes will discolor when exposed to the air or to carbon steel, so keep a bowl of water acidulated with lemon juice nearby, and use a non-carbon steel knife.

When preparing whole artichokes, first cut off about a ½ inch from the top of the bud, then carefully trim the pointy ends off the artichoke leaves. As you work, rub the cut ends with lemon or dip in the acidulated water. Cut the stem off at the base of the artichoke, and pull off any particularly tough leaves near the base. Drop the arti-choke into the bowl of acidulated water while you prepare the others.

Boil or steam in a nonreactive pan, and make sure the artichokes are completely submerged in the water to avoid discoloration. Do not add baking soda to the water—this will turn the artichokes an ugly green and decrease their nutritional value.

Cooking time can vary greatly depending on the size of the artichoke, but most large globes take 35 to 45 minutes to cook. Test them periodically. When the leaves separate easily from the bud and the edible base of the leaf is tender, the artichokes are ready.

Once they are cooked, you can scoop out the choke with a spoon (this is a smart idea if you plan to stuff the inside of the artichoke). Serve steamed or boiled artichokes with a dipping sauce, vinaigrette, or good quality olive oil.

To prepare just the artichoke bottom, remove the stem, and cut off the outer leaves. Cut off the top two-thirds of the artichoke, and scoop off any of the remaining choke with a spoon. Trim as necessary. Rub the artichoke bottom all over with lemon, or drop in acidulated water until it is ready to be cooked.

Precautions:

Artichokes are a rich source of potassium. People on potassium-restricted diets should consult a registered dietitian or doctor before eating artichokes.

ARUGULA

Serving size: 1 cup raw

Per serving:
Calories:.....................5
Carbohydrate:...............1 g
Protein:.....................1 g
Fat:........................0 g
Saturated fat:...............0 g
Cholesterol:..............0 mg
Sodium:....................5 g
Fiber:......................0 g

Good source of:
vitamin A, vitamin K, lutein

Description:
One bite of sharp, peppery arugula, and you'll know why it is sometimes called rocket—the flavor delivers an assertive zing straight to the taste buds, brightening salads and perking up pastas.

Arugula is native to the Mediterranean and to western Asia. It is prized in Italian, southern French, and Greek cuisine. Thanks in part to the rise of farmer's markets and an interest in world cuisines, arugula has attracted a following in the United States as well.

Health benefits:
Arugula is a perfect poster vegetable for the importance of studying phytonutrients. One cup of arugula has only 5 calories and mere traces of macronutrients and most micronutrients. But dismissing it as nutritionally void would be a huge mistake. A 2004 Brazilian study published in the *Journal of Agricultural and Food Chemistry* found that arugula contains a high concentration of flavonoids. Research indicates that these plant compounds appear to have anti-cancer and anti-inflammatory properties, among other health benefits.

Selection tips:
Look for deeply, evenly colored arugula with tender leaves. Avoid bunches that look waterlogged, or have wilted, yellowing leaves or spotty patches. Fresh arugula should have a sharp, peppery aroma.

Storage tips:
Arugula is very perishable, must be refrigerated, and is best used within 1 to 2 days of purchase. If necessary, you can extend its refrigeration for an extra day if you wrap the roots in a damp paper towel before placing the unwashed arugula in a plastic bag. Alternatively, place the arugula stems in a glass of water in the refrigerator, and cover the leaves with a plastic bag.

Preparation tips:

Bunches of arugula are often very sandy. Clean them thoroughly to avoid the unwelcome crunch of sand between your teeth. The easiest way to do this is to submerge the arugula in a large bowl of cold water and swish it around with your hands. (Don't allow it to soak, or it will become waterlogged.) Pull out the arugula and transfer it to a waiting colander. Dump the water out of the bowl, and rinse well to remove all traces of sand. Refill the bowl with cold water, add the arugula, and repeat the process until the water is clear and sand-free. Gently pat the arugula leaves dry, or spin out the water in a salad spinner.

Arugula's clean, peppery taste is especially nice in salads. Mix with various types of lettuce or add avocado, citrus, or thin shavings of Parmesan (or all three!) to soften arugula's sharp bite. Add arugula to sandwiches or wraps. Puree arugula into soups, or use it in place of basil to make pesto.

Arugula can also be wilted in a hot skillet and served in place of spinach or watercress or added to pastas, rice, or potato dishes.

Precautions:

Arugula is a good source of vitamin K. People who take warfarin (brand name Coumadin) should consult a doctor or registered dietitian before consuming arugula.

ASPARAGUS

Serving size: ½ cup cooked

Per serving:

Calories:	20
Carbohydrate:	4 g
Protein:	2 g
Fat:	0 g
Saturated fat:	0 g
Cholesterol:	0 mg
Sodium:	13 mg
Fiber:	2 g

Good source of:

folacin, potassium, thiamine, vitamin B6, rutin, glutathione

Description:

Aristocratic, aphrodisiacal asparagus hails from the Mediterranean region, and archaeological evidence suggests that humans have been eating the edible shoot for over 2,000 years. Green asparagus is most common, although a rarer purple variety exists. White asparagus is grown under soil in the absence of light so it can't produce chlorophyll. White asparagus tends to be expensive because it is labor-intensive to grow, yet it also tends to be less flavorful than green asparagus.

If you are new to asparagus, don't fret if you notice a very distinctive change in the odor of your urine. Asparagus contains a sulfur compound called methylmercaptan, which, when it breaks down, creates an unusual smell in the urine—often as quickly as 15 minutes after the vegetable's consumption. (Some researchers believe a different compound is responsible, but the principle is the same). If you don't smell anything funny, don't worry either. Thanks to genetics, some people lack the enzyme that produces the "asparagus urine" scent, and others actually lack the ability to smell it!

Health benefits:

Long perceived to be medicinal, asparagus is an excellent source of folic acid, which aids blood cell growth and helps prevent heart disease and neural tube birth defects. Asparagus contains glutathione, a powerful cancer-fighting antioxidant. Glutathione helps repair damaged DNA and helps recycle vitamins C and E to their active forms. Asparagus also contains rutin, an antioxidant that appears to exert a cardioprotective effect.

Selection tips:

Look for straight, firm spears with compact, closed tips. Tips may range from dark green to purple. Avoid blemished, slimy, wrinkly, or rubbery stalks or those with dried-out bottoms.

Storage tips:

Stand asparagus stalks upright in a glass with a half-inch of cold water and refrigerate for up to two days. Blanched asparagus can be frozen for up to nine months.

Preparation tips:

Snap off the fibrous ends of each asparagus stalk, then rinse well. (The closer to the base the ends snap off, the fresher the asparagus.) Thinner spears are best for delicate, quick-cooking preparations, while thicker spears can stand up to roasting or grilling.

Precautions:

Those on potassium-restricted diets should consult a doctor or registered dietitian before eating asparagus.

BEETS

Serving size: ½ cup cooked

Per serving:

Calories:.	37
Carbohydrate:	8 g
Protein:.	1 g
Fat:	0 g
Saturated fat:	0 g
Cholesterol:	0 mg
Sodium:.	65 mg
Fiber:.	2 g

Good source of:

potassium, vitamin A, folate, calcium, magnesium, anthocyanins, including betacyanin

Description:

Sweet beets are root vegetables that come in an astonishing variety of beautiful, intense colors. The red beet, with its fuchsia flesh, is familiar to most, but there are also white beets and heirloom varieties of golden, orange, and even red and white striped candy-cane beets.

Beets are cultivated widely for use in animal feed, while sugar and alcohol for human consumption are made from sugar beets.

Health benefits:

Red beets derive their color from anthocyanins, powerful antioxidants that protect the heart and help prevent cancer.

Perhaps because of their deep red color, beets were historically thought to fortify the blood and prevent anemia. Since they are sources of iron and folic acid, both of which are important to proper blood cell development, there might be some truth to the notion.

Selection tips:

Look for firm beets without bruises or wrinkles. If the beet greens are still attached, they should look robust, not dry or shriveled.

Storage tips:
If purchasing beets with the edible greens still attached, be sure to cut the greens from the beetroots, leaving about 1 to 2 inches of stem attached, before storing. Both greens and roots should be stored unwashed in separate plastic bags in the refrigerator, where the roots will keep for two to four weeks.

Preparation tips:
Beets can be consumed raw or cooked. For a colorful, unexpected addition to salads, use a mandoline or vegetable peeler to make ultra-thin beet ribbons. Beets can be pickled, boiled, or made into soups such as borscht. Beets make a stunning risotto, especially when served with the sautéed beet greens on top.

Beets are especially wonderful roasted. Wrap scrubbed, dried beets loosely in foil, and place on a cookie sheet in an oven preheated to 400°F. Roast for 45 minutes to an hour, until beets are tender. When the beets are cool enough to handle, slip their skins off, and serve halved or quartered. Although this might stain your hands temporarily, it is less potentially messy than disposing of the highly pigmented cooking water from boiled beets! A little lemon juice will help remove beet juice stains from the skin.

Precautions:
You might notice a harmless discoloration of the urine or stool after consuming beets. Those on potassium-restricted diets should consult a doctor or registered dietitian before consuming beets.

BEET GREENS

Serving size: ½ cup cooked

Per serving:
Calories:. 19
Carbohydrate: . . . . 4 g
Protein:. 2 g
Fat: . . . . 0 g
Saturated fat: . . . . 0 g
Cholesterol: . . . . 0 mg
Sodium:. . . . . 174 mg
Fiber:. . . . . 2 g

Good source of:
calcium, vitamin A, vitamin K, potassium, beta-carotene, lutein + zeaxanthin

Description:
Hearty beet greens are a fabulous but often overlooked bonus of many a beet purchase. They are most readily available atop young spring beets. Beet greens are extremely nutrient-dense and, unless they are very young, tend to work best cooked. They can stand alone or, because they have a subtle hint of beetlike flavor, they can be paired with the roots themselves.

Health benefits:
Beet greens are rich in calcium, which makes them an excellent choice for those who do not like or can't tolerate dairy products. They contain a great deal of the disease-fighting antioxidants beta-carotene and lutein + zeaxanthin, which might promote lung health. And as a rich source of vitamin A, beet greens can help protect healthy vision.

Selection tips:
Beet greens should be deep green and might have green or beet-red veins. Look

for unwilted specimens and avoid any that have yellowed or turned slimy.

Storage tips:
Store beet greens unwashed in a plastic bag in the refrigerator for three to five days. Rinse in several changes of cold water to remove all soil.

Preparation tips:
Beet greens can be eaten raw, although their nutrients are better absorbed if the greens are cooked. Try sautéing them with olive oil and garlic or braising them with a little vegetable stock or water.

Precautions:
Beet greens are high in vitamin K and potassium. Consult a doctor or registered dietitian before consuming beet greens if you are on warfarin (brand name Coumadin) therapy or a potassium-restricted diet.

BELL PEPPER

Serving size: 1 cup raw, ½ cup cooked

Per serving:
Calories:. 27
Carbohydrate: . . . . 6 g
Protein:. 1 g
Fat:. . . . . 0 g
Saturated fat: . . . . 0 g
Cholesterol: . . . . 0 mg
Sodium:. . . . . 2 mg
Fiber:. . . . . 2 g

Note: Values are given for red peppers. Values for green peppers are slightly lower, and they have a lower concentration of antioxidants and phytochemicals.

Good source of:
vitamin C, beta-carotene, beta-cryptoxanthin, lycopene

Description:
Bell peppers—which are sometimes called sweet peppers to distinguish them from their hot chili cousins—are a lot like the leaves on trees. They start off green, and as the season progresses and the peppers mature, they change to yellow, then orange, and then finally to red. They also get sweeter, and become more nutrient dense.

Peppers hail from Latin America. Spanish and Portuguese explorers helped spread the cultivated plant from South America; today, they are also grown in Asia, Europe, and the United States. Holland, Mexico, and Israel are among the biggest producers of bell peppers.

Bell peppers figure prominently in Mediterranean, Latin American, and Asian cuisine. Though technically a fruit, peppers are consumed as vegetables and have a nutrition profile similar to that of vegetables.

Health benefits:
Bell peppers are an excellent source of vitamin C and vitamin A. They contain large amounts of several carotenoids, which appear to play a role in the prevention of cancer, cardiovascular disease, and diabetes progression.

In 2005, the *American Journal of Clinical Nutrition* published new epidemiological research conducted at the University of

Queensland in Australia. The study revealed evidence that diets rich in these carotenoids may exert a significant protective effect in the prevention of diabetes. Therefore, both those with diabetes and family members at risk for developing it are likely to benefit from bell pepper consumption.

Selection tips:
Look for firm, brightly colored peppers that are heavy for their size. The skin should have a bit of a sheen and should be unwrinkled. Avoid peppers with soft spots or stems that show signs of mold.

Storage tips:
Peppers will keep in a plastic bag or in the crisper drawer in a refrigerator for up to a week. Raw peppers can be rinsed, cut, and frozen in an airtight container for later use. Roasted peppers can be marinated in oil and vinegar and stored in the refrigerator. Check individual recipes to determine how long marinated peppers may be kept.

Preparation tips:
Here is a simple method for removing the pepper flesh from the seeds and membranes with minimal waste: Hold a rinsed, dried pepper upright on a cutting board. Place a chef's knife or paring knife along one of the domed ridges at the top of the pepper, and slice downward toward the bottom. Repeat around the entire pepper. The seeds and most of the white membrane should still be attached to the stem, which can be discarded. The "walls" of the pepper can now be sliced or chopped as desired.

To prepare peppers for stuffing, use a paring knife to cut a circle around the stem, and pull the stem and seeds out. Use a spoon or your fingers to scoop out any remaining seeds or white membrane.

Peppers are great raw, with dips or guacamole. They work well in sandwiches and wraps. Roasted peppers have incredible depth and lend wonderful flavor to pasta, salsas, salads, grain dishes, or pizza. Try using pureed roasted peppers as a base for hot or cold soups, or stir into hummus.

Roasting peppers at home is quite easy. Rub washed and dried whole peppers with olive oil, and place on a cookie sheet lined with aluminum foil. Place peppers in an oven preheated to 425°F, and roast for about 30 to 40 minutes, turning the peppers periodically. When the skin is blackened and blistered all around, and the flesh is soft, the peppers are done. When they are cool enough to handle, slip off the skins, remove the seeds and membranes, and slice or chop.

On a side note, if you happen to find purple, brown, or black bell peppers at a farmer's market or gourmet shop, enjoy them raw—cooking will turn them green!

Precautions:
The Environmental Working Group (EWG) recommends purchasing organic bell peppers, based on its analysis of over 100,000 USDA and FDA tests for pesticides conducted between 1992 and 2001. Of all the vegetables evaluated, bell peppers had the greatest degree of pesticide contamination. The tests found pesticide contamination on 68% of the bell pepper samples. EWG also noted that 39 different pesticides were identified on the peppers, and that most bell peppers were contaminated with more than one pesticide.

If organic peppers are unavailable or prohibitively expensive, consider growing your own or shop at farmers markets, where you can ask farmers about their growing practices.

Serving size: ½ cup cooked or 1 large (approximately 7½ inches) raw

Per serving:
Calories:. 27
Carbohydrate: . . . . .6 g
Protein:. . . . . .1 g
Fat:. . . . . .0 g
Saturated fat: . . . . .0 g
Cholesterol: . . . . .0 mg
Sodium:. . . . . .45 mg
Fiber:. . . . . .2 g

Good source of:

vitamin A, alpha-carotene, beta-carotene

Description:

Carrots, which are related to fennel and parsley, are immensely popular and have been cultivated for centuries. Still, modern Americans are unlikely to recognize the root's dark purple ancestors. Carrots are native to the Middle East and Asia. There are hundreds of varieties of carrots, but the familiar orange cultivar wasn't bred until the 1800's.

Increasingly, some of the more interesting heirloom carrot varieties are turning up at farmer's markets, restaurants, and gourmet shops. There are round carrots, short and thin carrots, and golden or reddish-purple carrots.

Though marketed as "baby carrots," the small bagged carrots so ubiquitous in U.S. supermarkets aren't babies at all—they're actually full grown carrots, peeled and cut for easy snacking.

Health benefits:

Though they are remarkably nutritious, carrots have gotten a bad rap in certain popular diet books. These books claim carrots should never be eaten because of their medium-to-high glycemic index. In fact, carrots have a remarkably low glycemic load. University of Sydney researchers, who've spearheaded much of the work on the glycemic index, assert that those with diabetes should give low glycemic load vegetables the green light—even if those very vegetables have a higher glycemic index— and reap the benefit of all the micronutrients and antioxidants they contain. In the case of carrots, that includes a hefty dose of vitamin A, and sight-protecting, cancer-fighting beta-carotene. Carrots are regarded in Chinese medicine as a soothing digestive tonic and are said to have antidiarrheal properties.

Selection tips:

Look for firm, deeply colored carrots. Avoid those with soft spots or signs of "root rot," such as brown, shriveled ends. If the tops are still attached, they should be bright green and firm, without signs of moisture loss.

Storage tips:
Remove carrot tops before storing. Placed in a plastic bag, carrots will keep in the refrigerator for two to three weeks. Carrots should be blanched or cooked and pureed before freezing. They will keep for up to a year in a cold (0°F) freezer.

Preparations:
Carrots are one of the workhorses of the modern kitchen. They are used raw and cooked in a myriad of ways. They're an essential component of mirepoix, a mixture of finely diced onion, celery, and carrot that is used as a flavor base in French cuisine. They make their way into sauces, soups, stews, salads, and baked goods. They are ever-present on crudité platters and in kids' lunchboxes and can even be pickled. Julienned raw carrots, tossed with parsley, garlic, olive oil, and red wine vinegar make a wonderfully simple salad. Try whipping pureed carrots into mashed potatoes to lighten the tubers and give them a nutrient boost. Or sauté carrots with fresh ginger, onions, and garlic, cook in vegetable stock until tender, and puree for a delightful soup that can be served hot or cold.

Precautions:
Excessive carrot consumption can give the skin an orange cast, thanks to the pigment beta-carotene. This is harmless, although there are other conditions that can discolor skin. Consult a doctor if you notice unusual changes in skin color, but do mention it if you've been eating loads of carrots.

COLLARD GREENS

Serving size: ½ cup cooked

Per serving:
Calories:. 25
Carbohydrate: . . . . 5 g
Protein:. 2 g
Fat:. . . . . 0 g
Saturated fat: . . . . 0 g
Cholesterol: . . . . 0 mg
Sodium:. . . . . 15 mg
Fiber:. . . . . 3 g

Good source of:
calcium, vitamin A, vitamin K, vitamin C, thiamine, riboflavin, folate, manganese, potassium, lutein + zeaxanthin, beta-carotene

Description:
Collard greens are a member of the cabbage family, as one might guess from their large, hardy leaves and thick stems. Native to the Mediterranean and Asia, they became a Southern staple after African slaves brought them to America.

Collard greens are resilient and can endure even very cold temperatures, so they have a long growing season and are sometimes classified as "winter greens."

Collard greens figure prominently in Southern cuisine and soul food. They are a key accompaniment to Brazilian *feijoada* and the main ingredient in Portuguese *caldo verde*, a green broth often served during celebrations.

Health benefits:
One cup of cooked collard greens has 266 milligrams of calcium, making them an excellent source of this essential mineral and a great choice for those who dislike or don't tolerate dairy products. Besides being

essential for maintaining bone strength, calcium plays important roles in muscle and nerve function and appears to have a protective effect against colon cancer.

Collard greens are remarkably rich in disease-fighting phytochemicals and antioxidants. They are also a rich source of manganese, a component of many enzymes, and an important nutrient for bone health, nerve function, and nutrient use.

Selection tips:
Look for firm, deeply colored, unwilted collard greens without wet or slimy spots.

Storage tips:
Collard greens can be stored unwashed in a plastic bag in the refrigerator, where they will last for up to about five days. They are best, however, when used within two to three days of purchase.

Preparation tips:
Traditionally, collard greens are treated to long cooking times, and in the American South they are often prepared with ham hocks or other high-fat flavoring additions. Gentler cooking methods help preserve more of their nutrient value and distinctive flavor.

Wash collard greens well to remove any soil or sand and remove the large, tough rib that runs down the center of each leaf. (If the collards are young, you might be able to chop these stems and use them.) Collard greens are rarely served raw because the leaves are tough and hard to digest. They work nicely in soups, stews, or stir-fries and can be steamed or braised. If they are blanched and chopped beforehand, collard greens can be integrated into pilafs, omelets, or pasta dishes.

Precautions:
Collards provide an abundance of vitamin K and potassium. Those on warfarin (brand name Coumadin) therapy or those on a potassium-restricted diet should talk with their doctor or registered dietitian before consuming collards.

CORN

Serving size: ½ cup cooked kernels

Per serving:

Calories:	76
Carbohydrate:	18 g
Protein:	3 g
Fat:	1 g
Saturated fat:	0 g
Cholesterol:	0 mg
Sodium:	197 mg
Fiber:	2 g

Note: Nutrient values are slightly less for a typical small to medium-size ear of corn on the cob.

Good source of:
fiber, thiamine, folic acid, lutein + zeaxanthin, zinc

Description:
Archaeological evidence indicates that humans have used corn as a foodstuff for over 7,000 years. Corn, the only cereal grain indigenous to the Americas, was a vital component of the Mayan, Aztec, and Incan diet and culture. European explorers noted corn's growth throughout North, Central, and South America, and Spanish and Portuguese explorers helped spread corn cultivation to Europe and Africa, respectively.

European colonists benefited from the Native American's sophisticated corn cultivation techniques, although the advantage conferred to the colonists by ready access to a staple crop proved devastating to the indigenous Indians.

Today, the United States is one of the world's largest producers of corn. White, yellow, or bicolor corn are most widely available, although a range of colorful varieties—including red, blue, and black—exist.

Health benefits:
Corn is gluten-free, so it can be safely enjoyed by those with celiac disease or wheat allergies.

In a small cross-over study published in 2003 in *Diabetes Care,* researchers at a Mexican university found that overweight and obese people with diabetes had improved HbA_{1c} levels (a measure of blood glucose control) after changing to a traditional Mexican diet that emphasized low-glycemic-index food choices. Traditionally made corn tortillas fall into this category.

Few Americans' diets contain adequate amounts of whole grain, which can help lower cholesterol, improve blood pressure, and fight disease. Homemade air-popped popcorn is a great way to include whole grains in the diet. It's best to steer clear of microwave popcorns, which tend to contain *trans* fat (a type of fat best avoided).

Selection tips:
When picking fresh ears of corn, run a hand along the husk to feel for firm, plump, juicy kernels. The corn silk sprouting from the top of the ear should be golden, never blackened or shriveled. Ears that feel cool are allegedly sweeter, perhaps because the sugars in corn convert to starch more rapidly at warmer temperatures. Without question, the tastiest corn is the freshest; ears should be used within a couple of days of purchase.

Storage tips:
Refrigerate uncooked corn, preferably in its husk, in the coldest part of the refrigerator.

Preparation tips:
For corn on the cob, boiling is perhaps the most common preparation method. Remove the husk and silk, place cobs in a pot of cold water, and cook for one minute past the boiling point. Do not salt the water because this will harden the kernels. Corn on the cob can also be grilled or roasted. In both cases, peel back the husk to remove the silk but leave the husk attached. To roast, replace the husk, put the ears in a roasting pan, and cook in a 350°F oven for about 45 minutes. To grill, soak the de-silked ears in cold water for 30 minutes. Brush kernels with oil and season with spices, if desired. Replace the husks and grill for about 15 minutes, turning frequently.

For more formal meals, corn is generally served off the cob. Hold a cleaned cob upright on a cutting board and carefully run a sharp chef's knife from the top of the cob, near the base of the kernels, toward the cutting board. Rotate the cob and continue removing strips of kernels. Kernels can be boiled, roasted, or sautéed. Corn kernels make interesting additions to salsas and relishes.

Precautions:
Remember that although it is often consumed as a vegetable, corn is in fact a grain and is therefore primarily a source of carbohydrate. When planning meals, remember to account for the carbohydrate it contains and make a point of eating corn alongside nonstarchy vegetables.

According to the independent Pew Initiative on Food and Biotechnology, by 2004 nearly 45% of the corn planted in the United States was genetically modified. Those concerned about the application of genetic engineering technologies to foodstuffs should seek out certified organic corn and corn products.

Serving size: 1 clove

Per serving:

Calories:	4
Carbohydrate:	1 g
Protein:	0 g
Fat:	0 g
Saturated fat:	0 g
Cholesterol:	0 mg
Sodium:	1 mg
Fiber:	0 g
Calcium:	5 mg

Good source of:

antioxidants, organosulfur compounds (including allicin and diallyl sulfide).

Description:

Garlic is one of the oldest known plants in cultivation. For ages (and in many cultures), antibiotic, antiparasitic, antifungal, antiviral, and even antivampire powers have been ascribed to garlic. Science has borne out many of the medicinal properties of garlic (still no word on the vampires), and we've learned more about the bulb's antioxidant and cardioprotective capacities along the way.

Garlic seems to have originated in Asia, but its distinctive flavor and aroma have almost universal appeal, and it is an essential flavoring element in cuisines throughout the world. The bulb is even celebrated at California's annual Gilroy Garlic Festival, now in its 28th year.

Health benefits:

Garlic has been touted as a virtual cure-all, a factor that seems to have helped popularize garlic supplements. But the culinary use of garlic appears to be more effective, cheaper, and safer—not to mention far more delicious—than using garlic supplements.

The tremendous number of studies on garlic suggests that the common culinary flavoring helps promote cardiovascular health by reducing platelet clumping, improving blood lipid levels, and increasing the elasticity of the arteries. These effects may help reduce the risk of heart disease, stroke, and dementia.

Evidence from population studies suggests that garlic may reduce the risk of certain gastrointestinal cancers, including stomach and colon cancer, and may have antitumor effects.

A study published in the journal *Foodborne Pathogens and Disease* in 2005 found that garlic paste had the potential to kill or inhibit the growth of the potentially fatal strain of *E. coli* bacterium called *E. coli* O157:H7. (While some strains of *E. coli* are harmless, this particular strain, most commonly transmitted through undercooked ground beef, can cause kidney failure and death.) Other studies have found that garlic inhibits bacteria responsible for certain respiratory infections and that it appears to be effective against fungal, parasitic, and viral infections as well.

The common advice to pregnant and lactating women to avoid spicy foods, including garlic, is more old wives' tale than truth. If garlic doesn't cause heartburn or gastro-intestinal upset for the woman, it is absolutely fine to eat. In fact, one study found that infants who were breast-fed on demand nursed *more* after their mothers consumed garlic. The flavor of breast milk is influenced by the mother's diet; it seems that babies are fans of the so-called "stinking rose"!

Garlic has also been shown to inhibit the growth of *Streptococcus* bacteria. In 2004, *Midwifery Today with International Midwife* published a call to action to study the use of garlic as a preventative measure against *beta-hemolytic*, or *Group B Streptococcus* (GBS), for which pregnant women are routinely screened. Because GBS can be passed from mother to infant and can cause a rare but potentially fatal infection in the infant, GBS-positive mothers are dosed heavily with antibiotics during labor and delivery.

Unfortunately, this practice can cause dangerous side effects in the mother and is not always effective in treating the infant (who may not have developed GBS in the first place). Moreover, antibiotic-resistant strains of GBS have been identified, which means that actual infection can be extremely difficult to treat. While we don't yet know definitively if garlic is effective against GBS, mothers-to-be who enjoy garlic should consider consuming it regularly, especially from about 34 weeks of gestation until delivery.

Garlic-flavored toothpaste would probably have very limited appeal, but British researchers did find that, in the laboratory, an aqueous solution of garlic inhibited the growth of multiple pathogenic oral bacteria. Results of the study were published in the journal *Archives of Oral Biology* in 2005, and while further research in human subjects is necessary, the study results indicate that garlic may be therapeutic for oral health, especially for fighting periodontitis (gum disease). Gum disease is more prevalent among people with diabetes, so adding garlic to the diet may be a worthwhile preventative or therapeutic measure.

Selection tips:
While many people rely on dried, powdered garlic for convenience, fresh cloves of garlic deliver unsurpassed flavor and far more versatility. Look for heads of garlic with firm, tightly spaced cloves. The outer skin that holds the individual cloves together should be intact. Avoid heads that are sprouting or that show evidence of mold. Once peeled, the individual cloves should be plump and white—discard spongy cloves or those with soft brown or yellow spots.

Decorative garlic braids are fine for garlic fanatics who can go through several heads in a week. But for optimal freshness, less voracious consumers of garlic are better off buying individual bulbs.

Storage tips:
Store heads of garlic in a cool, dry, well-ventilated, and preferably dark place. Avoid storing them in the refrigerator, though, or your other foods will taste or smell of garlic! Properly stored, garlic will keep for several months, though over time it will dry out and lose its potency.

Preparation tips:
Crush or chop a clove of garlic and you'll immediately notice the increased intensity of the bulb's aroma. Those volatile aromatic compounds not only impart flavor to recipes, but they are also among the health-promoting components of garlic. In fact, chopping or crushing garlic actually makes those compounds available and active.

Rather than tossing freshly chopped garlic straight into the pan, it is best to prepare the garlic and allow it to sit for 5 to 10 minutes while you prepare other ingredients. That increases the activity and heat stability of garlic's beneficial compounds, which likely translates into greater health-protecting effects.

Garlic makes an appearance as a supporting player in so many recipes that its potential as a major ingredient is sometimes overlooked. That's a shame, because recipes that showcase garlic are really delightful. Crushed or minced garlic can be whisked directly into vinaigrettes or marinades. Add it to salsas, guacamole, tzatziki (cucumber and yogurt salad), or bean spreads such as hummus, or try it in sauces and soups.

Lots of chopped garlic is fantastic in simple salads—try it with julienned carrots, parsley, red wine vinegar, and extra-virgin olive oil, or with tomato chunks, balsamic vinegar, and extra-virgin olive oil. Bean salads benefit from a generous dose of chopped garlic, too—try it with white beans, lemon juice, extra-virgin olive oil, and oregano, or with black beans, lime, and chilis.

Sauté sliced garlic in olive oil (take care not to brown or burn the garlic, as this will cause bitterness) and add rinsed baby spinach, string beans, broccoli rabe, or any other favorite green vegetable. Toss together and cook until the vegetables are bright green and just cooked through. Add a splash of water or broth for vegetables that take a bit longer to cook.

Add chopped garlic to casseroles or toss with new potatoes or cubed sweet potatoes, drizzle with olive oil, and bake or roast until tender. To add extra flavor, cut a garlic clove in half and rub the inside of the baking dish with the cut side of the clove before proceeding with the recipe.

Roasting garlic mellows and sweetens its flavor. Drizzle a whole head of garlic (or several) with olive oil and give the garlic a rub to make sure the skin is well-coated. Place in a roasting dish or wrap loosely in foil, and roast the garlic in a 375°F oven for 45 minutes to an hour. The garlic is ready when the skin is lightly browned and the cloves feel soft. (Use an oven mitt or kitchen towel to protect your fingers when you check for doneness!)

Allow the garlic to cool, then cut off the top of the bulb with a sharp knife to expose the tops of the cloves. To use the roasted garlic, simply squeeze out the individual cloves. Spread them on bread, puree them into soups, sauces, or salad dressings, or add them to pasta, pizza, or fish dishes. Serve whole heads of roasted garlic at parties with crudités, roasted vegetables, and crusty bread, and allow guests to squeeze out the cloves themselves.

Feel a cold coming on? Add plenty of chopped garlic to your favorite vegetable soup or try a simple version of the soothing Spanish *sopa de ajo*—sauté six to eight whole cloves of garlic (or more, if you prefer) in olive oil, then mash the cloves lightly with a fork. Add four to six cups of vegetable or chicken stock and bring to a boil. Add cayenne or paprika if desired. Reduce the heat and simmer for ten minutes. Enjoy as is, or puree the soup for a thicker, smoother texture.

Precautions:
Do not attempt to bottle garlic-infused oil at home. Doing so can promote the growth of the deadly bacteria *Clostridium botulinum*, which produces the toxin that causes botulism. If you'd like to serve garlic oils for dipping, stick to commercially prepared oils, or pour plain extra-virgin olive oil over chopped garlic just before serving (refrigerate for up to a few hours if necessary), and discard any leftovers.

Take care with garlic-infused oils in restaurants, too. It's probably best to steer clear of any small bottles of oil on the table that contain garlic. If the waiter brings a dish of garlic and pours oil over it in front of you, the oil is fine to eat.

Numerous supplements have been developed to capitalize on garlic's health benefits without causing the characteristic "garlic breath" or body odors some people experience after consuming the fresh cloves. But scientists are still working to identify all of the active, health-promoting compounds in garlic, and in all likelihood the beneficial components work synergistically. Supplements, on the other hand, often provide only isolated compounds that are thought to confer benefit. Processing may also render them less effective or bioavailable.

Supplements can also interact with blood-thinning drugs such as warfarin (Coumadin), increasing the risk of bleeding. People on antiretroviral drug therapy for HIV should also avoid garlic supplements. Culinary use of garlic is likely to be safe, but people on blood-thinning or anti-retroviral drug therapy should discuss their personal garlic use with their doctor or a registered dietitian.

Anyone taking garlic supplements should discontinue them for at least 7 to 10 days before any surgery. People who eat large amounts of fresh garlic daily should also consider cutting down their garlic consumption for one week prior to surgery. Consuming smaller amounts of fresh garlic should be fine, and may even be beneficial since garlic appears to have infection-fighting properties. Balance is the key.

GINGER

Serving size: 1 teaspoon

Per serving:
Calories:. 2
Carbohydrate: . . . . 0 g
Protein:. 0 g
Fat:. . . . . 0 g
Saturated fat: . . . . 0 g
Cholesterol: . . . . 0 mg
Sodium:. . . . . 0 mg
Fiber:. 0 g
Calcium: . . . . 0 mg

Good source of:
gingerols, shogaols

Description:
Ginger is the knobby underground rhizome of a flowering plant indigenous to Asia. Ginger grows in tropical regions, and the fresh rhizome is important in Asian and Caribbean cuisines. Its thin, buff-colored skin conceals a cream-colored, fibrous flesh that has a warm spiciness.

Ginger is available in numerous forms, which is a testament to its long-prized status in culinary and medicinal applications. Beyond fresh ginger root, the versatile flavoring is available dried, powdered, pickled, candied in syrup, or crystallized in sugar. It is equally at home in savory and sweet recipes.

Health benefits:
Ginger has a host of health benefits, including antimicrobial, antioxidant, anticancer, and anti-inflammatory properties.

A study published in 2006 in the journal *Phytomedicine* found that certain compounds present in ginger inhibited the production of prostaglandin E(2), a mediator of inflammation. Therefore, ginger may have potential to help manage inflammation-related pain and mediate inflammatory conditions states such as arthritis, heart disease, and diabetes.

Other studies have found that ginger contains compounds that may help prevent and fight cancer. Ginger has antioxidant properties, and inhibits *angiogenesis*, or the development of new blood vessels from existing ones. This helps elucidate ginger's apparent tumor-fighting activity, since angiogenesis is an important factor in tumor growth.

A study published in the journal *Foodborne Pathogens and Disease* in 2005 found that ginger paste had the potential to kill or inhibit the growth of the potentially fatal strain of *E. coli* bacterium called *E. coli* O157:H7. (While some strains of *E. coli* are harmless, this particular strain, most commonly transmitted through undercooked ground beef, can cause kidney failure and death.) Other studies have also found powerful antimicrobial action associated with ginger.

Ginger has long been used to prevent motion sickness or treat nausea and vomiting associated with pregnancy, gastrointestinal infections, and chemotherapy. Several studies have borne out ginger's usefulness and safety for these gastrointestinal ills, including a meta-analysis published in 2006 in the *American Journal of Obstetrics and Gynecology*, which found that ginger is effective against postoperative nausea and vomiting.

Ginger also appears to benefit cardiovascular health by inhibiting blood platelet clumping.

Selection tips:
When purchasing fresh ginger, look for firm, plump specimens. Avoid ginger with wrinkled skin or evidence of mold.

Storage tips:
Fresh ginger can be stored at a cool room temperature in a dry place but will stay the freshest in the refrigerator, where it should keep for 2–3 weeks.

Preparation tips:
Break off a ginger knob, or cut the desired amount from the rhizome, and peel the skin from that section of ginger using a vegetable peeler or paring knife. Because the rhizome is fibrous, a larger chef's knife is often best for mincing or slicing peeled ginger or for cutting it into julienned matchsticks.

Asian markets and some specialty kitchen stores sell ginger graters that make quick work of pulverizing fresh ginger. Usually made from ceramic, the graters have tiny raised teeth and sometimes have a "moat" around the perimeter for capturing the ginger juice. To use a ginger grater, just run the peeled ginger back and forth over the teeth.

Use ginger in marinades—it is especially good with reduced-sodium soy sauce or tamari (another type of soy sauce), sesame oil, garlic, and a bit of maple syrup. Or make a ginger–citrus dressing—whisk together rice vinegar, a squeeze of orange, lemon, lime, and/or grapefruit juice, a splash of soy sauce, olive oil, a drop of toasted sesame oil, and freshly grated ginger. Try the dressing over baby greens with daikon radish, carrots, and avocado.

Add a little bit of grated fresh ginger to give smoothies a spicy kick—it's especially good with strawberries, melons, and tropical fruits like banana and mango. Or toss a fruit salad with a teaspoon or two of finely chopped crystallized ginger and a squeeze of lime juice for an elegant twist. Keep the salad in the refrigerator and allow the flavors to blend and intensify for a few hours before serving.

Ginger tea, served hot or iced, often helps those who are feeling queasy, but it tastes great in good health too! For each cup of water, use one to two teaspoons of grated, minced, or sliced ginger. Add the ginger to the boiling water, reduce the heat, and simmer for two to three minutes. Alternatively, simply place the ginger in a mug, pour boiling water over it, and allow the ginger to steep. Adjust the water or ginger quantities to achieve the preferred strength.

Ginger is great for colds, too, especially if a stuffy nose or chest makes it tough to enjoy food. Add a generous amount of ginger to chicken broth or vegetable soup to help break up congestion, fight infection, and impart some flavor that you may be able to taste!

Precautions:

Large amounts of ginger may slow blood clotting and may add to the effects of antiplatelet or anticoagulant ("blood-thin-ning") drugs. Ginger may also add to the effects of blood-pressure–lowering and diabetes drugs. The normal culinary use of ginger should be safe. However, people who take the above mentioned medicines should discuss ginger use—especially the use of ginger supplements—with a doctor or registered dietitian.

ONIONS

Serving size: ¼ cup chopped, or approximately one (¼-inch-thick) slice from a large onion

Per serving:

Calories:	17
Carbohydrate:	4 g
Protein:	0 g
Fat:	0 g
Saturated fat:	0 g
Cholesterol:	0 mg
Sodium:	1 mg
Fiber:	1 g
Calcium:	9 mg

Good source of:

quercetin

Description:

The origins of onions are unclear, as the plants grow wild in many climates and soils. Still, there is a consensus that they likely grew first in central Asia or in the "Fertile Crescent" of the Middle East, and that they have been cultivated for at least 5,000 years. Researchers suspect prehistoric humans were eating wild onions long before that.

Texts from India, Egypt, and Sumer document the importance of the onion in ancient cultures. Pharaohs were entombed with onions, and the bulbs were also used in mummification. The ancient Greeks and Romans appreciated onions on both culinary and medicinal levels and believed them to be a veritable panacea for everything from poor vision, gastrointestinal ills, and headaches to animal bites and insomnia.

The Romans helped spread onions throughout Europe, where they became one of the most important vegetable crops. The Pilgrims made a point of bringing them to North America, though they found that onions already grew wild in the New World and were regularly consumed by Native Americans.

Health benefits:

Onions are rich in the flavonoid antioxidant *quercetin,* which appears to help prevent cataracts. Quercetin also seems to play a role in preventing certain cancers, including breast, ovarian, lung, bladder, and some gastrointestinal cancers. In a large study published in 2005 in the *Asian Pacific Jour-*

nal of Cancer Prevention, researchers looked at onion consumption and stomach cancer rates in Shanghai and Qingdao, China, and reported that onion consumption was associated with lower rates of stomach cancer in these Chinese populations.

Onions may promote cardiovascular and cerebrovascular health by inhibiting platelet clumping and thinning of the blood. This may help reduce the risk of atherosclerosis ("hardening of the arteries"), heart attack, and stroke. It appears that the more pungent the onion, the stronger its effect.

Onions have antimicrobial properties as well, and appear to help fight respiratory and other infections.

Selection tips:

Look for firm, symmetrically-shaped onions with smooth, dry, intact outer skins. Avoid onions that are sprouting or have soft spots or evidence of mold.

Not sure which onion to pick? Yellow onions are an indispensable ingredient in most savory recipes. They have a nice balance of sharpness and sweetness, so their onion flavor comes through without being overwhelming.

Red onions have a beautiful, purplish tinge to their layers and have a sweet, sharp crunchiness that makes them especially versatile, whether served raw or cooked.

Vidalia onions are mild, juicy, and sweet. They are a great choice for eating raw on sandwiches or in salads. They are also a good choice for caramelizing (a technique that involves cooking the onions slowly to bring out their natural sweetness). Because of their higher moisture content, Vidalias are more perishable than other varieties, so be sure to use them quickly.

White onions are mild and sweet, yet they have a straightforward flavor that makes them a good all-purpose onion choice.

Spanish onions tend to be more pungent than other varieties and are often cooked to tame their sharpness. They also tend to keep well, because the sulfur compounds that give them their strong flavor help to preserve them.

Green (or "spring") onions are immature young onions. They have small bulbs and are harvested with their green tops still attached. They can be used interchangeably with scallions. In fact, green onions are sometimes picked early, before the bulb develops fully, and sold as scallions. "True" scallions are a member of the onion family that has a mild flavor and doesn't grow a bulbous bottom. However, most shoppers wouldn't notice the difference between true scallions and young green onions.

Fresh onions will deliver the best flavor, culinary versatility, and health benefits, though dried onion flakes and powder are also available. Avoid onion salt however, which is very high in sodium and low on onion.

Storage tips:

Store onions in a cool, dry, well-ventilated place. Do not leave whole onions in plastic bags, as they will trap moisture and cause the onions to rot. Do not store whole onions in the refrigerator either, or their scent will permeate the other foods.

Once they are peeled and sliced or chopped, onions should be stored in the refrigerator to prevent spoilage. Just be sure to put them in a well-sealed container to prevent them from drying out and to keep the volatile onion compounds from flavoring other items in the refrigerator.

Peeled and chopped onions can be stored in the freezer for later use. Be aware, however, that the onions will become softer and their flavor milder with freezing. Place them in a well-sealed container and freeze for up to six months.

Preparation tips:

There's no need to cry when chopping onions. Prevent teary eyes by chilling the onion in the refrigerator for 15–20 minutes before cutting, or cut the onion under cold running water. Use a sharp knife, and leave the root end, where the tear-inducing sulfurous compounds concentrate, intact.

Consider using a separate cutting board for pungent foods like onions and garlic to prevent transferring their flavors to other foods. For the same reason, be sure to wash the knife you use for preparing onions before moving on to other foods. If it proves difficult to wash away the onion smell from cutting boards or hands, try rubbing them with the cut side of a lemon half. The juice does a good job of neutralizing onion scent.

Onions make an appearance in so many recipes that it's tough to think of what *not* to do with them. Chopped and sautéed, onions contribute great flavor to grains, potatoes, and vegetables. Roast them alongside meats, or add chopped onion to your favorite turkey or veggie burger recipe. Toss chopped onions into omelets, or slice them thinly and use in a quiche.

Try onions in salsas and chutneys—white or yellow onions are great in tomato salsa, while red onion is delicious in mango chutney, guacamole, or a salsa made of pineapple, red pepper, and tomato.

For an unconventional barbeque or picnic offering, try a cold rice salad. Spread cooked brown rice in a large serving dish. Top with chopped tomatoes, peppers, red onions, and cucumber, arranged in stripes of color if you like, and drizzle with red wine vinaigrette. Cover and chill until ready to serve.

Next time you fire up the grill, throw on some thick slices of red onion, then use them to top burgers, grilled chicken, or fish. Or thread chunks of red onion, pineapple, cherry tomatoes, mushrooms, and fish or tofu on skewers, brush with sesame-soy vinaigrette, barbecue sauce, or olive oil and herbs, and grill the kabobs.

Caramelizing onions is remarkably easy to do, and gives them a complex, sophisticated flavor, enhances their sweetness, and imparts a meltingly luscious texture. Peel and slice onions thinly. In a large skillet, heat 1–2 tablespoons of olive oil over medium heat. Add the sliced onions and stir until they are well-coated with oil. Cook the onions, stirring occasionally, for about 15–20 minutes. Adjust the heat if necessary to keep the onions from burning or becoming crisp. When they've become soft and the color deepens to a rich brown, they are done. Serve caramelized onions over a spinach salad, add them to roasted vegetable sandwiches, or serve atop fish or chicken.

When there are onions on hand but the pantry is nearly bare, improvise a lightened version of French onion soup—the recipe is forgiving, so tinkering with it is just fine. Sauté four to six large, sliced onions in 2–3 tablespoons of olive oil, until they soften and begin to caramelize. Add garlic, herbs, and cracked black pepper, if desired. Pour in ½–1 cup of white wine, if desired, and reduce until the wine has nearly evaporated. Pour in chicken or vegetable stock (or even plain water will do in a pinch!) and simmer for 15–20 minutes. Ladle the soup into ovenproof crocks or bowls and top each crock with a slice of sourdough or a multigrain baguette spread with goat cheese or topped with a sprinkle of shredded Swiss or Gruyère cheese. Place the crocks on a cookie sheet and bake or broil for 2–3 minutes, until the cheese melts and bubbles.

Precautions:
Green onions (scallions) harvested in Mexico were implicated in multiple hepatitis A outbreaks in the United States in 2003. The FDA recommends avoiding raw or undercooked green onions, especially for people who are undergoing chemotherapy or are immune compromised or have chronic liver disease, or for anyone else who may be susceptible to more severe illness from hepatitis A exposure.

PARSLEY

Serving size: ¼ cup

Per serving:

Calories:.....................5
Carbohydrate: ....1 g
Protein:....................0 g
Fat: ....0 g
Saturated fat: ....0 g
Cholesterol: ....0 mg
Sodium:..................8 mg
Fiber:.....................1 g
Calcium: ....21 mg

Good source of:

polyacetylenes, potassium, vitamin C, vitamin A, vitamin K, beta-carotene, lutein + zeaxanthin

Description:

Bright green with curly or flat leaves, parsley is an indispensable herb in many cuisines. Parsley is used so often as a decorative garnish that its pleasant, refreshing flavor is often overlooked. That's a shame, because parsley is surprisingly high in nutrients. Recipes that showcase parsley's unique flavor are like a virtual taste of spring.

Health benefits:

Parsley has long been touted as a diuretic, digestive aid, and breath freshener. Now, a study published in 2005 in the *World Journal of Gastroenterology* suggests parsley may help inhibit infection with the peptic ulcer causing bacteria *H. pylori*. While further research is needed, an aqueous extract of parsley was among the plants that both killed *H. pylori* and inhibited its adhesion to stomach cells.

In an Austrian study published in 2005 in the *Journal of Agricultural and Food Chemistry,* researchers concluded that parsley, which contains high amounts of bioactive compounds called *polyacetylenes,* may be helpful in cancer prevention. The authors also noted that polyacetylenes have antifungal and antibacterial properties, which suggests other possible health benefits from regular parsley consumption.

Parsley is rich in vitamin C, which has antioxidant properties of its own and is vital to collagen synthesis, wound healing, gum health, and tissue, bone, and tooth maintenance.

The vitamin A in parsley is important for vision and proper immune function, and also displays antioxidant capabilities, while the vitamin K in parsley is important for proper blood clotting and bone health.

Selection tips:

Select fresh-looking, evenly-colored parsley that is deep, bright green. Avoid parsley that is brown, yellowed, or wilted or that has slimy spots.

Choose curly parsley for garnishing dishes. Flat leaf (or Italian) parsley is a better choice for cooking, as its flavor stands up better when subjected to heat.

Dried parsley is less flavorful than its fresh counterpart, although some people like to use it in dressings and breading. Look for deep green, evenly colored dried parsley in an airtight container. Try to purchase it in a store with high turnover to ensure that it isn't too old. Flavorwise, dried herbs tend to be past their prime after about six months.

Storage tips:
Store fresh parsley in the refrigerator. Wrap the stems in a damp paper towel and place the parsley in a plastic bag. Alternatively, stand the stems in a glass of water and place a plastic bag loosely over the leaves. Properly stored, parsley should keep in the refrigerator for 4–5 days.

Dried parsley should be kept in an airtight container in a cool, dry, preferably dark place. Dried parsley can be kept for up to six months.

Preparation tips:
Parsley can be sandy, so be sure to wash it well before using. If it is very dirty, it may help to swish it around in a bowl of cool water. Use as many changes of water as necessary until the parsley no longer releases sand or dirt into the water.

Gently blot the washed parsley dry with paper towels or a tea towel before chopping.

Try chopped parsley on tomato or carrot soup. Mix it into goat cheese and spread on sandwiches or use as a dip for crudités. Add a generous amount of parsley to omelets or frittatas, or use it in sauces, pestos, salsas, and salad dressings.

Toss new potatoes with olive oil, parsley and lemon zest, and roast, or mix chopped parsley into rice or grain dishes like *tabbouleh* (a salad of bulgur, parsley, and other vegetables).

Try using parsley in place of some of the greens in salads to really highlight the herb's bright, assertive flavor.

Parsley is a key ingredient in several sauces and condiments. Make an Italian *gremolata* with finely chopped parsley, lemon or orange zest, and garlic, and serve with roasted meats, fish, or even potatoes.

Argentinean *chimichurri* is fantastic drizzled over meat, poultry, grilled fish, vegetables, or tofu. It even works well over salad. Recipes vary, but most include red wine vinegar, olive oil, hot pepper, and generous amounts of garlic and parsley.

Precautions:
Parsley is abundant in vitamin K. People who take blood-thinning drugs such as warfarin (brand name Coumadin) should talk with a doctor or registered dietitian before adding parsley to their diet.

Serving size: ½ cup cooked

Per serving:
Calories:. 41
Carbohydrate: . . . . 10 g
Protein:. . . . . 1 g
Fat: . . . . 0 g
Saturated fat: . . . . 0 g
Cholesterol: . . . . 0 mg
Sodium: . . . . 3 g
Fiber:. 2 g

Good source of:
vitamin D, pantothenic acid, potassium, zinc

Description:
Shiitake mushrooms are native to East Asia, where they have been cultivated for over 2,000 years. They have been equally valued medicinally and culinarily, particularly in China and Japan, where they remain the most popularly cultivated mushroom. Shiitakes are typically grown on dead tree trunks or logs; recently, shiitake logs have sprung up in specialty gift catalogs for those who want to try growing their own small crops of shiitakes at home.

The venerated mushrooms have dark brown caps that tend to peak toward the center, while the gills on the underside are a pale vanilla color. The stems are quite woody and are usually discarded. Shiitakes are available fresh or dried; the flavor of the latter is more intensely savory.

Health benefits:
In a 2006 in-vitro study published in the *Journal of Alternative and Complementary Medicine*, researchers at the University of Arkansas found that the "mycochemicals" in shiitakes appear to have an antiproliferative effect against several types of human tumor cells. Although studies of these mycochemicals have yet to be conducted in humans, shiitakes contain other components that appear to have beneficial effects, including antifungal and immune-enhancing properties. Shiitakes have many compounds that might confer benefit and that likely work synergistically. Therefore, as is generally the case, the greatest health benefits are probably obtained by eating whole shiitakes. This is typically more effective and safer than taking extracts or supplements derived from the mushrooms.

Selection tips:
Look for firm, dry mushrooms with a pleasant aroma. Very flat or wrinkled mushrooms are past their prime and should be avoided.

Storage tips:
Shiitakes are a bit hardier than other mushrooms, so if they are purchased when very

fresh, they might last about a week in the refrigerator. They should be stored unwashed, either in a paper bag or in a single layer in a bowl covered with a slightly damp dishtowel. For the best flavor, however, they should be used as soon after purchase as possible.

Preparation tips:
Fresh shiitakes should be wiped with a damp cloth or cleaned with a mushroom brush. They can be rinsed very briefly if necessary, but be sure to dry them well so they don't absorb too much water. Slice the shiitakes and sauté or add to soups, pilafs, or risotto.

Dried shiitakes should be soaked in warm water for about an hour, until they are soft enough to use. Keep the soaking water—it is an excellent base for soups or sauces and imparts a lovely flavor when added to the cooking water for grains.

Precautions:
Normal consumption of whole shiitakes does not appear to cause adverse reactions. However, dermatitis, photosensitivity, eosinophilia (a blood condition), and gastrointestinal symptoms have been reported among those taking high doses of shiitake supplements.

SWEET POTATOES

Serving size: ½ cup cooked (without skin)

Per serving:
Calories:................... 120
Carbohydrate: .... 28 g
Protein:..................... 2 g
Fat: .... 0 g
Saturated fat: .... 0 g
Cholesterol: .... 0 mg
Sodium:.................. 44 mg
Fiber:..................... 4 g

Good source of:
vitamin A, beta-carotene, vitamin C, iron, potassium, anthocyanins

Description:
Though they share half a moniker and have a similar appearance, sweet potatoes aren't actually potatoes at all. Nor are they true yams—white tubers native to Africa, Asia, and the West Indies—although "yam" and "sweet potato" are often used interchangeably. In fact, Louisiana sweet potato growers have something to do with the confusion. Decades ago, eager to set their root vegetable apart from East Coast sweet potatoes, they dubbed their variety "yams." Like potatoes and yams, however, sweet potatoes appear to have originated in Central and South America and have a remarkably long history of cultivation. True sweet potatoes belong to the same family as the morning glory. There are many varieties of sweet potatoes on the market. The flesh may range from light yellow to a deep, intense pumpkin color. Skins may be thin or thick; both are edible, although many people prefer to peel the thicker-skinned variety.

Health benefits:
Sweet potatoes contain a hefty dose of immunity-boosting, cancer-fighting beta-carotene. Despite their sweet taste, sweet potatoes have a lower glycemic index than white potatoes,

which might have a beneficial effect on overall blood glucose control for those who substitute sweet potatoes for potatoes.

A 2001 article published in the *Asia Pacific Journal of Clinical Nutrition* notes that residents of Okinawa's Ryukyu Island chain have some of the longest life expectancies and lowest disease rates in the world and that sweet potatoes are a staple of their traditional cuisine. Although many factors contribute to the Okinawan's excellent health, antioxidant-packed and nutrient-rich sweet potatoes likely exert a helpful effect. And, thanks in part to the sweet potato's nutrient density, NASA recommended inclusion of the root in its vegetarian meal options for astronauts on lunar and Mars missions.

Selection tips:
Look for firm, dry, sweet potatoes without cracks, bruises, or dark spots. Small to medium-size sweet potatoes are most desirable. Avoid refrigerated raw sweet potatoes.

Storage tips:
Raw sweet potatoes will keep in a cool, dark, well-ventilated area (between approximately 55–60°F). They are best used within 7 to 10 days, although they can be stored for up to four weeks under proper conditions. Higher temperatures might compromise the root's texture or cause it to sprout. Once cooked, sweet potatoes may be refrigerated for about a week or frozen.

Preparation tips:
If the words "sweet potato" conjure visions of the ubiquitous cinnamon-laced, marshmallow-topped casserole that lands on Thanksgiving tables everywhere, you've probably been missing out on a host of delicious preparations. Sweet potatoes are remarkably versatile. In terms of flavor enhancements, cinnamon is just the tip of the iceberg—sweet potatoes have an affinity for fresh or dried herbs and spices like thyme, rosemary, and chilies.

They can be baked in their skins or boiled and mashed. They make great oven fries, or they can be cubed, tossed with olive oil and herbs or spices, and roasted in a hot oven. Substitute boiled, cubed sweet potatoes for white potatoes in your favorite potato salad recipe or try grilling them. Shredded or cooked and mashed, they enhance baked goods.

Scrub, rinse, and dry sweet potatoes thoroughly before using. Remove any blemishes before cooking and leave the skin on to preserve the most nutrient value.

Precautions:
Sweet potatoes are a rich source of potassium. People on potassium-restricted diets should consult a registered dietitian or doctor before eating sweet potatoes and should discuss whether "leaching" them of their potassium is recommended. Leaching is accomplished by peeling and dicing the sweet potatoes into small pieces (about ⅛ inch thick), rinsing, then covering the pieces with a generous amount of warm water, and allowing them to soak in the refrigerator for a minimum of four hours. (The water should be changed every four hours if the potatoes will be soaked longer). The sweet potatoes should then be rinsed well before cooking in a fresh change of water.

Serving size: 1 cup raw, ½ cup cooked

Per serving:
Calories:. 27
Carbohydrate: . . . . 6 g
Protein:. 1 g
Fat: . . . . 0 g
Saturated fat: . . . . 0 g
Cholesterol: . . . . 0 mg
Sodium:. . . . . 7 mg
Fiber:. . . . . 2 g

Good source of:

lycopene, phytosterols, beta-carotene, potassium, vitamin K, vitamin A

Description:

When it comes to tomato trivia, many people know that the familiar "vegetable" is actually a fruit (it's a berry, to get even more specific), and may even know it is a member of the nightshade family, which also includes potatoes and eggplants. Though tomatoes have a long history of human consumption and are now cultivated for food throughout the world, there were several periods during which they were regarded with suspicion and believed to be poisonous.

When tomatoes were introduced to Italy, the plants' resemblance to other nightshades—some of which truly are poisonous—was noted, and the plants were grown ornamentally for nearly two centuries. In a pattern that was repeated in England and America, once people got wise to the fact that tomatoes were safe to eat—not to mention delicious—they rapidly became a cornerstone of their cuisine.

Perhaps because they were typically used in savory preparations, tomatoes came to be known as vegetables. In any case, despite their botanical classification as fruits, they do have a nutrition profile more akin to vegetables. They also went from being feared as poisonous to being touted as medicinal. Modern research is confirming the health-protective benefits of tomatoes.

There are over 1,000 varieties of tomato. The fruits range from tiny to large and come in a range of colors and shapes. There are red cherry and grape tomatoes, oddly-shaped yellow specimens, green and white-striped heirloom tomatoes, pear-shaped orange tomatoes, as well as the familiar red plum and beefsteak tomatoes. The list, of course, goes on, but it's hard to get tired of these versatile, nutrient-packed beauties.

Health benefits:

That tomatoes are rich in lycopene, a powerful antioxidant, is well publicized. Lycopene consumption from food sources, such as tomatoes, appears to reduce the risk of prostate, cervical, breast, and lung cancer. It should be noted, however, that this protective effect is probably not from lycopene alone—tomatoes are rich in a host of carotenoids, of which lycopene is one.

Preliminary research from a University of California study published in 2006 suggests that consumption of tomato sauce may also help protect against disease progression in those already diagnosed with prostate cancer.

A 2005 study from the Cardiovascular Research Center at the University of Connecticut School of Medicine found that tomato juice (though not isolated lycopene) conferred cardioprotective benefits. There is also preliminary research showing that lycopene may have a positive impact on the cells responsible for bone growth. While we don't yet have a clear picture about the role tomatoes may play in bone health, it can't hurt to eat them if you enjoy them.

Selection tips:
Because ripe tomatoes are easily bruised, many growers pick them early and ship them before they are ripe. But although they may look nicer on the supermarket shelf, but they may not taste as good. Tomatoes will ripen at room temperature, so if they were handled well in shipping and at the store, they may be just fine. Look for plump, heavy, unbruised fruits. Smell them, too—the smell of a good tomato is unmistakable, while those with no aroma usually have no taste.

Increasingly, even supermarkets stock locally grown tomatoes during their growing season. These are often the best bet for optimally flavorful, fresh, and properly ripened tomatoes.

Storage tips:
Until they are ripe, tomatoes should be kept at room temperature (55°F to 70°F). To speed ripening, put tomatoes in a closed paper bag. This traps the ethylene gas they naturally emit as they ripen, speeding the process. If you have totally ripe tomatoes that you can't use right away, it is fine to refrigerate them for up to three days, but beyond that, their condition tends to deteriorate.

Preparation tips:
Robust, garden-ripe tomatoes are best treated simply. Just rinse and slice as desired. Remove the stem if it is large or woody by cutting a small cone out of the top of the tomato with a paring knife.

Add ripe tomatoes to salads or sandwiches, or slice thick, layer with fresh mozzarella and basil, and drizzle with extra virgin olive oil. For a quick side dish or impromptu pasta topping, chop tomatoes in large chunks and marinate with extra virgin olive oil, balsamic vinegar, and fresh chopped garlic. Blend tomatoes in a blender with cucumber, bell peppers, and tomato juice for a refreshing gazpacho. Use tomatoes as a base for salsa, and get creative with the add-ins. If your tomatoes look ripe but are a little lackluster, you may be able to improve their flavor by cooking—turn them into a sauce, or roast them with herbs, garlic, and olive oil.

If a recipe calls for peeled tomatoes, the simplest way to peel them is as follows: Bring a large pot of water to a boil. Rinse tomatoes and cut a small "x" in the bottom with a paring knife. Once the water comes to a boil, drop the tomatoes in, and be prepared to fish them out as soon as the skins start to peel away, usually within about 15 to 30 seconds. Immediately rinse under cold water to loosen the skins and prevent the tomatoes from cooking. Alternatively, drop the tomatoes in a bowl of icy water. The skins should slip off easily.

To seed tomatoes, cut them in half and gently squeeze out the seeds, or remove them by hand.

Precautions:
Tomatoes are a rich source of potassium. People on potassium-restricted diets should consult a registered dietitian or doctor before eating tomatoes.

VITAMINS AND MINERALS

Vitamins and minerals don't directly provide energy to the body, but they assist the body in processing the energy it gets from dietary protein, fat, and carbohydrate. A diet that is deficient in certain vitamins and minerals can make it more difficult to control blood glucose levels and can lead to other serious medical conditions. High blood glucose levels can cause the body to lose large amounts of some vitamins and minerals in the urine, leading to deficiencies. For both blood glucose control and general good health, following a nutritious diet with adequate amounts of vitamins and minerals is key.

The Food and Nutrition Board of the National Academy of Sciences gives the following recommendations for daily vitamin and mineral intake. These amounts include vitamins and minerals from both food and supplements. The recommended dietary allowance (RDA) is the amount found to be sufficient to meet the nutrient requirements of nearly all (98%) individuals in a group. In cases where RDAs have not been established, the adequate intake (AI) is the amount believed to cover the needs of all individuals in a group. The tolerable upper intake level (UL) is the maximum level of daily nutrient intake that is unlikely to pose a risk of adverse health effects in almost all individuals in a group. Unless otherwise noted, the amounts listed in the table are recommendations for adults.

In this table, the word "milligram" is abbreviated as "mg," and the word microgram is abbreviated as "µg." In some cases, amounts are given in international units, abbreviated "IU."

FAT-SOLUBLE VITAMINS

Fat-soluble vitamins require a certain amount of dietary fat to be absorbed by the body.

VITAMIN	FUNCTION	DEFICIENCY	FOOD SOURCES
Vitamin A* The RDA for vitamin A includes vitamin A as retinol and precursors to vitamin A known as carotenoids: Men 900 µg Women 700 µg	Normal vision, healthy skin and mucous membranes, defense against infections.	Night blindness; dry eye, sometimes progressing to ulcerations and blindness; dry, scaly skin or inflammation of skin, leading to increased susceptibility to infection.	Liver, fortified milk and other fortified foods, fish, liver oil, butter, cream, egg yolks. Plants containing carotenoids, which convert to vitamin A in the body, include carrots and other red, orange, or yellow fruits and vegetables, and green, leafy vegetables.
Vitamin D (calciferol) AI for men and women aged: 19–50: 5 µg (200 IU) 50–70: 10 µg (400 IU) over 70: 15 µg (600 IU)	Promotes absorption of calcium and phosphorus; helps deposit these minerals in bones and teeth.	In children, faulty bone and tooth development and rickets. In adults, a higher risk of osteomalacia (softening of the bones) and osteoporosis (porous bones).	Fortified milk and other fortified foods, fatty fish. The body also makes its own vitamin D with direct exposure of skin to sunlight.

*Do not take more than 3,000 IU of vitamin A as retinol in a daily supplement.

VITAMIN	FUNCTION	DEFICIENCY	FOOD SOURCES
Vitamin E (alpha-tocopherols) Men 15 mg (22.5 IU) Women 15 mg (22.5 IU) Pregnancy 15 mg (22.5 IU) Lactation 19 mg (28.5 IU)	Protects body cells from oxidation, which can lead to cell damage.	Hemolytic anemia (anemia caused by premature destruction of red blood cells), nerve damage. Deficiency is rare.	Vegetable oils and margarine or salad dressing made with vegetable oils, whole grains, wheat germ, nuts, seeds, green, leafy vegetables.
Vitamin K AI: Men 120 μg Women 90 μg	Makes proteins that cause normal blood clotting.	Abnormal blood clotting.	Green vegetables, pork, liver, vegetable oils, eggs, wheat bran. Vitamin K is also produced by bacteria in the intestines.

WATER-SOLUBLE VITAMINS

Most water-soluble vitamins cannot accumulate in the body; any extra is simply excreted in the urine.

VITAMIN	FUNCTION	DEFICIENCY	FOOD SOURCES
Vitamin C (ascorbic acid) Men 90 mg Women 75 mg Pregnancy 85 mg Lactation 120 mg	Collagen formation; strong blood vessels, healthy skin, healthy gums, wound healing; formation of red blood cells: absorption of iron, conversion of folacin to its active form.	Weakness; swollen gums; dry hair; rough, dry skin; slow wound healing; anemia. Severe deficiency leads to scurvy.	Citrus fruits, broccoli, strawberries, cantaloupe, guava, mango, papaya, bell peppers, tomatoes, potatoes.
Thiamine (vitamin B_1) Men 1.2 mg Women 1.1 mg Pregnancy 1.4 mg Lactation 1.4 mg	Energy metabolism; synthesis of DNA, RNA.	Fatigue, irritability, loss of appetite, constipation, heart rhythm abnormalities, peripheral neuropathy, heart failure.	Vegetables, whole grains, wheat germ, legumes, pork, nuts.
Riboflavin (vitamin B_2) Men 1.3 mg Women 1.1 mg Pregnancy 1.4 mg Lactation 1.6 mg	Energy and protein metabolism.	Sensitivity to light, eye irritation, sores in the corners of the mouth, cracks in the lips, sore, red tongue.	Milk and other dairy products, organ meats, meat, fish, eggs, enriched breads and cereals, green, leafy vegetables.

Vitamin	Function	Deficiency	Food sources
Niacin (vitamin B$_3$) Men 16 mg Women 14 mg	Energy metabolism; production of fatty acids, cholesterol, steroid hormones.	Fatigue, poor appetite, anxiety, and pellagra, whose symptoms include diarrhea, skin problems, and deteriorated mental state.	High-protein foods such as liver, meat, fish, poultry, peanuts, legumes, and whole-grain breads and cereals.
Vitamin B$_6$ (pyridoxine) Men 19–30: 1.3 mg 50 and older: 1.7 mg Women 19–30: 1.3 mg 50 and older: 1.5 mg Pregnancy: 1.9 mg Lactation: 2.0 mg	Amino acid metabolism involving protein synthesis; synthesis of regulatory substances such as serotonin; niacin production; hemoglobin synthesis.	Anemia; nerve damage; sore, red tongue; nausea; dermatitis; irritability, depression, confusion. In infants, convulsions.	Liver, kidneys, red meat, whole-grain cereals, legumes, bananas, potatoes, green, leafy vegetables.
Pantothenic acid AI: Men 5 mg Women 5 mg	Energy metabolism; synthesis of amino acids, fatty acids, cholesterol, steroid hormones, hemoglobin.	Unlikely unless part of a deficiency of all B vitamins.	Organ meats, fish, shellfish, eggs, broccoli, mushrooms, whole grains, legumes.
Vitamin B$_{12}$ (cobalamin) Men 2.4 mg Women 2.4 mg Pregnancy 2.6 mg Lactation 2.8 mg	Protein metabolism; synthesis of DNA, production of red blood cells; healthy nervous system; carbohydrate metabolism, myelin formation (intrinsic factor of gastric secretions is required for absorption).	Poor appetite, weakness, fatigue, diarrhea, numbness and tingling of hands and feet, anemia.	Meat, fish, poultry, fortified cereals and soy products.
Folate (folic acid, folacin) Men 400 µg Women 400 µg Pregnancy 600 µg Lactation 500 µg	Protein metabolism; synthesis of DNA and RNA, red blood cell formation.	Decrease in numbers of all blood cells, anemia, higher risk of giving birth to an infant with neural tube defects such as spina bifida.	Green, leafy vegetables, fruits, liver, kidney, meats, fish, nuts, legumes, whole grains.

MINERALS AND TRACE ELEMENTS

MINERAL OR ELEMENT	FUNCTION	DEFICIENCY	FOOD SOURCES
Calcium AI for men and women aged: 19–50: 1,000 mg Over 50: 1,200 mg Pregnancy: 1,000 mg Lactation: 1,000 mg UL 2,500 mg	Bone and teeth formation, blood clotting, muscle contractions, normal heart rhythm, normal functioning of numerous enzymes, nerve stimulation.	In children, stunted growth and rickets. In adults, osteoporosis (porous bones), low blood calcium levels, which over time can affect the brain.	Milk and other dairy products such as yogurt and cheese, fortified soy milk or cultured soy, tofu, made with calcium sulfate, tempeh, dried figs, dried beans, certain green, leafy vegetables (including broccoli, bok choy, collard greens, kale, mustard greens, and turnip greens), okra, fish with edible bones.

Chromium
AI:
Men 19–50: 35 µg
  over 50: 30 µg
Women 19–50: 25 µg
  over 50: 20 µg
Pregnancy: 30 µg
Lactation: 45 µg
	Necessary for carbohydrate and fat metabolism.	Impaired glucose tolerance, elevated circulating insulin.	Fruits, vegetables, seeds, brewer's yeast, bran cereals.

Copper AI: Men 900 µg Women 900 µg Pregnancy 1,000 µg Lactation 1,300 µg	Involved in many bodily processes, including the absorption, storage, and metabolism of iron.	Anemia.	Nuts, shellfish, organ meats, legumes, grains, chocolate.
Fluoride AI: Men 4 mg Women 3 mg	Mineralization and remineralization of of tooth enamel. Reduces incidence of dental decay.	Tooth decay in young children.	Fluoridated water.
Iodine Men 150 µg Women 150 µg Pregnancy 220 µg Lactation 290 µg	Synthesis of thyroid hormones that regulate basal metabolic rate.	Goiter, impaired growth and neurological development, cretinism.	Iodized salt, seafood, food grown near the sea.

MINERAL OR ELEMENT	FUNCTION	DEFICIENCY	FOOD SOURCES
Iron Men 8 mg Women aged 19 to menopause 18 mg Postmenopausal women 8 mg Pregnancy 27 mg Lactation 9 mg UL 45 mg	Component of the oxygen-carrying proteins hemoglobin (in blood) and myoglobin (in muscle) as well as numerous enzymes.	Anemia, impaired physical work performance, developmental delay, cognitive impairment, adverse pregnancy outcomes, abnormal temperature regulation.	Meat, poultry, fish, fortified grains and cereals, legumes, dried fruits, green, leafy vegetables.
Magnesium Men 19–30: 400 mg over 30: 420 mg Women 19–30: 310 mg over 30: 320 mg	Component of bones and teeth; activates any enzymes, including those involved in energy metabolism; nerve stimulation; muscle contraction.	High blood pressure, heart arrhythmias, neuromuscular manifestations, personality changes. Deficiencies commonly seen in alcoholism or kidney disease.	Green, leafy vegetables, legumes, nuts, whole grains, meat, milk, seafood, cocoa.
Manganese AI: Men 2.3 mg Women 1.8 mg	A component of several enzyme systems in the body; essential for bone structure.	Deficiency is rare but may cause skin problems and high cholesterol.	Pecans, peanuts, pineapple, oatmeal, Shredded Wheat and raisin bran, dried beans, rice, spinach, sweet potatoes, whole wheat bread.
Molybdenum Men 45 μg Women 45 μg Pregnancy 50 μg Lactation 50 μg	A component of several enzymes in the body.	Deficiency is rare.	Organ meats, whole-grain cereals, legumes, green, leafy vegetables.
Phosphorus Men 700 mg Women 700 mg	Bone and tooth formation; energy metabolism; component of DNA and RNA; fat transport; acid-base balance; enzyme formation.	In infants and children, stunted growth and rickets (due to excessive excretion rather than to dietary deficiency). Low blood phosphorus and depleted phosphorus stores may be associated with gastrointestinal malabsorption, diabetes, kidney dysfunctions, antacid overuse, and premature birth.	Distributed widely in foods, including milk, meat, poultry, fish, eggs, cheese, nuts, legumes, whole grains.

Mineral or element	Function	Deficiency	Food sources
Potassium AI: Men 4700 mg Women 4700 mg Pregnancy 4700 mg Lactation 5100 mg	Plays major roles in cell metabolism and nerve and muscle function.	Moderate deficiency can lead to high blood pressure, increased salt sensitivity, increased risk of kidney stones, and increased bone turnover. Severe deficiency can cause heart arrhythmias, muscle weakness, and glucose intolerance.	Fruits, vegetables, dried beans, bran cereal, meats.
Selenium Men 55 μg Women 55 μg Pregnancy 60 μg Lactation 70 μg	A component of enzymes involved in antioxidant protection and thyroid hormone metabolism. May have an anticancer effect.	Deficiency is rare.	Meat, fish, grains, Brazil nuts.
Sodium AI for men and women aged: 19–50: 1500 mg 51–70: 1300 mg 71 and older: 1200 mg UL 2300 mg	Maintains fluid and acid-base balance, important for nerve and muscle function.	Nausea, vomiting, giddiness, exhaustion, cramps.	Processed foods and condiments, table salt, milk, meat, fish, poultry, eggs.
Zinc Men 11 mg Women 8 mg Pregnancy 11 mg Lactation 12 mg	Constituent of many enzyme systems, including those involved in protein digestion and synthesis, carbon dioxide transport, and vitamin A utilization.	Delayed wound healing, recurring infections, impaired sense of taste, loss of appetite. Chronic deficiency can cause retarded sexual development and dwarfism.	Meat, liver, poultry, seafood (especially herring and oysters), eggs, legumes, seeds, wheat germ.

HERBS AT A GLANCE

Some herbal products can have beneficial effects, but most are unproven therapies, and many can have dangerous side effects or drug interactions. See Chapter 11 for a fuller discussion of the uses of these botanical products.

NAME	COMMON USES	PRECAUTIONS
Alfalfa (*Medicago sativa*)	Lowering cholesterol and blood glucose.	Little supporting evidence; plants may induce the growth of estrogen-dependent cancers; seeds may cause relapse of lupus symptoms in people with systemic lupus erythematosus.
Aloe (*Aloe barbadensis, Aloe vera*)	Gel used topically to heal minor wounds; juice used as laxative.	Aloe juice is a potent laxative and is not considered safe. Ingestion of gel has no proven benefits.
Artichoke (*Cynara scolymus*)	Indigestion and improved liver health.	None.
Banaba (*Lagerstroemia speciosa*)	Lowering blood glucose.	Not well studied.
Barley (*Hordeum vulgare*)	Lowering cholesterol and blood glucose.	None.
Bilberry (*Vaccinium myrtillus*)	Fruits used for improved blood circulation, treatment of diarrhea.	Fruits may interact with anticoagulant medicines. Chronic use of bilberry leaves can be toxic.
Bitter melon (*Momordica charantia*)	Lowering blood glucose.	Could cause hypoglycemia.
Black cohosh (*Actaea racemosa, Cimicifuga racemosa*)	Symptoms of menopause.	May have an estrogenic effect, so it should be used under the supervision of a physician.
Boneset (*Eupatorium perfoliatum*)	Colds, flus, fever.	Bitter taste can cause vomiting. Little known about long-term safety.
Buchu (*Barosma betulina, Barosma serratifolia, Barosma crenulata*)	Urinary tract problems, high blood pressure, congestive heart failure.	Herbal diuretics such as buchu can irritate the kidneys.

NAME	COMMON USES	PRECAUTIONS
Burdock (*Arctium lappa, Arctium minus*)	Numerous, unproven medicinal uses.	Risk of contamination of supplements with belladonna considered high. Safe to eat as a vegetable.
Capsicum (*Capsicum frutescens, Capsicum annuum*)	Used topically to treat painful neuropathy.	Hurts if it comes in contact with eyes or mucous membranes.
Chamomile (*Matricaria recutita*)	Relaxation, soothing skin irritations.	Can cause allergic reactions in people who are allergic to ragweed, asters, or chrysanthemums.
Cinnamon (*Cinnamomum verum, Cinnamomum cassia*)	Lowering blood glucose.	Large doses can cause fast heartbeat, increased sweating, and rapid breathing, followed by sedation.
Cranberry (*Vaccinium macrocarpon*)	Preventing and treating urinary tract infections.	Cranberry juices may contain large amounts of sugar.
Dandelion (*Taraxacum officinale*)	Diuretic (leaves) and laxative (roots) effects.	Should not be used by people with bile duct obstruction, bowel obstruction, or gallstones.
Echinacea (*Echinacea purpurea, Echinacea angustifolia, Echinacea pallida*)	Cold symptoms.	Should not be taken by people with autoimmune diseases, multiple sclerosis, tuberculosis, HIV, or AIDS, or by people taking immunosuppressant drugs.
Elder (*Sambucus nigra*)	Flowers and fruits used for colds, flu, and fever.	Leaves and stems are toxic.
Eucalyptus (*Eucalyptus globulus*)	Respiratory ailments, mouth rinses.	Pure eucalyptus oil taken by mouth can have severe and deadly reactions.
Evening primrose oil (*Oenothera biennis*)	Premenstrual syndrome, arthritis, multiple sclerosis, eczema, and painful neuropathy.	Can precipitate seizures in people taking phenothiazines, a class of drugs used to treat schizophrenia and other mental disorders.
Fenugreek (*Trigonella foenum-graecum*)	Lowering blood glucose, laxative effect.	May interact with anticoagulant medicines and alter absorption and effectiveness of other medicines taken at the same time.

NAME	COMMON USES	PRECAUTIONS
Feverfew (*Tanacetum parathenium*)	Preventing and treating migraine headaches.	Should not be used by people taking aspirin or anticoagulant medicines.
Fo-ti (*Polygonum multiflorum*)	Laxative effect.	Using laxatives frequently can lead to dependence on them.
Garlic (*Allium sativum*)	Lowering blood pressure, blood cholesterol, and tendency of blood to clot.	May increase the risk of bleeding in people who take aspirin or anticoagulant medicines.
Ginger (*Zingiber officinale*)	Nausea, other gastrointestinal complaints, cold symptoms.	Very large doses may cause heart arrhythmias and central nervous system depression. Ginger supplements should not be taken by people taking anticoagulant medicines.
Ginkgo (*Ginkgo biloba*)	Circulatory problems, including problems with memory and concentration.	Should not be taken by people taking aspirin or anticoagulant medicines.
Ginseng (*Panax ginseng, Panax quinquefolius*)	Bolstering mood and immunity, lowering blood glucose.	Long-term use associated with skin rash, diarrhea, sore throat, increased blood pressure, excitability, anxiety, depression, and insomnia. May increase the risk of bleeding when taken with aspirin or anticoagulant medicines.
Glucosamine	Osteoarthritis pain relief.	May raise blood glucose levels in people with diabetes.
Goldenseal (*Hydrastis canadensis*)	Upper respiratory infections.	Plant in short supply, raising the possibility that other herbs may be substituted for goldenseal in supplements.
Grape seed extract (*Vitis vinifera*)	Lowering blood pressure, preventing atherosclerosis, improving cholesterol levels.	May increase the risk of bleeding when taken with anticoagulant medicines.
Green tea (*Camellia sinensis*)	Lowering the risk of heart disease, improved bone and dental health.	Contains caffeine, can cause jitteriness or sleeplessness.

Herbs at a Glance

Name	Common uses	Precautions
Guar gum (Cyamopsis tetragonoloba)	Lowering blood pressure, blood cholesterol, and blood glucose.	Can cause esophageal, gastric, and intestinal obstruction if taken with inadequate fluids. May reduce absorption of some other drugs if taken at the same time.
Gymnema (Gymnema sylvestre)	Lowering blood glucose, lowering intake of sweets.	Few large studies have been done.
Hawthorn (Crataegus laevigata, Crataegus oxycantha, and Crataegus monogyna)	Lowering blood pressure, treating angina.	Self-treatment of serious heart problems not recommended. May interact with prescription drugs taken for heart conditions.
Holy basil (Ocimum sanctum)	Controlling blood glucose and blood cholesterol levels.	Not well studied.
Hoodia (Hoodia gordinii)	Suppressing appetite.	Not well studied.
Horsetail (Equisetum arvense)	Diuretic effects, kidney stones, urinary tract infections.	People with kidney disorders or edema due to heart problems should avoid horsetail.
Licorice (Glycyrrhiza glabra, Glycyrrhiza uralensis)	Cough remedy, stomach ulcers, anti-inflammatory effects.	Potential toxic effects include headache, sodium and water retention, excessive excretion of potassium, high blood pressure, heart failure, and cardiac arrest.
Maitake mushrooms (Grifola frondosa)	Preventing cancer, lowering blood glucose and cholesterol.	None, when eaten as a food. Supplement use not well studied.
Milk thistle (Silybum marianum)	Liver problems.	Can cause upset stomach or diarrhea and allergic reactions in people allergic to ragweed.
Nettle (Urtica dioica)	Benign prostatic hypertrophy, diuretic effects.	May raise blood glucose as well as cause stomach upset, sweating, and skin irritation.
Nopal cactus (Opuntia streptacantha)	Lowering blood glucose levels.	Same side effects as would be expected from increasing fiber intake from any source.

NAME	COMMON USES	PRECAUTIONS
Passionflower (*Passiflora incarnata*)	Sedative, tranquilizer, and treatment for insomnia.	Not well studied.
Peppermint (*Mentha x piperita*)	Coughs, colds, nasal congestion, heartburn, irritable bowel syndrome.	Pure peppermint oil can cause heartburn and irritate the skin. Pure menthol, the active ingredient in peppermint, is toxic; ingestion can be fatal.
Psyllium (*Plantago ovata, Plantago isphagula*)	Constipation, lowering blood cholesterol.	Should not be taken by people with bowel obstructions. People with delayed stomach emptying should consult a physician before taking psyllium.
Raspberry (*Rubus idaeus* and *Rubus strigosus*)	Diarrhea, menstrual pain, diabetes, and as a mouthwash.	Generally considered safe.
St. John's wort (*Hypericum perforatum*)	Depression, externally for wounds and skin infections.	Interacts with numerous prescription drugs, herbs, and supplements.
Saw palmetto (*Serenoa repens*)	Benign prostatic hypertrophy.	Self-prescription not advised without a doctor's diagnosis of problem.
Shiitake mushrooms (*Lentinula edodes*)	Cancer prevention, lowering blood cholesterol.	None, when consumed as a food. Prolonged consumption of shiitake mushroom powder may result in dermatitis, photosensitivity, and gastrointestinal upset.
Soy (*Glycine max*)	Lowering cholesterol, symptoms of menopause, preventing cancer and cardiovascular disease.	May encourage the growth of estrogen-dependent cancers or interfere with drugs used to treat such cancers. Moderate consumption of soy foods considered safe.
Stevia (*Stevia rebaudiana*)	Sweetening foods.	Believed safe when consumed in moderate amounts.
Valerian (*Valeriana officinalis* or *Valerianae radix*)	Sedative.	May cause headache, morning drowsiness, and impaired alertness. Long-term use associated with liver toxicity.

BODY-MASS INDEX (BMI) CHART FOR ADULTS

Determine your BMI by locating your height along the left side of the chart and your weight across the top. Note that BMI may overestimate body fat in athletes and others with a muscular build and may underestimate body fat in older people who have lost muscle mass.

Weight	100	105	110	115	120	125	130	135	140	145	150	155	160	165	170
Height															
4'10"	21	22	23	24	25	26	27	27	29	30	31	32	33	35	36
4'11"	20	21	22	23	24	25	26	27	28	29	30	31	32	33	34
5'0"	20	21	22	23	23	24	25	26	27	28	29	30	31	32	33
5'1"	19	20	21	22	23	24	25	26	26	27	28	29	30	31	32
5'2"	18	19	20	21	22	23	24	25	26	27	27	28	29	30	31
5'3"	18	19	20	20	21	22	23	24	25	26	27	28	28	29	30
5'4"	17	18	19	20	21	22	22	23	24	25	26	27	28	28	29
5'5"	17	18	18	19	20	21	22	23	23	24	25	26	27	28	28
5'6"	16	17	18	19	19	20	21	22	23	23	24	25	26	27	27
5'7"	16	16	17	18	19	20	20	21	22	23	24	24	25	26	27
5'8"	15	16	17	18	18	19	20	21	21	22	23	24	24	25	26
5'9"	15	16	16	17	18	19	19	20	21	21	22	23	24	24	25
5'10"	14	15	16	17	17	18	19	19	20	21	22	22	23	24	24
5'11"	14	15	15	16	17	17	18	19	20	20	21	22	22	23	24
6'0"	14	14	15	16	16	17	18	18	19	20	20	21	22	22	23
6'1"	13	14	15	15	16	17	17	18	19	19	20	20	21	22	22
6'2"	13	14	14	15	15	16	17	17	18	19	19	20	21	21	22
6'3"	12	13	14	14	15	16	16	17	18	18	19	19	20	21	21
6'4"	12	13	13	14	15	15	16	16	17	18	18	19	20	20	21
6'5"	12	12	13	14	14	15	15	16	17	17	18	18	19	20	20
6'6"	12	12	13	13	14	14	15	16	16	17	17	18	19	19	20

BMI below 18.5 = Underweight
BMI 18.5–24.9 = Healthy weight
BMI 25–29.9 = Overweight
BMI over 30 = Obese

In addition to checking your BMI, check your waist circumference. Men whose waist circumference is larger than 40 inches and women whose waist circumference is larger than 35 inches probably have excess abdominal fat.

175	180	185	190	195	200	205	210	215	220	225	230	235	240	245	250	255
37	38	39	40	41	42	43	44	45	46	47	48	49	50	51	52	53
35	36	37	38	39	40	41	42	43	44	45	47	48	49	50	51	52
34	35	36	37	38	39	40	41	42	43	44	45	46	47	48	49	50
33	34	35	36	37	38	39	40	41	42	43	44	44	45	46	47	48
32	33	34	35	36	37	38	38	39	40	41	42	43	44	45	46	47
31	32	33	34	35	35	36	37	38	39	40	41	42	43	43	44	45
30	31	32	33	34	34	35	36	37	38	39	39	40	41	42	43	44
29	30	31	32	32	33	34	35	36	37	37	38	39	40	41	42	42
28	29	30	31	32	32	33	34	35	36	36	37	38	39	40	40	41
27	28	29	30	31	31	32	33	34	35	35	36	37	38	38	39	40
27	27	28	29	30	30	31	32	33	33	34	35	36	37	37	38	39
26	27	27	28	29	30	30	31	32	33	33	34	35	35	36	37	38
25	26	27	27	28	29	29	30	31	32	32	33	34	34	35	36	37
24	25	26	27	27	28	29	29	30	31	31	32	33	34	34	35	36
24	24	25	26	26	27	28	29	29	30	31	31	32	33	33	34	35
23	24	24	25	26	26	27	28	28	29	30	30	31	32	32	33	34
23	23	24	24	25	26	26	27	28	28	29	30	30	31	32	32	33
22	23	23	24	24	25	26	26	27	28	28	29	29	30	31	31	32
21	22	23	23	24	24	25	26	26	27	27	28	29	29	30	30	31
21	21	22	23	23	24	24	25	26	26	27	27	28	29	29	30	30
20	21	21	22	23	23	24	24	25	25	26	27	27	28	28	29	30

FOOT-CARE CHECKLIST

Post this checklist in your bedroom or bathroom to help you remember daily foot care.

DAILY

- ■ Check your feet for blisters, sores, cuts, swollen areas, or infections. Use a mirror if necessary.
- ■ Wash your feet with warm water and mild soap. Dry them completely, especially between the toes.
- ■ Moisturize the tops and bottoms of your feet with lotion or petroleum jelly.
- ■ Smooth rough calluses with a pumice stone.
- ■ Check your shoes and socks for foreign objects before putting them on.

WEEKLY

- ■ Trim your toenails, cutting or filing them straight across or following the natural curve of the toe.

EVERY YEAR

- ■ Have your feet examined by a podiatrist or your primary health-care provider.

NEVER

- ■ Soak your feet, unless instructed to by your doctor.
- ■ Get moisturizer between your toes.
- ■ Cut the corners of your toenails.
- ■ Go barefoot.
- ■ Let your feet get too hot or too cold.

USEFUL NAMES, ADDRESSES, AND WEB SITES

These organizations can help you learn more about the topics introduced in this book. Many of them can help you find a teacher, therapist, or other professional.

Acupuncture & Acupressure
ACUPRESSURE INSTITUTE
1533 Shattuck Avenue
Berkeley, CA 94709
(800) 442-2232
www.acupressure.com

AMERICAN ACADEMY OF MEDICAL ACUPUNCTURE
4929 Wilshire Boulevard, Suite 428
Los Angeles, CA 90010
(323) 937-5514
www.medicalacupuncture.org

AMERICAN ASSOCIATION OF ORIENTAL MEDICINE
P.O. Box 162340
Sacramento, CA 95816
(866) 455-7999
www.aaom.org

NATIONAL CERTIFICATION COMMISSION FOR ACUPUNCTURE AND ORIENTAL MEDICINE
11 Canal Center Plaza, Suite 300
Alexandria, VA 22314
(703) 548-9004
www.nccaom.org

Alexander Technique
ALEXANDER TECHNIQUE INTERNATIONAL
1692 Massachusetts Avenue, 3rd Floor
Cambridge, MA 02138
(888) 668-8996
www.ati-net.com

AMERICAN SOCIETY FOR THE ALEXANDER TECHNIQUE
P.O. Box 60008
Florence, MA 01062
(800) 473-0620
www.alexandertech.com

Aromatherapy
NATIONAL ASSOCIATION FOR HOLISTIC AROMATHERAPY
3327 W. Indian Trail Road PMB 144
Spokane, WA 99208
(509) 325-3419
www.naha.org

Asian Bodywork
AMERICAN ORGANIZATION FOR BODYWORK THERAPIES OF ASIA
1010 Haddonfield-Berlin Road, Suite 408
Voorhees, NJ 08043-3514
(856) 782-1616
www.aobta.org

Ayurvedic Medicine
AMERICAN INSTITUTE OF VEDIC STUDIES
P.O. Box 8357
Santa Fe, NM 87504-8357
(505) 983-9385
www.vedanet.com

THE AYURVEDIC INSTITUTE
P.O. Box 23445
Albuquerque, NM 87912-1445
(505) 291-9698
www.ayurveda.com

Biofeedback
ASSOCIATION FOR APPLIED PSYCHOPHYSIOLOGY AND BIOFEEDBACK
10200 West 44th Avenue, Suite 304
Wheat Ridge, CO 80033
(800) 477-8892
www.aapb.org

Bowen Technique
BOWEN RESEARCH & TRAINING
INSTITUTE, INC.
245 North Seminole Avenue
Lake Alfred, FL 33850
(863) 956-3538
www.bowen.org

Chiropractic
AMERICAN CHIROPRACTIC
ASSOCIATION
1701 Clarendon Boulevard
Arlington, VA 22209
(703) 276-8800
www.amerchiro.org

Chronic Pain
AMERICAN CHRONIC PAIN
ASSOCIATION
P.O. Box 850
Rocklin, CA 95677
(800) 533-3231
www.theacpa.org

Cognitive-Behavioral Therapy
NATIONAL ASSOCIATION OF
COGNITIVE-BEHAVIORAL
THERAPISTS
P.O. Box 2195
Weirton, WV 26062
(800) 853-1135
www.nacbt.org

Complementary and Alternative Medicine
NATIONAL CENTER FOR
COMPLEMENTARY AND
ALTERNATIVE MEDICINE
National Institutes of Health
P.O. Box 7923
Gaithersburg, MD 20898
(888) 644-6226
http://nccam.nih.gov

Craniosacral Therapy
THE UPLEDGER INSTITUTE, INC.
11211 Prosperity Farms Road, Suite D-325
Palm Beach Gardens, FL 33410-3487
(800) 233-5880
www.upledger.com

Dance Therapy
AMERICAN DANCE THERAPY
ASSOCIATION
2000 Century Plaza, Suite 108
Columbia, MD 21044
(410) 997-4040
www.adta.org

Diabetes
AMERICAN ASSOCIATION OF
CLINICAL ENDOCRINOLOGISTS
1000 Riverside Avenue, Suite 205
Jacksonville, FL 32204
(904) 353-7878
www.aace.com

AMERICAN ASSOCIATION OF
DIABETES EDUCATORS
100 W. Monroe Street, Suite 400
Chicago, IL 60603
(800) 338-3633
www.aadenet.org

AMERICAN DIABETES ASSOCIATION
1701 North Beauregard Street
Alexandria, VA 22311
(800) DIABETES (342-2383)
www.diabetes.org

CHILDREN WITH DIABETES
5689 Chancery Place
Hamilton, OH 45011
www.childrenwithdiabetes.com

JUVENILE DIABETES RESEARCH
FOUNDATION INTERNATIONAL
120 Wall Street
New York, NY 10005-4001
(800) 533-CURE (2873)
www.jdrf.org

NATIONAL CENTER FOR CHRONIC
DISEASE PREVENTION AND HEALTH
PROMOTION
Division of Diabetes Translation
Centers for Disease Control and
Prevention
4770 Buford Highway NE, Mailstop K-10
Atlanta, GA 30341-3717
(800) CDC-INFO (232-4636)
www.cdc.gov/diabetes

Useful Names, Addresses and Web Sites

NATIONAL INSTITUTE OF DIABETES
& DIGESTIVE & KIDNEY DISEASES
National Institutes of Health
Building 31, Room 9A04
31 Center Drive, MSC 2560
Bethesda, MD 20892-2560
www.niddk.nih.gov

Dietary Supplements
OFFICE OF DIETARY SUPPLEMENTS
National Institutes of Health
6100 Executive Boulevard, Room 3B01,
MSC 7517
Bethesda, MD 20892-7517
(301) 435-2920
www.ods.od.nih.gov

UNITED STATES PHARMACOPEIA
12601 Twinbrook Parkway
Rockville, MD 20852-1790
(800) 227-8772
www.usp.org

Feldenkrais
FELDENKRAIS EDUCATIONAL
FOUNDATION OF NORTH AMERICA
3611 SW Hood Avenue, Suite 100
Portland, OR 97239
(800) 775-2118
www.feldenkrais.com

Guided Imagery
ACADEMY FOR GUIDED IMAGERY
30765 Pacific Coast Highway, Suite 369
Malibu, CA 90265
(800) 726-2070
www.academyforguidedimagery.com

Healing Touch
HEALING TOUCH INTERNATIONAL
445 Union Boulevard, Suite 105
Lakewood, CO 80228
(303) 989-7982
www.healingtouchinternational.org

Hellerwork
HELLERWORK INTERNATIONAL
www.hellerwork.com

Herbal Medicine
AMERICAN BOTANICAL COUNCIL
6200 Manor Road
Austin, TX 78723
(512) 926-4900
www.herbalgram.org

AMERICAN HERBALISTS GUILD
141 Nob Hill Road
Cheshire, CT 06410
(203) 272-6731
www.americanherbalistsguild.com

AMERICAN HERBAL
PHARMACOPOEIA
P.O. Box 66809
Scotts Valley, CA 95067
(831) 461-6318
www.herbal-ahp.org

HERB RESEARCH FOUNDATION
4140 15th Street
Boulder, CO 80304
(303) 449-2265
www.herbs.org

Holistic Medicine
AMERICAN HOLISTIC HEALTH
ASSOCIATION
P.O. Box 17400
Anaheim, CA 92817-7400
(714) 779-6152
www.ahha.org

AMERICAN HOLISTIC MEDICAL
ASSOCIATION
12101 Menaul Boulevard, NE, Suite C
Albuquerque, NM 87112
(505) 292-7788
www.holisticmedicine.org

AMERICAN HOLISTIC NURSES
ASSOCIATION
P.O. Box 2130
Flagstaff, AZ 86003-2130
(800) 278-2462
www.ahna.org

HOLISTIC DENTAL ASSOCIATION
P.O. Box 5007
Durango, CO 81301
www.holisticdental.org

Homeopathy
AMERICAN INSTITUTE OF
HOMEOPATHY
801 North Fairfax Street, Suite 306
Alexandria, VA 22314
(888) 445-9988
www.homeopathyusa.org

NORTH AMERICAN SOCIETY OF
HOMEOPATHS
P.O. Box 450039
Sunrise, FL 33345-0039
(206) 720-7000
www.homeopathy.org

Horticultural Therapy
AMERICAN HORTICULTURAL
THERAPY ASSOCIATION
3570 E. 12th Avenue, Suite 206
Denver, CO 80206
(800) 634-1603
www.ahta.org

Hypnosis
AMERICAN COUNCIL OF HYPNOTIST
EXAMINERS
700 S. Central Avenue
Glendale, CA 91204
(818) 242-1159
www.hypnotistexaminers.org

AMERICAN SOCIETY OF CLINICAL
HYPNOSIS
140 North Bloomingdale Road
Bloomingdale, IL 60108-1017
(630) 980-4740
www.asch.net

Labyrinth
THE LABYRINTH SOCIETY
P.O. Box 144
New Canaan, CT 06840
(877) 446-4520
www.labyrinthsociety.org

Massage
AMERICAN MASSAGE THERAPY
ASSOCIATION
500 Davis Street
Evanston, IL 60201
(877) 905-2700
www.amtamassage.org

Music Therapy
AMERICAN MUSIC THERAPY
ASSOCIATION, INC.
8455 Colesville Road, Suite 1000
Silver Spring, MD 20910
(301) 589-3300
www.musictherapy.org

Naturopathy
AMERICAN ASSOCIATION OF
NATUROPATHIC PHYSICIANS
4435 Wisconsin Avenue NW, Suite 403
Washington, DC 20016
(866) 538-2267
www.naturopathic.org

Nutrition and Diet
AMERICAN DIETETIC ASSOCIATION
120 South Riverside Plaza, Suite 2000
Chicago, IL 60606-6995
(800) 877-1600
www.eatright.org

DEPARTMENT OF HEALTH & HUMAN
SERVICES
National Heart, Lung, and Blood Institute
National Institutes of Health
DASH (Dietary Approaches to Stop
Hypertension) Eating Plan
(301) 592-8573
www.nhlbi.nih.gov/health/public/heart/
hbp/dash

U.S. DEPARTMENT OF AGRICULTURE
U.S. Department of Health & Human
Services
Dietary Guidelines for Americans 2005
(866) 512-1800
www.healthierus.gov/dietaryguidelines

Orthomolecular Medicine
ORTHOMOLECULAR MEDICINE
ONLINE
www.orthomed.org

Osteopathy
AMERICAN ACADEMY OF
OSTEOPATHY
3500 DePauw Boulevard, Suite 1080
Indianapolis, IN 46268
(317) 879-1881
www.academyofosteopathy.org

AMERICAN OSTEOPATHIC
ASSOCIATION
142 East Ontario Street
Chicago, IL 60611
(800) 621-1773
www.osteopathic.org

Polarity Therapy
AMERICAN POLARITY THERAPY
ASSOCIATION
P.O. Box 19858
Boulder, CO 80308
(303) 545-2080
www.polaritytherapy.org

Qigong
QIGONG INSTITUTE
561 Berkeley Avenue
Menlo Park, CA 94025
www.qigonginstitute.org

Quackery
www.quackwatch.org

Reflexology
AMERICAN ACADEMY OF
REFLEXOLOGY
725 E. Santa Anita Avenue, Suite B
Burbank, CA 91501-2964
(818) 841-7741
www.americanacademyofreflexology.com

REFLEXOLOGY ASSOCIATION OF
AMERICA
P.O. Box 26744
Columbus, OH 43266-0744
(740) 657-1695
www.reflexology-usa.org

Reiki
INTERNATIONAL CENTER FOR
REIKI TRAINING
21421 Hilltop Street, Unit #28
Southfield, MI 48034
(800) 332-8112
www.reiki.org

Rolfing
INTERNATIONAL ASSOCIATION OF
STRUCTURAL INTEGRATORS
P.O. Box 8664
Missoula, MT 59807
(877) THE-IASI (843-4274)
www.theiasi.org

ROLF INSTITUTE OF STRUCTURAL
INTEGRATION
5055 Chaparral Court, Suite 103
Boulder, CO 80301
(800) 530-8875
www.rolf.org

Rosen Method
ROSEN METHOD: THE BERKELEY
CENTER
825 Bancroft Way, Suite A
Berkeley, CA 94710
(510) 845-6606
www.rosenmethod.com

THE ROSEN INSTITUTE
www.rosenmethod.org

Sleep Medicine
AMERICAN ACADEMY OF SLEEP
MEDICINE
One Westbrook Corporate Center, Suite
920
Westchester, IL 60154
(708) 492-0930
www.aasmnet.org

NATIONAL SLEEP FOUNDATION
1522 K Street NW, Suite 500
Washington, DC 20005
(202) 347-3471
www.sleepfoundation.org

Sound Therapy
SOUND LISTENING & LEARNING
CENTER
301 E. Bethany Home Road, Suite A107
Phoenix, AZ 85012
(602) 381-0086
www.soundlistening.com

Therapeutic Touch
NURSE HEALERS-PROFESSIONAL
ASSOCIATES INTERNATIONAL
P.O. Box 158
Warnerville, NY 12187-0158
(877) 32NHPAI (326-4724)
www.therapeutic-touch.org

Thought Field Therapy
CALLAHAN TECHNIQUES, LTD.
P.O. Box 1220
La Quinta, CA 92247
(800) 359-CURE (2873)
www.tftrx.com

Trager
TRAGER INTERNATIONAL
P.O. Box 3246
Courtenay, British Columbia, Canada
V9N 5N4
(250) 337-5556
www.trager.com

UNITED STATES TRAGER
ASSOCIATION
13801 W. Center Street, Suite C
Burton, OH 44021
(440) 834-0308
www.trager-us.org

Yoga
AMERICAN YOGA ASSOCIATION
P.O. Box 19986
Sarasota, FL 34276
(941) 927-4977
www.americanyogaassociation.org

BIBLIOGRAPHY

The following resources were consulted in the preparation of this book:

GENERAL REFERENCES

Balch, J.F. and M. Stengler. *Prescription for Natural Cures: A Self-Care Guide for Treating Health Problems with Natural Remedies Including Diet and Nutrition, Nutritional Supplements, Bodywork, and More.* Hoboken, NJ: John Wiley & Sons, 2004.

Benson, H. and E.M. Stuart. *The Wellness Book: The Comprehensive Guide to Maintaining Health and Treating Stress-Related Illness.* Secaucus, NJ: Carol Publishing Group, 1992.

Childs, B.P., M. Cypress, and G. Spollett, eds. *Complete Nurse's Guide to Diabetes Care.* Alexandria, VA: American Diabetes Association, 2005.

Dossey, B.M., L. Keegan, and C.E. Guzzetta. *Holistic nursing: A Handbook for Practice.* Sudbury, MA: Jones and Bartlett Publishers, 2005.

Hale, Teresa. *The Hale Clinic Guide to Good Health: How to Choose the Right Complementary Therapy.* Woodstock, NY: The Overlook Press, 1998.

Huebscher, R., and P.A. Shuler. *Natural, Alternative, and Complementary Health Care Practices.* St. Louis, MO: C.V. Mosby, 2004.

Ivker, R.S., R.A. Anderson, and L. Trivieri, Jr. *The Complete Self-Care Guide to Holistic Medicine: Treating Our Most Common Ailments.* New York: Jeremy P. Tarcher/Putnam, 1999.

Null, Gary. *The Complete Encyclopedia of Natural Healing: A Comprehensive A–Z Listing of Common and Chronic Illnesses and Their Proven Natural Treatments.* Stamford, CT: Bottom Line, 2003.

Rakel, David, ed. *Integrative Medicine.* Philadelphia: W.B. Saunders Company, 2003.

Shealy, C. Norman, ed. *The Complete Illustrated Encyclopedia of Alternative Healing Therapies: A Complete Guide to Natural Healing.* Boston: Element Books, 1999.

Weil, Andrew. *Healthy Aging: A Lifelong Guide to Your Physical and Spiritual Well-Being.* New York: Alfred A. Knopf, 2005.

Weil, Andrew. *Natural Health, Natural Medicine: A Comprehensive Manual for Wellness and Self-Care.* New York: Houghton Mifflin, 2004.

ACUPRESSURE

Forem, Jack. *Healing with Pressure Point Therapy: Simple, Effective Techniques for Massaging Away More than 100 Common Ailments.* Paramus, NJ: Prentice Hall Press, 1999.

ALTERNATIVE MEDICINE

Shanbhag, Vivek. *A Beginner's Introduction to Ayurvedic Medicine.* New Canaan, CT: Keats Publishing, Inc., 1994.

Williams, Tom. *The Complete Illustrated Guide to Chinese Medicine: A Comprehensive System for Health and Fitness.* Rockport, MA: Element Books Limited, 1996.

AROMATHERAPY

Buckle, Jane. *Clinical Aromatherapy: Essential Oils in Practice,* 2nd ed. New York: Churchill Livingstone, 2003.

Essential Oils: Desk Reference, 3rd ed. Orem, UT: Essential Science Publishing, 2004.

BREATHING

Zi, Nancy. *The Art of Breathing: Six Simple Lessons to Improve Performance, Health and Well-Being,* 4th ed. Berkeley, CA: North Atlantic Books, 2000.

ENERGY HEALING

Bright, Mary Anne. *Holistic Health and Healing*. Philadelphia: F.A. Davis Company, 2002.

Burmeister, Mary. *Jin Shin Jyutsu: Getting to Know Myself*. Scottsdale, AZ: Jin Shin Jyutsu, Inc., 1994.

Dwoskin, Hale. *The Sedona Method: Your Key to Lasting Happiness, Success, Peace and Emotional Well-Being*. Sedona, AZ: Sedona Press, 2003.

Gerber, Richard. *Vibrational Medicine: The #1 Handbook of Subtle-Energy Therapies*, 3rd ed. Rochester, VT: Bear & Company, 2001.

Gilkeson, Jim. *Energy Healing: A Pathway to Inner Growth*. New York: Marlowe & Company, 2000.

Goldberg, B., J.W. Anderson, and L. Trivieri, Jr. *Alternative Medicine: The Definitive Guide*, 2nd ed. Berkeley, CA: Ten Speed Press, 2002.

Gordon, Richard. *Quantum-Touch: The Power to Heal*, rev. Berkeley, CA: North Atlantic Books, 2002.

Kam-Chuen, Lam. *Everyday Chi Kung with Master Lam: 15-Minute Routines to Build Energy, Boost Immunity, and Banish Stress*. Hammersmith, London: Thorsons, 2004.

Karagulla, S., and D. van Gelder Kunz. *The Chakras and the Human Energy Fields*. Wheaton, IL: The Theosophical Publishing House, 1989.

Krieger, Dolores. *The Therapeutic Touch: How to Use Your Hands to Help or to Heal*. New York: Prentice Hall Press, 1979.

McGee, C.T., and E.P.Y. Chow. *Qigong: Miracle Healing From China*. Coeur d'Alene, ID: Medipress, 1994.

HYPNOSIS

Hathaway, Michael R. *The Everything Hypnosis Book: Safe, Effective Ways to Lose Weight, Improve Your Health, Overcome Bad Habits, and Boost Creativity*. Avon, MA: Adams Media Corporation, 2003.

LIGHT AND COLOR THERAPY

Lilly, Sue. *Color Healing*. New York: Lorenz Books, 2002.

MEDITATION

Marriott, Susannah. *Get Fit Meditation*. London: MQ Publications Limited, 2005.

NUTRITION

Agatston, Arthur. *The South Beach Diet*. New York; Random House, 2003.

Bernstein, Richard K. *Dr. Bernstein's Diabetes Solution: The Complete Guide to Achieving Normal Blood Sugars*. Boston: Little, Brown and Company, 1997.

Brand-Miller, J., et al. *The New Glucose Revolution: The Authoritative Guide to the Glycemic Index—the Dietary Solution for Lifelong Health*. New York: Marlowe & Company, 2003.

Cloutier, M., and E. Adamson. *The Mediterranean Diet*. New York: Avon Books, 2004.

D'Adamo, Peter J. *Eat Right 4 Your Type*. New York: G.P. Putnam's Sons, 1996.

D'Elgin, Tershia. *What Should I Eat?: A Complete Guide to the New Food Pyramid*. New York: Ballantine Books, 2005.

Gerwick, Clara L. *Calorie-Carbohydrate Controlled Diet*, rev. Overland Park, KS: C.L. Gerwick & Associates, Inc., 2005.

Guttersen, Connie. *The Sonoma Diet: Trimmer Waist, Better Health in Just 10 Days*. Des Moines, IA: Meredith Books, 2005.

Harrar, Sari. *The Sugar Solution: Balance Your Blood Sugar Naturally to Avoid Diabetes, Lose Weight, Gain Energy, and Feel Great.* Emmaus, PA: Rodale, 2004.

Kushner, R.F., and N. Kushner. *Dr. Kushner's Personality Type Diet.* New York: St. Martin's Press, 2003.

Miller, M., and D. Miller. *Reversing the Weight Gain Spiral: The Groundbreaking Program for Lifelong Weight Management,* 2nd ed. Independence, MO: Harrison Publishers, 1997.

Ornish, Dean. *Dr. Dean Ornish's Program for Reversing Heart Disease: The Only System Scientifically Proven to Reverse Heart Disease Without Drugs or Surgery.* New York: Random House, 1990.

Perricone, Nicholas. *The Perricone Weight-Loss Diet: A Simple 3-Part Plan to Lose the Fat, the Wrinkles, and the Years.* New York: Ballantine Books, 2005.

Pritikin, Nathan. *The Pritikin Promise: 28 Days to a Longer, Healthier Life.* New York: Simon and Schuster, 1985.

Pritikin, Robert. *The Pritikin Weight Loss Breakthrough: Five Easy Steps to Outsmart Your Fat Instinct.* New York: Dutton, 1998.

Rolls, Barbara. *The Volumetrics Eating Plan: Techniques and Recipes for Feeling Full on Fewer Calories.* New York: Morrow Cookbooks, 2005.

Rubin, Jordan. *The Great Physician's Rx for Health & Wellness: Seven Keys to Unlock Your Health Potential.* Nashville, TN: Nelson Books, 2006.

Schwarzbein, Diana. *The Schwarzbein Principle, The Program: Losing Weight the Healthy Way: An Easy, 5-Step, No-Nonsense Approach.* Deerfield Beach, FL: Health Communications, Inc., 2004.

Sears, Barry. *A Week in the Zone: A Quick Course in the Healthiest Diet for You.* New York: Regan Books, 2004.

Steward, H.L., et al. *The New Sugar Busters: Cut Sugar to Trim Fat.* New York: Ballantine Books, 2003.

Tribole, E., and E. Resch. *Intuitive Eating: A Revolutionary Program That Works.* New York: St. Martin's Griffin, 2003.

Wolcott, W.L., and T. Fahey. *The Metabolic Typing Diet: The Ultimate Guide to Permanent Weight Loss and Optimum Health, High Energy and Peak Athletic Performance, Preventing and Reversing Disease, Staying Young at Any Age.* New York: Doubleday, 2000.

Zinczenko, David. *The Abs Diet Get Fit, Stay Fit Plan: The Exercise Program to Flatten Your Belly, Reshape Your Body, and Give You Abs for Life.* Emmaus, PA: Rodale, 2006.

PSYCHOLOGY

Rubin, R.R., J. Biermann, and B. Toohey. *Psyching Out Diabetes: A Positive Approach to Your Negative Emotions,* 3rd ed. Chicago: Lowell House, 1999.

Snoek, F.J., and T.C. Skinner, eds. *Psychology in Diabetes Care.* New York: John Wiley & Sons, 2000.

SPIRITUALITY

Artress, Lauren. *Walking a Sacred Path: Rediscovering the Labyrinth as a Spiritual Tool.* New York: The Berkley Publishing Group, 1995.

Dossey, Larry. *Be Careful What You Pray For: You Just Might Get It.* New York: HarperCollins, 1997.

O'Brien, Mary E. *Spirituality in Nursing: Standing on Holy Ground,* 2nd ed. Boston: Jones and Bartlett Publishers, 2002.

Young, C., and C. Koopsen. *Spirituality, Health, and Healing.* Thorofare, NJ: Slack Inc., 2004.

STRESS MANAGEMENT

Seaward, Brian L. *Managing Stress: Principles and Strategies for Health and Well-Being*, 4th ed. Boston: Jones and Bartlett Publishers, 2004.

VITAMINS, MINERALS, AND HERBAL THERAPY

Brinker, Francis. *Herb Contraindications and Drug Interactions*, 2nd ed., ed. N. Stodart. Sandy, OR: Eclectic Medical Publications, 2000.

Duke, James A. *Handbook of Medicinal Herbs*, 2nd ed. Boca Raton, FL: CRC Press, 2002.

Foster, S., and V.E. Tyler. *Tyler's Honest Herbal: A Sensible Guide to the Use of Herbs and Related Remedies*, 4th ed. Binghamton, NY: Haworth Herbal Press, 1999.

Huang, Kee Chang. *The Pharmacology of Chinese Herbs*, 2nd ed. Boca Raton, FL: CRC Press, 1999.

McGuffin, M., et al, eds. *American Herbal Products Association's Botanical Safety Handbook*. Boca Raton, FL: CRC Press, 1997.

Murray, Michael. *The Pill Book Guide to Natural Medicines: Complete Information on More Than 250 Popular Natural Remedies for Over 70 Common Health Conditions, From Acne to Varicose Veins*. New York: Bantam Books, 2002.

Packer, L., and C. Colman. *The Antioxidant Miracle*. New York: John Wiley & Sons, Inc., 1999.

PDR for Herbal Medicines, 3rd ed. Montvale, NJ: Thomson PDR, 2004.

PDR for Nonprescription Drugs, Dietary Supplements, and Herbs. Montvale, NJ: Thomson PDR, 2006.

PDR for Nutritional Supplements. Montvale, NJ: Thomson PDR, 2001.

Wichtl, Max, ed. *Herbal Drugs and Phytopharmaceuticals*. Boca Raton, FL: CRC Press, 1994.

INDEX